W9-CVW-783

Contemporary Challenges to the Rehabilitation Counseling Profession

Contemporary Challenges to the Rehabilitation Counseling Profession

edited by

Stanford E. Rubin, Ed.D., CRC
Professor and Coordinator of the
Doctor of Rehabilitation Program
Rehabilitation Institute
Southern Illinois University at Carbondale

and

Nancy M. Rubin, M.Ed., Ed.S.
School Psychologist
Tri-County Special Education District
Murphysboro, Illinois

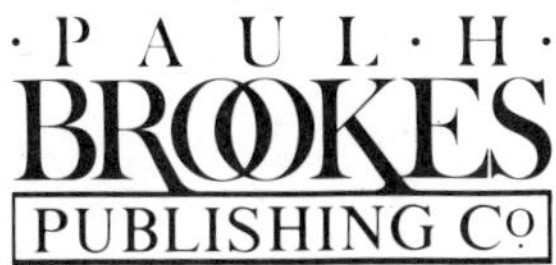

Baltimore · London · Toronto · Sydney

Paul H. Brookes Publishing Co.
P.O. Box 10624
Baltimore, Maryland 21285-0624

Typeset by The Composing Room, Grand Rapids, Michigan.
Manufactured in the United States of America by
The Maple Press Company, York, Pennsylvania.

Library of Congress Cataloging-in-Publication Data

Contemporary challenges to the rehabilitation counseling profession.

Includes bibliographies and index.
1. Rehabilitation counseling. 2. Rehabilitation—United States. I. Rubin, Stanford E. II. Rubin, Nancy M., 1945– . [DNLM: 1. Counseling. 2. Handicapped. 3. Rehabilitation, Vocational.
HD 7255.5 C761]
HD7255.5.C65 1988 362′.0425 87-26890
ISBN 0-933716-85-0

Contents

Contributors vii
Preface xi

Contemporary Challenges: An Introduction
Edna Mora Szymanski, Stanford E. Rubin, and Nancy M. Rubin 1

1 Organizational Accommodation and Rehabilitation Values
John H. Noble, Jr., and Colleen M. McCarthy 15

2 The Rehabilitation Counselor and the Disabled Client: Is a Partnership of Equals Possible?
Phyllis Rubenfeld 31

3 Independent Living and Rehabilitation Counseling
Margaret A. Nosek 45

4 Life-threatening Disabilities: Barriers to Rehabilitation
Harry A. Allen, John D. Dolan, Doreen Miller, and Richard Millard 61

5 The Role of the Rehabilitation Counselor in the Provision of Transition and Supported Employment Programs
Marvin L. Tooman, W. Grant Revell, Jr., and Richard P. Melia 77

6 Transition from School to Work for Individuals with Learning Disabilities: A Comprehensive Model
Patricia Schmitt, Bruce Growick, and Michael Klein 93

7 Rehabilitation Counseling in Supported Employment: A Conceptual Model for Service Delivery and Personnel Preparation
Edna Mora Szymanski, Jay Buckley, Wendy S. Parent, Randall M. Parker, and John D. Westbrook 111

8 Rehabilitation Counseling and Client Transition from School to Work
Tennyson J. Wright, William G. Emener, and Joseph M. Ashley 135
9 Rehabilitation Counseling Considerations with Sensory-Impaired Persons
Sue E. Ouellette and James A. Leja 153
10 Neoplastic Disease: Considerations for the Rehabilitation Profession
John D. Dolan, Harry A. Allen, and Terry Tregle Bell 183
11 Basic Issues and Trends in Head Injury Rehabilitation
Brian T. McMahon and Robert T. Fraser 197
12 Vocational Rehabilitation Counseling with Head-Injured Persons
Robert T. Fraser, Brian T. McMahon, and Donald R. Vogenthaler 217
13 The Family and the Rehabilitation Process: Counselor Roles and Functions
Paul W. Power 243
14 Computer Applications and Issues Related to Their Use in Rehabilitation Counseling
Fong Chan, Ralph E. Matkin, Harry J. Parker, and Paul S. McCollum 259
15 Challenges for Rehabilitation Counselor Education
Marvin D. Kuehn, Ralph M. Crystal, and Alex Ursprung 273
16 Preparing Rehabilitation Counselors to Deal with Ethical Dilemmas: A Major Challenge for Rehabilitation Education
Stanford E. Rubin, Jorge Garcia, Richard Millard, and Henry Wong 303
17 The Study of the Future: A Contemporary Challenge for the Rehabilitation Counseling Profession
Charles Victor Arokiasamy, James A. Leja, Gary Austin, and Stanford E. Rubin 317

Index 331

Contributors

Harry A. Allen, Ed.D.
Professor
Rehabilitation Institute
Southern Illinois University at Carbondale
Carbondale, IL 62901

Charles Victor Arokiasamy, M.S.
Rehabilitation Institute
Southern Illinois University at Carbondale
Carbondale, IL 62901

Joseph M. Ashley, M.Ed.
Coordinator
Project PERT
Woodrow Wilson Rehabilitation Center
Fishersville, VA 22939

Gary Austin, Ph.D.
Director
Rehabilitation Institute
Southern Illinois University
Carbondale, IL 62901

Terry Tregle Bell, B.S.
School of Allied Health Professions
Louisiana State University Medical Center
Rehabilitation Counseling Program
1900 Gravier St.
New Orleans, LA 70112

Jay Buckley, Ed.D.
Research Associate
Specialized Training Program
University of Oregon
135 College of Education
Eugene, OR 97403

Fong Chan, Ph.D.
Assistant Professor and
Director of Vocational Evaluation Services
Department of Rehabilitation Science
University of Texas Health Science Center at Dallas
5323 Harry Hines Boulevard
Dallas, TX 75235-9088

Ralph M. Crystal, Ph.D.
Associate Professor and
Director, Graduate Program in Rehabilitation Counseling
Graduate School
124 Taylor Education Building
University of Kentucky
Lexington, KY 40506

John D. Dolan, Rh.D.
Assistant Dean
School of Allied Health Professions
Louisiana State University Medical Center
1900 Gravier St.
New Orleans, LA 70112

William G. Emener, Ph.D.
Professor
Department of Rehabilitation Counseling
University of South Florida
Tampa, FL 33620

Robert T. Fraser, Ph.D.
Associate Professor
University of Washington
Departments of Neurological Surgery and Rehabilitation Medicine
Harborview Medical Center ZA-50
Seattle, WA 98104

Jorge Garcia, M.A.
Doctoral Candidate
Doctor of Rehabilitation Program
Rehabilitation Institute
Southern Illinois University at Carbondale
Carbondale, IL 62901

Bruce Growick, Ph.D.
Associate Professor and
Coordinator, Rehabilitation Services Program
Ohio State University
356 Arps Hall
1945 N. High Street
Columbus, OH 43210-1390

Michael Klein, Ph.D.
Assistant Professor
Rehabilitation Services Program
Ohio State University
356 Arps Hall
1945 N. High Street
Columbus, OH 43210-1390

Marvin D. Kuehn, Ed.D.
Professor and
Director, Rehabilitation Programs
Division of Counselor Education and Rehabilitation Programs
Visser Hall, 1200 Commercial
Emporia State University
Emporia, KS 66801

James A. Leja, M.S.
Assistant Professor
Department of Blind Rehabilitation and Mobility
Western Michigan University
Kalamazoo, MI 49008-3899

Ralph E. Matkin, Rh.D.
Compensated Work Therapy
Rehabilitation Medicine Services
V.A. Medical Center: West Los Angeles
Wilshire and Sautlelle Boulevards
Los Angeles, CA 90073

Colleen M. McCarthy, M.S.W. Candidate
School of Social Work
SUNY Buffalo
191 Alumni Arena
Buffalo, NY 14260

Paul S. McCollum, Ph.D.
3510 North St. Mary's
San Antonio, TX 78212

Brian T. McMahon, Ph.D.
Executive Director
New Medico Rehabilitation Center of Wisconsin
1701 Sharp Road
Waterford, WI 53185

Richard P. Melia, Ph.D.
Rehabilitation Program Specialist
National Institute on Disability and Rehabilitation Research
Room 3428 Switzer Building
330C Street, S.W.
Washington, DC 20202

Richard Millard, M.A.
Doctoral Candidate
Rehabilitation Institute
Southern Illinois University at Carbondale
Carbondale, IL 62901

Doreen Miller, Rh.D.
Assistant Professor
Psychology Department
Southern University
Baton Rouge, LA 70813

John H. Noble, Jr., Ph.D.
School of Social Work
SUNY Buffalo
191 Alumni Arena
Buffalo, NY 14260

Margaret A. Nosek, Ph.D.
ILRU Research and Training Center on Independent Living at TIRR
3233 Weslayan, Suite 100
Houston, TX 77027

Sue E. Ouellette, Ph.D.
Professor
Department of Communicative Disorders
Northern Illinois University
DeKalb, IL 60115-2899

Wendy S. Parent, M.S.
Assistant Director
Employment Services Division
Rehabilitation Research and Training Center
Virginia Commonwealth University
Richmond, VA 23284

Harry J. Parker, Ph.D.
Professor
Departments of Physical Medicine and Rehabilitation, Psychiatry, and Rehabilitation Science
University of Texas Health Science Center at Dallas
5323 Harry Hines Boulevard
Dallas, TX 75235-9088

Randall M. Parker, Ph.D.
Professor of Special Education
College of Education
University of Texas at Austin
Austin, TX 78712

Paul W. Power, Sc.D.
Director
Rehabilitation Counseling Program
College of Education
University of Maryland
College Park, MD 20742

W. Grant Revell, Jr., M.S., M.Ed.
State Program Supervisor for Supported Employment
Virginia Department of Rehabilitative Services
Richmond, VA 23230

Phyllis Rubenfeld, Ed.D.
Assistant Professor
Department of Academic Skills/SEEK Program
Hunter College of the City University of New York
695 Park Avenue
New York, NY 10021

Nancy M. Rubin, M.Ed., Ed.S.
School Psychologist
Tri-County Special Education District
1725 Shomaker Drive
Murphysboro, IL 62966

Stanford E. Rubin, Ed.D.
Professor and Coordinator of the Doctor of Rehabilitation Program
Rehabilitation Institute
Southern Illinois University at Carbondale
Carbondale, IL 62901

Patricia Schmitt, M.A.
Graduate Research Associate
Rehabilitation Services Program
356 Arps Hall
1945 N. High Street
Columbus, OH 43210-1390

Edna Mora Szymanski, M.S.
Senior Vocational Rehabilitation Counselor
New York State Office of Vocational Rehabilitation
Utica, NY 13501

Marvin L. Tooman, Ed.D.
Chief of Placement
Iowa Division of Vocational Rehabilitation Services
510 East 12th St.
Des Moines, IA 50319

Alex Ursprung, Ph.D.
Assistant Professor
Division of Counseling and Educational Psychology
327 Cedar Building
The Pennsylvania State University
University Park, PA 16802

Donald R. Vogenthaler, Rh.D.
Rehabilitation Institute
Southern Illinois University at Carbondale
Carbondale, IL 62901

John D. Westbrook, Ph.D.
Director
Regional Rehabilitation Exchange
Southwest Educational Development Laboratory
Austin, TX 78701

Henry Wong, M.S.
Doctoral Candidate
Doctor of Rehabilitation Program
Rehabilitation Institute
Southern Illinois University at Carbondale
Carbondale, IL 62901

Tennyson J. Wright, Ph.D.
Associate Professor
Department of Rehabilitation Counseling
University of South Florida
Tampa, FL 33620

Preface

CONTEMPORARY CHALLENGES TO the Rehabilitation Counseling Profession focuses on the philosophical and operational challenges facing the contemporary rehabilitation counselor. It includes chapters on many of the "hottest" and most significant areas of concern in the profession, such as: supported employment, transition, independent living, head injury, cancer, learning disabilities, sensory impairment, computer technology, the role of the family in rehabilitation, consumer issues, paternalistic professional attitudes, stresses and strains in rehabilitation counselor education, dealing with ethical dilemmas, and looking toward the future.

Contemporary Challenges was a sponsored project of the American Rehabilitation Counseling Association (ARCA). The project began in 1985 as a major effort on the part of ARCA to stimulate improvement of the quality and range of rehabilitation counseling services provided to persons with disabilities. The then-president of ARCA, Edna Mora Szymanski, formed task groups to examine current and emerging areas of concern for the profession. Each task group contained nationally recognized educators and/or researchers in the area it was charged to address. A number of practicing rehabilitation counselors and rehabilitation administrators with substantial expertise were also spread among the task groups to ensure that the resultant products would be relevant to current field practice. Each task group was expected to develop a chapter for this book. One or more members of each task group took responsibility for writing the chapters.

In sponsoring this book, ARCA saw as one of its major roles the fostering of the development of the rehabilitation counseling profession by bringing together known rehabilitation researchers, academicians, administrators, and service delivery professionals to address current knowledge needs of the profession. The book was proactively planned to contain state-of-the-art information in highly relevant content areas, in order to provide significant additions to the literature of the field.

Contemporary Challenges to the Rehabilitation Counseling Profession can play a significant role in both preservice and continuing rehabilitation education. In preservice education, it should be very suitable as a primary text in seminar courses at the undergraduate and graduate levels where emphasis is placed on issues and considerations in serving persons with severe disabilities. It should also prove useful as a supplemental text in many of the nonseminar courses found in rehabilitation education curricula. In regard to continuing education, it can play a major role in providing suggestions for innovative practice, as well as stimulating attitudinal and philosophical self-analysis. Although the book is somewhat selective in what it covers, it contains much practical information for both the current and the aspiring rehabilitation counseling professional.

We wish to express our thanks to the many contributors to this book, who without any financial incentive spent numerous days developing the chapters. For their cooperative attitude throughout the development of this book we will be forever grateful. Special recognition is due to Edna Mora Szymanski who, while president of ARCA, conceived the idea for this book and who provided ongoing assistance as we carried it through to completion. Special thanks is also due to Randy Parker, who as president-elect and president of ARCA strongly supported the development of this volume. We also express our appreciation to the members of the ARCA Board of Directors for their support. Finally, our thanks go out to Angela Jones and Rosemary Nelson at the Rehabilitation Institute, and to Linda Patrick and her staff at the College of Human Resources at Southern Illinois University at Carbondale, for their careful typing and/or general handling of the manuscript.

To our parents,
Ruth and Frank and Ruth and Leonard,
for their never-ending support

Contemporary Challenges to the Rehabilitation Counseling Profession

Contemporary Challenges
An Introduction

Edna Mora Szymanski,
Stanford E. Rubin, and Nancy M. Rubin

THE REHABILITATION COUNSELING profession is currently being challenged to reconceptualize its identity, its value structure, and its mission. Several identifiable trends have produced a series of challenges; these trends and an overview of the resulting challenges are the subjects of this introduction. The chapters of this book elaborate on the challenges and how they can be addressed.

TRENDS

Five identifiable trends have affected the rehabilitation counseling profession in recent years. These are: 1) legislative action, 2) social movements, 3) the emergence of new or newly recognized disability groups, 4) recognition of the importance of environment and of intervention strategies, and 5) changing disability models and rehabilitation approaches. Each of these trends has had a profound influence on the current status of disability policy and rehabilitation in the United States.

Legislative Action

A review of history and legislation has shown systematic discrimination against persons with disabilities in many areas affecting basic human rights, including education, employment, and full participation in society. In the 1970s, major laws began a trend to reverse such discrimination and to create a mandate for full integration of persons with disabilities into all aspects of society. The Education for All Handicapped Children Act (PL 94-142), the

Rehabilitation Act of 1973 (PL 93-112), especially Sections 501–504, the 1978 Rehabilitation Act amendments (PL 95-602), and the Developmental Disabilities and Bill of Rights Act (PL 94-103) combine to guarantee persons with disabilities the same rights granted to any other citizen (Hohenshil & Humes, 1984; Nosek, Chapter 3, this volume; Rubin, Garcia, Millard, & Wong, Chapter 16, this volume). Rubin et al. provide a discussion of the full integration mandate and barriers to its implementation.

Social Movements

The disability rights movement has given rise to the minority group orientation and the independent living movement, both of which present significant challenges to the rehabilitation counseling profession (Hahn, 1985; Nosek, Chapter 3, this volume).

The independent living movement emerged in the 1970s from the disability rights movement. It incorporated principles and strategies from other social movements, including civil rights, consumerism, self-help, demedicalization/self-care, and deinstitutionalization/normalization. Its focus has been on independence and self-determination. Traditional rehabilitation approaches along with environmental barriers have been seen as impediments to the full integration mandate. Advocacy, removal of environmental barriers, and consumer control have been seen as the primary solutions (DeJong, 1979). Nosek (Chapter 3, this volume) captures the essence of the movement in her challenge to rehabilitation counselors: Affirm an unwavering commitment to the development of productive and cooperative relationships focusing on the enhancement of human potential, and also support this affirmation with personal action.

Concomitant with the emergence of the independent living movement has been the emergence of the interpretation of second class citizenship for disabled persons as a result of their minority group status. This minority group orientation has focused on prejudice and discrimination as major barriers for persons with disabilities, and has attempted to promote change through unified political action (Hahn, 1985). It has been an empowering orientation with approaches similar to those of the civil rights movement.

New or Newly Recognized Disability Groups

Several chapters of this book deal with disabilities that are either new or are newly recognized in rehabilitation services. The rehabilitation of persons with head injury, the topic of Chapters 11 and 12, this volume, is a major area of interest today, whereas it was rarely heard of ten years ago. Life-threatening illnesses (Chapter 4, this volume) and neoplastic diseases (Chapter 10, this volume) represent another group of disabilities that are only beginning to receive recognition and service from rehabilitation counselors. Specific learning disabilities (Chapter 6, this volume) were not recognized in rehabilitation legislation until 1978.

The significance of the family in rehabilitation has received increased attention in recent years. This recognition has been accelerated by the attention given to these "new" disability groups. This point is driven home in the aforementioned chapters on specific disabilities and in Chapter 13, this volume, which deals with the role of the family in the rehabilitation process.

Recognition of the Importance of Environment and Intervention Strategies

In recent years, increasing evidence has accumulated on the influence of environments on individual behaviors (Bruininks & Lakin, 1985). The independent living movement (Chapter 3, this volume) has a strong environmental emphasis. The ecobehavioral approach to service delivery has recently evolved as an attempt to connect behavioral training strategies with environmental effects. This approach, which is fundamental to supported employment (Chapters 5 and 7, this volume) enhances the congruence between individuals and their environment by interventions focused simultaneously on the individual and the environment (Chadsey-Rusch, 1986).

Changing Disability Models and Rehabilitation Approaches

Disability is a central focus of the profession of rehabilitation counseling. Although at first it may seem to be a simple concept, its complexity is demonstrated by the existence of competing conceptual models of disability that have produced different approaches to rehabilitation.

Hahn (1985) identified three models of disability—medical, economic, and sociopolitical. The medical model has defined disability in terms of physical impairment. The economic model has focused on the individual's vocational limitations. The sociopolitical model has defined disability as the product of the interaction between the individual and the environment. Thus, in the sociopolitical model, the handicap is produced by the environment and experienced in the interaction between the person and the environment. For example, a person who is deaf and uses manual communication would not be handicapped in a job where everyone was fluent in manual communication and where adaptations were made for those job functions that required hearing.

The three models of disability emerged sequentially during the 20th century. At present, all three models are reflected in disability policy. Therefore, the particular form or thrust of services for disabled persons is dependent on which model holds a position of dominance in a particular service system at a given point in time.

The medical and economic models, by virtue of their definition of disability as something that is inherent within the person, have consequences that run counter to the dignity of and achievement of independence by persons with disabilities (Scott, 1969). In this volume, Rubenfeld (Chapter 2), Nosek (Chapter 3), Noble and McCarthy (Chapter 1), and Allen, Dolan, Miller, and Millard (Chapter 4) discuss the negative impact of these models as experienced by persons with disabilities who interact with professionals and service delivery systems.

The three models of disability, in interaction with recent social movements, have given rise to two competing approaches to rehabilitation—the *functional limitations approach* and the *environmental/interactional approach.* The functional limitations approach locates the disability within the person. This approach is compatible with the medical and economic models of disability and focuses intervention on the remediation of individual deficits (Hahn, 1985). Common interventions include prevocational training, personal or work adjustment counseling, and job readiness training.

Scott (1969) criticizes the functional limitations approach in agencies serving persons who are blind as ignoring "an important fact about the problems of blindness, namely, that they are as much a product of social definition and societal reactions as they are of intrapsychic forces" (p. 8). In this volume, Rubenfeld (Chapter 2) and Nosek (Chapter 3) point to the negative impact of the functional limitations approach upon the counselor-client relationship. Allen et al. (Chapter 4, this volume) and Dolan, Allen, and Bell (Chapter 10, this volume) refer to the exclusionary effect this approach can have with respect to services for persons with life-threatening illnesses or neoplastic diseases.

The environmental/interactional approach encompasses principles and strategies of the independent living movement (Nosek, Chapter 3, this volume), the minority group interpretation (Hahn, 1985), and the ecobehavioral approach (Chadsey-Rusch, 1986). Based on the socio-political model of disability, the environmental/interactional approach works toward optimizing the interaction between individuals and environments through support to the individual and/or the modification of environment. The goals of this approach are: independence, self-determination (Nosek, Chapter 3, this volume), political change to alleviate discrimination (Hahn, 1985), and full participation in society. Although individual interventions are provided, they are referenced to specific current or future environments. Examples of environmental/interactional interventions include job modification, interpreter service, cognitive training, and job coaching. This approach to rehabilitation is exemplified by the environmentally referenced interventions characteristic of supported and transitional employment services (Tooman, Revell, & Melia, Chapter 5, this volume; Szymanski, Buckley, Parent, Parker, & Westbrook, Chapter 7, this volume), school-to-work transition (Schmitt, Growick &

Klein, Chapter 6, this volume; Wright, Emener, & Ashley, Chapter 8, this volume), and head injury rehabilitation (McMahon & Fraser, Chapter 11, this volume; Fraser, McMahon, & Vogenthaler, Chapter 12, this volume).

THE CHALLENGES

Some challenges require a reexamination of the very core of our professional existence and identity. Other challenges involve the function of the profession with diverse constituencies and environments. All of these require conscious resolution by individual professionals as well as by the profession as a whole. This section poses some questions to facilitate such resolution.

Is the Profession Consistent with Respect to Values, Goals, Practices, and Outcomes?

On the one hand, the profession perceives its mission as helping persons with disabilities to become active productive members of society (Rubin et al., Chapter 16, this volume). On the other hand, Noble and McCarthy (Chapter 1, this volume), Rubenfeld (Chapter 2, this volume), Nosek (Chapter 3, this volume), and Scott (1969) indicate that the attitudes of professionals represent major barriers to full integration and independence.

Is it possible that the traditional rehabilitation process itself contributes to this inconsistency? Does the process as practiced imply a paternalistic and devaluing relationship and orientation for persons with disabilities? Social reaction theory as explained by Gove (1976) has provided one explanation for the apparent inconsistencies noted by Rubin et al. (Chapter 16, this volume). According to Gove, deviance is not a characteristic of individual action or characteristics, but rather of the application by others of rules or sanctions. He identified three stages in the change of an individual's social status from normal to deviant. They are 1) confrontation, 2) announcement of judgment, and 3) social placement. Screening procedures in the first stage, confrontation, can "take on the characteristics of a degradation ceremony, and the institutional role in which the individual is placed may act to strip him of his former identity and to produce a sense of stigmatization and incompetence" (Gove, 1976, p. 64). In a further elaboration on change of status, Gove summarized an argument of social reaction theorists.

> Persons who have passed through a degradation ceremony and who have been forced to become members of a deviant group have experienced a profound and frequently irreversible socialization process. They have acquired an inferior status and have developed a deviant self-image which is rooted in the image of themselves reflected by the actions of others. (p. 59)

Rubenfeld's comments (Chapter 2, this volume) on the potentially unequal and paternalistic orientation of the counseling relationship and its devaluing effect suggest that the profession may need to examine thoroughly the unintended consequences of some of its practices. A difficult question for the rehabilitation counseling profession is the extent to which Gove's process parallels parts of the rehabilitation process. Do our diagnostic and evaluative procedures parallel the confrontation stage and degradation ceremony just described? Can announcing judgment be analogous to determining eligibility for rehabilitation services? Is the remainder of the rehabilitation process related to Gove's concept of social placement? Are rehabilitation counselors among those professionals in society charged with identifying deviancy and enforcing perceived social roles? Resolution of these questions is necessary if the profession is to work effectively toward the full integration mandate. Such resolution is also a prerequisite for establishment of a complementary rather than adversarial relationship between the profession and the independent living movement.

Does the Profession Need a Change in Definition?

The response to this question depends on which of the many available definitions are employed. In addressing the general membership of the American Rehabilitation Counseling Association (ARCA) Szymanski (1985) proposed the following definition:

> Rehabilitation counseling is a profession that assists individuals with disabilities in adapting to the environment, assists environments in accommodating the needs of the individual, and works toward full participation of persons with disabilities in all aspects of society, especially in work. (p. 3)

If we employ this definition, the question becomes one of emphasis rather than definition. Has the profession focused too heavily on individual intervention at the expense of environmental action, including societal change? In this book, Rubenfeld (Chapter 2), Nosek (Chapter 3), and Allen et al. (Chapter 4) have suggested that this may be the case. There is no doubt that disability causes a profound effect on the individual so labeled. Certainly some individually oriented intervention can be provided in an empowering context that supports the individual's self-determination. Perhaps it is the context of this intervention that needs examination.

Is a Change in Emphasis Needed?

It is suggested that the profession needs to shift its emphasis from the individual to the environment. While individually oriented interventions may continue to be appropriate, their intent should always be to increase client independence and self-determination.

Major problems faced by persons with disabilities are influenced by the environment. Societal attitudes are an environmental factor that presents major barriers for persons with disabilities (Livneh, 1984). The debilitating effect of negative attitudes held by professionals and society in general are discussed in this book by a number of authors, including Noble and McCarthy (Chapter 1); Rubenfeld (Chapter 2); Nosek (Chapter 3); Allen et al. (Chapter 4); Dolan, Allen, and Bell (Chapter 10); and Power (Chapter 13). Other environmental barriers include architectural and transportation inaccessibility (Nosek, Chapter 3), communication barriers (Ouellette & Leja, Chapter 9), and debilitating contingencies within service delivery (Rubenfeld, Chapter 2; Allen et al., Chapter 4; Szymanski et al., Chapter 7) and income maintenance systems (Rubin et al., Chapter 16).

Will the Rehabilitation Counselor's Role Change?

Changes in emphasis and orientation will be accompanied by changes in service delivery. In this volume, Nosek, in Chapter 3, emphasizes the changes in role that accompany an independent living orientation. Chapters 5 (Tooman et al.) and 7 (Szymanski et al.) explore rehabilitation counselor roles and activities in supported employment. Chapters 6 (Schmitt et al.) and 8 (Wright et al.) describe the role rehabilitation counselors can play in enabling successful school-to-work transition for adolescents with disabilities. Power (Chapter 13) addresses the role of the rehabilitation counselor in working with families of persons with disabilities. Chan, Matkin, Parker, and McCollum (Chapter 14) examine the impact of computer technology on the role of the rehabilitation counselor. Arokiasamy, Leja, Austin, and Rubin (Chapter 17) stress the importance of futures studies in helping the profession to prepare for future roles.

Will Rehabilitation Counselor Education Be Affected?

The challenges presented in this volume have clear implications for the preparation of rehabilitation counselors. Effective service delivery requires a complex combination of facilitative attitudes, comprehensive knowledge, and strong skills. The content of the chapters by Noble and McCarthy, Rubenfeld, Nosek, Allen et al., and Rubin et al. suggest that greater emphasis should be placed on shaping facilitative attitudes during the rehabilitation counselor education process. The need for expanding the knowledge and skills of the professionals who work with persons with severe disabilities is driven home by the chapters on head injury, sensory disability, cancer, independent living, and rehabilitation education. As Kuehn, Crystal, and Ursprung point out in Chapter 15, rehabilitation counselor education is challenged to accommodate the training needs dictated by diverse disability groups and by different and changing service delivery approaches. This challenge is complicated by cutbacks in federal funding and changing funding priorities.

SOME ADDITIONAL THOUGHTS

Many challenges to the profession are presented by changing models of disability and rehabilitation approaches along with new or improved methods of service delivery and new or newly recognized groups of consumers. From these discussions, it is obvious that rehabilitation counselors must become societal change agents if they are to assist persons with disabilities in achieving full participation in society. It also follows from this discussion that rehabilitation counselors must be conscious of the potential effects of their intervention. They can be potent enablers of societal change, assisting persons with disabilities in achieving full participation. Or, they can themselves be handicapping conditions whose values, negative attitudes, or limited perception of potential pose additional impediments for persons with disabilities. Rehabilitation counselors are challenged to adopt a respectful and equal partnership with persons with disabilities, a partnership that recognizes and advocates for their rights to self-determination, independent living, and full participation in all aspects of society, especially employment.

Adopting a disability rights approach will bring the professional face to face with new ethical dilemmas caused by scarcity of resources, debilitating contingencies in service delivery and income maintenance, and societal perceptions of the value of life with respect to a devalued class (Noble, 1985). Ethics education will be paramount as rehabilitation counseling faces these contemporary challenges (Rubin et al., Chapter 16, this volume).

In reviewing these challenges to the rehabilitation counseling profession, there is an emerging sense that these challenges have somehow caught the profession largely unprepared. Hence, Arokiasamy et al. in Chapter 17 discuss the need for a systematic study of the future to enable the profession to be better prepared for the challenges of the 21st century and beyond. Throughout its history, rehabilitation counseling for the most part has been reactive in its program planning and policy development. It is an ongoing challenge to the profession to anticipate and preempt future challenges through a serious exploration of the future that leads to successful, proactive planning.

CHAPTER CONTENT OVERVIEW

Chapter 1, by John Noble and Colleen McCarthy, forcefully drives home the point that rehabilitation professionals must not only harbor ethical values that are compatible with accommodating the needs of persons with disabilities, but also must act in accordance with those values. To investigate the degree to which this may be the case, Noble and McCarthy surveyed a random sample of ARCA members regarding the extent to which their employers had made accommodations for the special needs of employees with disabilities through the modification of contract authority, hiring policies, and in-service and other professional training opportunities. The results of the survey suggest that there is room for improvement in both the attitudes and the behavior of rehabilitation professionals in regard to accommodating the needs of persons with disabilities. The chapter concludes with a discussion of issues related to promoting a more accommodating future for persons with disabilities.

In Chapter 2, Phyllis Rubenfeld identifies factors that affect the rehabilitation counseling relationship and result in disabled persons being less than equal partners in that relationship. She argues that both counselors and disabled persons must change their roles. For example, counselors should focus on client potential rather than limitations, and newly disabled clients have to move beyond dependency, anger, and lack of motivation to become active participants in the rehabilitation process. The chapter concludes with the proposal of a co-management alternative for rehabilitation services.

In Chapter 3, Margaret Nosek provides a historical review of the independent living movement, service, and profession. Independent living (IL) arose early in the 1970s from a grassroots movement of severely disabled persons. When Congress added independent living programs to the Rehabilitation Services Administration discretionary programs in 1978, IL became an acceptable goal for rehabilitation services. However, Nosek points out that most practicing rehabilitation counselors and recent college graduates have not been prepared to deal with client IL needs. Given the fact that independent living has become a permanent part of the system that serves disabled persons, Nosek sees the failure to remedy this deficit in the education of rehabilitation counselors as having serious effects in the near future.

Chapter 4, by Harry Allen, John Dolan, Doreen Miller, and Richard Millard, discusses barriers to rehabilitation for clients with life-threatening disabilities—diseases, illnesses, or physical conditions that will probably result in untimely death. The authors contend that these individuals are not receiving the services for which they are eligible, due to such factors as client physical condition, state/federal rehabilitation system policies, employer attitudes, individual psychosocial adjustment to the disease, and the level and appropriateness of rehabilitation counselor training.

New options in service delivery such as transition and supported employment present challenges to the role of the rehabilitation counselor. In Chapter 5, Marvin Tooman, Grant Revell, and Richard Melia discuss the roles of various service providers involved in supported employment programs. They stress the importance of a multidisciplinary team approach that recognizes potential role changes during the service delivery process. The authors discuss rehabilitation counselor roles in relation to the roles of other providers involved in supported employment services. They suggest that the rehabilitation counselor is in the best position to comprehend the importance of the various roles. In ensuring successful supported employment outcomes, the rehabilitation counselor is challenged with the coordination of these roles into a focused effort that is both understood by the service consumer and valued by the employer.

Learning disabilities present yet another challenge to rehabilitation counselors. In Chapter 6, Patricia Schmitt, Bruce Growick, and Michael Klein address the difficulties and frustrations encountered by these individuals and their families in making successful transitions from school to work. They stress the unique problems arising from the invisible nature of the disability and resultant incongruence between societal expectations and individual performance. A comprehensive service delivery model is introduced with the following phases: 1) development of an individualized transition plan based on a comprehensive assessment, 2) learning skills identification, 3) vocational exploration and career education, 4) employability skills training, 5) supported job search/placement/follow-up, and 6) parent and agency cooperation and involvement. The flexibility of the model in addressing individual needs and aspirations is stressed.

Supported employment is the result of a recognition of barriers to employment occurring in the environment and in the interaction between the individual and the environment. In Chapter 7, Edna Szymanski, Jay Buckley, Wendy Parent, Randall Parker, and John Westbrook address the challenge of this focus through a conceptual model for supported employment service delivery and personnel preparation. The model suggests potential rehabilitation counselor activities at each of the following service delivery phases: 1) initial assessment of both individual clients and potential job sites, 2) plan development, 3) job placement, 4) initial training, 5) ongoing support, and 6) periodic assessment. The chapter compares these potential activities with rehabilitation counselor education program content areas and makes recommendations for preservice and in-service training. The authors discuss common questions and misconceptions regarding supported employment. They stress the importance of supported employment in increasing employment opportunities and options for persons with severe disabilities.

Transition from school to work presents a series of challenges for adolescents with disabilities, their families, and involved professionals. In Chapter 8, Tennyson Wright, William Emener, and Joseph Ashley discuss the problems encountered in transition and the role of the rehabilitation counselor in their resolution. They emphasize the need for a coordinated, multidisciplinary, outcome-oriented approach. The authors provide a comprehensive discussion of the rehabilitation counselor's role in transition, and discuss related needs in personnel preparation and professional development. They identify a number of issues and challenges for the profession of rehabilitation counseling and other disciplines involved in enabling successful school-to-work transitions for adolescents with disabilities.

In Chapter 9, Sue Ouellette and James Leja focus on sensory impairments: visual impairment, hearing impairment, and deaf-blindness. While these have been low-incidence impairments, they are expected to increase as the average age of the population of the United States increases. The authors define these disabilities and discuss their prevalence. In addition, they focus on the importance to successful rehabilitation of early identification of these clients before they leave school. Parents may tend to be overprotective of children with these impairments. Therefore, there is a need to promulgate the value of group homes and independent living facilities for persons with sensory impairments.

John Dolan, Harry Allen, and Terry Tregle Bell state in Chapter 10 that cancer is the most feared disease in the United States today. Cancer has devastating effects on both the individual with the disease and family members. The authors discuss the costs of cancer and its treatment, the psychological impact on the family, and vocational considerations such as retention of jobs and loss of health insurance. Behavioral interventions to lessen the effects of the illness and treatment are proposed. The growing need for rehabilitation counselors to become involved with cancer patients as treatment leads to prolonged life, and in some cases, to the "curing" of the disease, is stressed. The authors conclude with a discussion of how diagnosis and treatment of cancer affect family roles and communication.

Chapters 11 and 12 focus on head injuries. The rehabilitation of persons with head injuries is stressed as one of the major rehabilitation service trends of the 1980s. While persons with head injuries have normal life spans, more than 50,000 of the nearly one-half million individuals sustaining such injuries each year cannot return to previous work and/or independence levels. In Chapter 11, Brian McMahon and Robert Fraser note that this area requires not only a reemphasis of age-old rehabilitation themes, but also a thorough understanding of some new ones. Thus, the team approach and case management concepts are stressed as extremely important for working with this group. Emphasis is placed on the need for a unique treatment environment as a behavioral consequence of brain injury. The authors also stress the preference for behavioral interventions rather than psychiatric treatment, and discuss the effects of brain injury on the family—the "true victims." The change in the family constellation often leads to denial of the effects of the injury and a need for family education to deal with the head-injured person and the new family situation. McMahon and Fraser conclude with a discussion of standards to evaluate head-injury programs, employment feasibility for the client, and the opportunities for rehabilitation counselors to work with this population.

Chapter 12, by Robert Fraser, Brian McMahon, and Donald Vogenthaler, provides a broad overview of the consequences subsequent to head injury, with an emphasis on vocational issues. Specifically, this chapter begins with a description of the biomechanics of head injury; some of the sequelae of mild, moderate, and severe head injuries; an overview of the rehabilitation staffing patterns that occur at various periods during the postinjury period; and a brief description of cognitive retraining. The presentation of the vocational rehabilitation process with this population includes discussion of: 1) eligibility determination, 2) evaluation (e.g., sociodemographic, medical, neuropsychological), 3) the planning and counseling process, 4) job placement approaches, and 5) postemployment services. Case examples are also presented.

Paul Power, in Chapter 13, defines disability as moving from a medical concept to a sociocultural concept as a product of the interaction between the individual and his or her environment. He proposes focusing attention on external influences that affect a person with a disability, such as the family. Thus, Power suggests that the rehabilitation counselor–client relationship should move to a rehabilitation counselor–client-family triad. Family support or lack of support can have an important impact on the success of vocational rehabilitation. Family counseling can not only provide support to the family, but also challenge the family to confront unrealistic expectations, and encourage family members to facilitate the client's rehabilitation.

In Chapter 14, Fong Chan, Ralph Matkin, Harry Parker, and Paul McCollum delineate how disabled persons and rehabilitation counselors can utilize computers. Rehabilitation counselors are seen as using computer data bases, spreadsheets, and word processing programs to handle much of the paper work that currently consumes their time, thus allowing them to focus more on counseling. But to reap the full benefits, counselors must become "computer literate." Persons with disabilities are seen as benefitting from computer technology through enhanced independent living and increased employment opportunities. In addition, functional limitations can be reduced through assistive and augmentative communication devices that enable disabled persons to acquire greater control of their environment.

Chapter 15, by Marvin Kuehn, Ralph Crystal and Alex Ursprung, reviews factors that have shaped the development of rehabilitation counselor education (RCE) programs (e.g., federal policy, rehabilitation counselor role and function research, certification and accreditation, definitions of the terms *disability* and *handicap,* and employment trends in rehabilitation). The authors also discuss challenges confronting RCE. These include: 1) effectively preparing potential rehabilitation practitioners to meet the rehabilitation service needs of a population containing a diversity of disability groups; 2) developing valid criteria for assessing the quality of training for new service areas such as independent living, transition from school to work, and supported employment; and 3) expanding the focus of training in spite of cutbacks in RCE program funding. In addition, the chapter stresses the importance and contribution of RCE to the profession for the development of rehabilitation professionals, and provides suggestions for the modification of training curricula that could lead to more qualified graduates.

Chapter 16, by Stanford Rubin, Jorge Garcia, Richard Millard, and Henry Wong, discusses the conflict created by federal legislation mandating the full integration of individuals with disabilities into the mainstream of American life in the face of coexisting attitudinal barriers, limited resources, and counterincentives within public policy. The chapter describes the potential effect of this conflict on rehabilitation counselors providing services for people with disabilities—that is, the emergence of ethical dilemmas in the service delivery process. The authors discuss the need for rehabilitation counselors to be sensitive to ethical dilemmas inherent in their job role, and to be able to analyze them critically and resolve them. In addition, the chapter discusses the need for more emphasis on ethics in rehabilitation education, guidance on methods of teaching ethics, and approaches to teaching ethics appropriate for rehabilitation counselors.

An obvious phenomenon in contemporary society is rapid change. In Chapter 17, Charles Arokiasamy, James Leja, Gary Austin, and Stanford Rubin describe the need for the rehabilitation profession to come to terms with this modern reality. The chapter stresses the need for the rehabilitation profession to engage in the study of the future and its implications for disabled persons and for the profession. The authors briefly describe the current status of and reasons for the study of the future, review the rehabilitation literature on futures study, provide an overview of techniques used, and present sample scenarios of rehabilitation in the next century. Emphasis is placed on the need for rehabilitation counselors to be able to plan desirable futures and to avoid undesirable futures. The reality of accelerative change through proactive planning has to be considered in rehabilitation programs and in policy development. Techniques described for the study of the future include trend extrapolation, the Delphi method, qualitative historical observation, and scenario writing.

REFERENCES

Bruininks, R. H., & Lakin, K. C. (Eds.). (1985). *Living and learning in the least restrictive environment.* Baltimore: Paul H. Brookes Publishing Co.

Chadsey-Rusch, J. (1986). Identifying and teaching valued social behaviors. In F. R. Rusch (Ed.), *Competitive employment issues and strategies* (pp. 273–287). Baltimore: Paul H. Brookes Publishing Co.

DeJong, G. (1979). Independent Living: From social movement to analytic paradigm. *Archives of Physical Medicine and Rehabilitation, 60,* 435–446.

Gove, W. R. (1976). Social reaction theory and disability. In G. L. Albrecht (Ed.), *The sociology of physical disability and rehabilitation* (pp. 57–71). Pittsburgh: University of Pittsburgh.

Hahn, H. (1985). Changing perception of disability and the future of rehabilitation. In L. G. Perlman & G. F. Austin (Eds.), *Social influences in rehabilitation planning: Blueprint for the 21st century* (pp. 53–64). [A report of the ninth Mary E. Switzer Memorial Seminar.] Alexandria, VA: National Rehabilitation Association.

Hohenshil, T. H., & Humes, C. W. (1984). Roles of counseling in ensuring the rights of the handicapped. In R. P. Marinelli & A. E. Dell Orto (Eds.), *The psychological and social impact of physical disability* (2nd ed., pp. 14–29). New York: Springer-Verlag.

Livneh, H. (1984). On the origins of negative attitudes toward people with disabilities. In R. P. Marinelli & A. E. Dell Orto (Eds.), *The psychological and social impact of physical disability* (2nd ed., pp. 167–184). New York: Springer-Verlag.

Noble, J. H. (1985). Ethical considerations facing society in rehabilitating severely disabled persons. In L. G. Perlman & G. F. Austin (Eds.), *Social influences in rehabilitation planning: Blueprint for the 21st century* (pp. 71–79). [A report of the ninth Mary E. Switzer Memorial Seminar.] Alexandria, VA: National Rehabilitation Association.

Scott, Robert A. (1969). *The making of blind men: A study of adult socialization.* New York: Russell Sage Foundation.

Szymanski, E. M. (1985). Rehabilitation counseling: A profession with a vision, an identity, and a future. *Rehabilitation Counseling Bulletin, 29,* 2–5.

1

Organizational Accommodation and Rehabilitation Values

John H. Noble, Jr.
and Colleen M. McCarthy

PASSAGE OF SECTIONS 501, 503, and 504 of the Rehabilitation Act of 1973, as amended, was greeted with widespread resistance from organizations who felt that their economic interests would be adversely affected. Section 504 prohibits discrimination on the basis of handicap in programs and activities conducted by the federal government or by recipients of federal financial assistance. Section 503 requires federal government contractors to take affirmative action to employ and advance workers with disabilities.[1] Section 501 places a similar affirmative action duty on the federal government as an employer. Sections 503 and 504 require the federal government to use the "power of the purse" to ensure compliance by recipients of federal grant or contract funds.

The federal legislation is consistent with numerous resolutions of the United Nations (UN) and its member organizations, including the International Labor Organization (ILO), the United Nations Educational, Scientific and Cultural Organization (UNESCO), the World Health Organization (WHO), and The United Nations Children's Emergency Fund (UNICEF). These include the General Assembly resolutions relating to the Universal

[1]The terms *disability* and *handicap* are used interchangeably here, recognizing at the same time the distinction between them made by the World Health Organization (1980). In this distinction, *disability* refers to reduced role functioning caused by physical or mental impairments arising from anatomical loss or disease. *Handicap* refers to problems that result from society's adverse judgments or behaviors toward those whose functional limitations interfere with the role functioning considered normative by society.

Declaration of Human Rights (No. 217 A [III]), the International Covenants on Human Rights (No. 2200 A [XXI]), the Declaration of the Rights of the Child (No. 1386 [XIV]), the Declaration on the Rights of Mentally Retarded Persons (No. 2856 [XXVI]), and the Declaration on Social Progress and Development (No. 2542 [XXIV]). The UN General Assembly Resolution 3447 (XXX), adopted December 9, 1975, proclaimed a Declaration on the Rights of Disabled Persons, and called for national and international action to ensure that it be used as a common frame of reference for the protection of the rights of persons with disabilities. Among the declared rights of persons with disabilities are entitlement to:

1. Measures designed to enable them to become as self-reliant as possible
2. Economic and social security and a decent level of living, including the right to secure and retain employment or to engage in a useful, productive and remunerative occupation and to join trade unions
3. To have their special needs taken into consideration at all stages of economic and social planning
4. An environment and living conditions as close as possible to those of the normal life of a person of his or her age in the event that the stay of a person with a disability in a specialized establishment becomes indispensable

In essence, the UN resolutions call for societal accommodation of the special needs of persons with disabilities. Sections 501, 502, and 503 of the Rehabilitation Act of 1973, as amended, specify what is meant by *accommodation* in the United States; namely, that unfair and unnecessary barriers and discrimination be eliminated so that persons with disabilities can achieve the goals of independence and equal access to all the opportunities afforded by citizenship.

The National Council on the Handicapped (1986), established first as an advisory body by the U.S. Congress in 1978 (PL 95-602) and later transformed into an independent federal agency (PL 98-221), has spelled out what accommodation should include:

> The nondiscrimination requirement should expressly include a duty to make reasonable accommodations, which should be defined as providing or modifying devices, services, or facilities, or changing practices or procedures in order to allow a particular person to participate in a particular program, activity, or job. The duty not to discriminate should also include an obligation to remove architectural, transportation, and communication barriers, including meeting . . . accessibility requirements. (p. 20)

Health and social welfare provider agencies—especially those that cater to the needs of persons with disabilities—and the professionals and other staff whom they employ would be expected to identify closely with the professed values of nondiscrimination and accommodation. Indeed, education for the professions that typically serve persons with disabilities—medicine, nursing, physical therapy, occupational therapy, speech therapy, education, rehabilitation counseling, and social work—has inculcation of values as one of its primary goals.

Personal responsibility and a commitment to humane values have long been the hallmarks of a profession. By themselves, distinctive knowledge and techniques that can be taught to others do not define a profession. There must be personal responsibility for the application of knowledge and technique with the intent of serving the best interests of those being served. Since Flexner (1910) first defined the criteria for professional medical education as the distinctive knowledge and techniques that can be taught to others and a commitment to ethical practice, these have remained the basis for newly emerging groups of practitioners to proclaim themselves as a "profession" deserving societal recognition and sanction. Restating Flexner's criteria, Wilensky and Lebeaux (1958) formulate the commitment to ethical practice as "adherence to a set of professional norms, involving impersonal objectivity, impartiality, and devotion to the client's interests more than profit . . . when the two are in conflict" (p. 285).

In considering the relationship between knowledge, technique, and ethical practice, Reamer (1979) emphasizes the supremacy of values. Regardless of what intuition, or practice wisdom, or the results of empirical research would suggest, at issue is always judgment about how "the freedom and well-being of clients will best be safeguarded and promoted" (Reamer, 1979, p. 242). As interpreted by such thinkers as Plant (1970), this commitment to the individual's well-being also requires that the ethical professional make every effort to change society in ways that make it more compatible with individual needs.

In summary, the "bottom line" for a profession is the value placed on seeking the client's interests above all other considerations—advocating and even politicizing needed societal reforms to increase the welfare of clients.

But what is the reality? Do members of the profession actually perform according to the dictates of their professed values? More specifically, do rehabilitation professionals and the organizations for which they work actualize the values that they profess within their sphere of influence?

To answer these questions, a mail survey was undertaken of a 10% random nonreplacement sample of the members of the American Rehabilitation Counseling Association (ARCA) and their employers. It was assumed that ARCA members had received a healthy dose of professional values in the course of their professional education, including exposure to the major pronouncements of the United Nations and its member organizations. It was further assumed that frequent, if not daily, involvement with clients with disabilities and a familiarity with, if not a strong support for, the federal legislation relating to their clients would influence how the ARCA members and their employers comport themselves in accommodating the special needs of persons with disabilities.

The findings of the ARCA membership survey are compared and interpreted in light of the findings of the Berkeley Planning Associates (1982) survey of 2,000 federal contractors about accommodations provided to persons with disabilities. In addition, one of the authors of this chapter, who has a significant disability, gives a consumer perspective on what she encountered in trying to obtain responses from ARCA members who failed to reply to the first mailing of the survey questionnaire.

ARCA SURVEY

A 10% random nonreplacement sample (N = 293) of the national ARCA membership was surveyed in July, 1986 by mail questionnaire with stamped return envelopes provided. Nonrespondents were contacted by a repeat mailing in October, 1986. Efforts to contact nonrespondents by telephone continued through March, 1987, when telephone numbers could be obtained. The first mailing yielded a 32.2% response rate; the second mailing increased the rate to 37.2%, more than twice the 17% rate of return for the Berkeley Planning Associates (1982) survey of 2,000 federal contractors. Follow-up telephone calls brought the response rate for completed questionnaires up to 43.3%.

The brief questionnaire sought largely close-ended answers to 21 questions, with some branching among questions, depending on given responses. Information was sought about the personal characteristics of respondents, including whether they had a handicapping condition as defined by Section 504 of the Rehabilitation Act of 1973, as amended, and any accommodations they might have received from their employer. The rest of the questionnaire focused on the extent to which the ARCA members' employers had made accommodations to meet the special needs of other employees with disabilities through the use of personnel hiring policies, contract authority, and in-service and other professional training opportunities.

Personal Characteristics

The majority (66.9%) of the ARCA respondents were over 35 years old. The majority (54.3%) were male. About 92% of the respondents were Caucasian.

About 61% had a master's degree; 29.1% held a doctorate; and 7.1% possessed a bachelor's degree.[2] In rank order, 49.3% held a degree in rehabilitation counseling; 11.3% in psychological counseling; 7.3% in psychol-

[2]Unless otherwise indicated, the difference between the sum of the percentages reported and 100% consists of the percentage of missing data that results from the failure of respondents to provide the requested information.

ogy; 6.0% in educational counseling; and the remainder reported degrees in a variety of other disciplines.

Almost 56% of the respondents occupied supervisory positions with their employer; 41.7% supervised 1–10 employees; 7.1%, between 11 and 20; and another 7.1%, more than 20 employees.

The majority (81.9%) of the respondents had no handicapping condition as defined by Section 504. Of the 21 respondents with a handicapping condition, 9 (42.9%) reported that their employer had made an accommodation for them. Five of the accommodations required an outlay of money—$25, $45, $500, $1,500, and $2,000, respectively. The types of accommodation reported were special equipment (44.4%); special training opportunities (22.2%); and each of the remainder (33.3%) was given either special hours, a reduced work load, or other type of accommodation.

Employer Characteristics

The random nonreplacement sampling procedure provided an unduplicated national sample of organizations employing ARCA members. No two respondents were employed by the same organization. Thus, respondent reports, if accurate, characterize organizational attributes and behaviors.

Exactly 31% of the ARCA respondents were employed by private, for-profit organizations; 27.6% by private nonprofit agencies; 34.5% by federal, state, county, or municipal government.

The principal types of service provided by these organizations were vocational rehabilitation (19.8%), education (19.8%), mental health (11.2%), workers' compensation (9.5%), substance abuse (7.7%), mental retardation/developmental disabilities (5.2%), and a remainder of miscellaneous other services.

The principal employers were post-secondary school and higher education institutions (19.0%), private practice (16.4%), rehabilitation facilities (11.2%), private businesses (10.3%), hospitals (8.6%), professional associations (4.3%), high schools (4.3%), and advocacy organizations (4.3%).

In terms of size, 57.8% of the organizations employed 1–200 employees; 12.1%, 201–1,000; and 10.3%, more than 1,000. The majority (52.6%) of the ARCA respondents could not give the size of their employer's most recent annual budget.

Accommodation Policies

Employment Just over 50% of the organizations for which the ARCA respondents worked employed persons with a handicap—12.6% employed 1 such person; 18.1%, 2–5; 3.1%, 6–10; 3.9%, 11–20; and 12.6% employed more than 20 persons with a handicap. Almost 42% of these employees are classified as holding a professional position; 24.7%, a clerical position; and 33.7%, some other position.

Purchases Only 27.6% of the organizations purchased goods and services from sheltered workshops and other vendors whose workforce consists largely of persons with handicaps. Slightly more than 16% of the respondents did not indicate what their organization's policy was in this regard. The most common reason given for not making such purchases (48.2%) was the lack of suitable vendors for needed purchases. After this, the most common reason was "never considered the possibility," which was reported by 13.0% of the respondents. "No such need" was mentioned by 9.3%, and 11.1% cited "government purchasing rules" as the reason for not making such purchases.

Work Site Accommodations Almost 53% of the organizations made some degree of work site accommodation for employees with handicapping conditions. The majority (26.8%) were reported as providing a single kind of accommodation; 14.9% provided two; 22.4%, three; 19.4%, four; 10.5%, five; 1.5%, six; and 3.0%, seven kinds of accommodation. The most frequently given reason for not making such accommodations was the lack of need because of the minimal handicaps involved (48.0%), or the lack of employees with handicapping conditions (16.0%). Where work site accommodations were made, 22.1% involved architectural barrier removal; 21.1%, special equipment; 14.7%, special hours; 12.1%, reduced work load; 11.6%, special transportation; 10.0%, special training; and 5.8%, relaxation of sick leave policies.

Special Funds ARCA respondents were asked whether their organization had a policy of setting aside funds to accommodate the special travel, housing, or other needs of employees with handicaps who may wish to attend professional conferences, training courses, and the like. Only 25.2% reported the availability of special funds for this purpose. The most frequently given reason for the lack of special funds (38.6%) was "none needed for minimal handicaps," followed by 21.1% responding, "never considered the possibility"; 10.5%, "no employees with handicaps"; and 8.8%, "too expensive to afford."

The same question was asked with respect to participants with handicaps who may wish to attend professional conferences, training courses, and the like either directly provided or paid for by the respondent's organization. Nearly 25% reported the availability of special funds for this purpose. Again, the most frequently given reason for the lack of special funds (32.7%) was "none needed for minimal handicaps"; followed by 19.3% responding, "never considered the possibility,"; and 14.5%, "too expensive to afford."

Not unexpectedly, ARCA respondents with handicaps had knowledge of the costs incurred by their organization to accommodate their own special needs, but virtually no knowledge of the costs of accommodating the special needs of fellow employees or participants with handicaps.

FEDERAL CONTRACTORS AND EMPLOYERS OF ARCA MEMBERS COMPARISONS

How do the organizations for which the ARCA respondents work compare with the federal contractors in accommodating the special needs of persons with handicaps?

Putting aside for the moment differences in survey procedures, the response rate of 37.2% before telephone follow-up of the ARCA membership sample was more than twice as high as the 17.0% reported by Berkeley Planning Associates (1982) for its sample of 2,000 federal contractors. While this higher response rate may suggest a greater commitment by rehabilitation professionals and their organizations to the goal of accommodation, it should also be noted that 52.8% of the ARCA members reported that their employers make specific work site accommodations for their employees—almost the same percentage as the 52.2% figure reported by federal contractors.

Accommodation and Values

The specific work site accommodations provided by 52.8% of the employers of ARCA members and by 52.2% of the federal contractors are compared in Table 1.

The uniformly higher percentages reported by the ARCA respondents of specific work site accommodations by their employers compared to those reported by the federal contractors are probably the result of multiple accommodations made by given employers of ARCA members. In terms of percentage, this means that employers of ARCA members compared to the federal contractors made more extensive accommodations for their employees with handicapping conditions.

The ARCA respondents could not estimate the costs of making these accommodations except where they were personally involved. Berkeley Plan-

Table 1. Specific work site accommodations, employers of ARCA members, and federal contractors compared

Type of accommodation	ARCA member employers (%)	Federal contractors (%)
Architectural barrier removal	22.1	5.7
Special equipment	21.1	8.6
Special training	10.0	5.2
Special hours	14.7	5.2
Special transportation and mobility assistance	11.6	3.2
Reduced work load	12.1	8.8
Relaxed sick leave policy	5.8	
Adapted work environment		2.8

ning Associates (1982), however, found that 51% of the accommodations by federal contractors cost nothing; 30.4% cost less than $500; 10.5%, $500 to less than $2,000; 4.8%, $2,000 to less than $10,000; and 3.2% cost more than $10,000. Of the nine ARCA respondents who reported that their employer had made an accommodation for them, four required no outlay; three, $500 or less; and two, $2,000 or less. If anything, the cost of the accommodations made by employers of ARCA members for their employees was less than the cost of accommodations made by the Berkeley Planning Associates' sample of federal contractors. For both sets of employers, the cost burden of accommodation was not very large in most instances.

From these statistics can be inferred a greater extent of multiple accommodations made by employers of ARCA members as compared to federal contractors. This could be construed as evidence of the greater commitment of employers of ARCA members to the goal of accommodation. In this regard, it should be noted that if there is bias toward overstatement of the true extent of accommodation by virtue of respondent knowledge of and willingness to report their organization's superior track record, the bias should run in the same direction among the federal contractors, who were also free to respond or not in light of similar knowledge about their own situation.

But before reaching the self-eulogizing conclusion that employers of ARCA members show greater commitment to accommodating the special needs of persons with disabilities, consider two additional facts. First, the majority of the ARCA sample did not respond; hence, the statistics on accommodation among employers of ARCA members are partial and probably accent the positive just as much as do the statistics on federal contractors. Second, follow-up telephone calls to nonrespondents reveal a less than complimentary side of the rehabilitation counseling profession that should be factored into such inferences.

THE TELEPHONE FOLLOW-UP

The telephone follow-up of nonrespondents provided some evidence of a gap between the professed values and behavior of members of the ARCA sample. After the first mailing of the questionnaire, the response rate was 32.2%. Efforts to obtain the numbers of nonrespondents yielded 70.9% of 199 needed telephone numbers. All but 38 (27.0%) of the ARCA members with an identifiable telephone number were contacted and asked to provide answers to the questionnaire over the phone if for any reason they could not return the mail questionnaire. The telephone calls produced 18 additional completed questionnaires.

The responses obtained from the 103 nonrespondents contacted by telephone confirmed the suspicion that the consumers of the services of some

ARCA professionals are still fighting an uphill attitudinal battle. The experience and impressions of the author who conducted the telephone follow-up are presented below.

Seven (6.8%) of the 103 ARCA members contacted by telephone were "positive" in expressed attitudes and remarks; they apologized for not having responded to the mail questionnaire and made every effort to provide ample information and commentary about their agency's policies and practices. Eleven (10.7%) were classified as "resistant," although they eventually did provide what information they could over the phone. The majority (82.5%) of those reached by telephone were "rejecting" in expressed attitudes and remarks.

It is easy to conclude that the attitudes of many rehabilitation professionals are indifferent at best, based on the low response to the ARCA membership survey and the unexpected rejecting responses received from the majority of the respondents reached by telephone. Remarks by rejecting ARCA members included: "I resent being called on my day off"; "no handicapped person ever applied here"; "we work with the retarded"; "my agency would not want me to provide this kind of information"; and "I never received the mailings." The latter response was surprising, since the method used to obtain the home telephone numbers of nonrespondents was the cross-indexing of the ARCA membership labels, the area codes, and the information operator's listing of telephone numbers.

There were also some rather unique insights offered by several respondents who revealed themselves as being either presently or previously handicapped, as defined by Section 504. These ARCA members had received services from their state Office of Vocational Rehabilitation, secured their professional degrees, and remained unemployed. They were candid about their frustration with able-bodied counselors who accepted salaries for providing services to "rehabilitate me but were unable or unwilling to help me secure decent employment." Two of these individuals now subcontract with their state Office of Vocational Rehabilitation to provide services to other persons with disabilities, with an emphasis on employment. The old cliché "walk a mile in my shoes" holds true.

If the expressions of indifference and hostility encountered in the nonrespondent ARCA members are representative of a substantial proportion of rehabilitation professionals, then it must be said that the disability rights movement's greatest adversary is not ignorance, inexperience, or the environment. Its adversary is the prejudicial attitude of many rehabilitation professionals, who should know and behave better. Such attitudes are part of the substance of that passively imposed form of discrimination, described by Hahn (1985), that ultimately stigmatizes and oppresses persons with disabilities in our society.

CHALLENGES FOR THE FUTURE

The survey of the ARCA membership directly or indirectly raises four major issues that seem likely to challenge the future of the counseling professions. First, the value placed on respecting and even aggressively pursuing the client's interests above all other considerations—the "bottom line" for a profession—may not be as strong a motivating force in practice as it should be. From the perspective of many consumers, it hardly exists.

Second, the weakness of client advocacy among both the able-bodied laity and the counseling professions has politicized consumers and stimulated development of a civil rights movement among persons with disabilities. Is not the next logical step the development of professional associations with memberships consisting exclusively of persons with disabilities bent on self-development?

Third, the prevailing ethic of utilitarianism in rehabilitation circles, as manifested by the rhetoric of human resource investment and a long-standing preoccupation with benefit-cost analysis, may not provide an adequate foundation for educating and preparing students for professional practice. If this is the case, are there alternative systems of ethics that may better serve the purposes of professional education?

Fourth, even with an appropriate ethic there is need for a technology that can translate values into effective action. Do the counseling professions possess such a technology? If so, are they motivated to use it, given the structure of rewards in the counseling marketplace?

Each of these issues is discussed in turn, and some suggestions are made.

Professional Values

All professions profess humane values and at least give lip service to altruism as the principal motivation for their endeavors. Existing practices are defended and proposed changes are supported or resisted—all in the name of serving the best interests of clients. Self-interest, however, can lurk close to the surface of proclaimed beneficence. While this rhetoric is often convincing to the laity, the more honest members of a profession know what it is all about, but often remain silent lest they be ostracized by their peers. When large numbers of clients become disillusioned, however, the professions face a crisis. What will become of their livelihoods if clients are free to, and choose to, refuse their services?

Professional education may not be imparting the values needed to sustain practitioners throughout their careers. Whether the problem is the rising commercialism of the 1980s, reaction to the idealism of the 1960s, or the insecurity of a nation whose dominance in international affairs and trade is under attack makes no difference. Somehow the balance between knowledge, technology, and values in the professions has been upset.

What can be done to right the balance? Actively recruiting more persons with disabilities into the counseling professions would be a good beginning. There is also a need to engage clients in a dialogue about counseling technology and its underlying knowledge base. It will be important to listen closely to what clients have to say about its utility to them in their daily lives. A critical part of this dialogue will be a discussion of the role of professional values in the choice of service options for persons with disabilities. As unsettling an experience as it is likely to be for the professionals who engage in the dialogue, the growing crisis of confidence in the counseling professions argues for such strong countermeasures.

Advocacy and Community Action

The role of advocacy and community action in the counseling professions needs attention. As Plant (1970) indicates, the commitment to an individual's well-being requires that the ethical professional make every effort to change society in ways that make it more compatible with individual needs.

The point has been reached where many persons with disabilities can "name the game." Disillusioned, they look increasingly for alternatives to traditional service providers. To many of these persons, independent living centers, peer counseling, and other forms of self-help are attractive alternatives to reliance on the counseling professions.

Thus, the logical next step for disabled consumers who have overcome the odds and obtained a professional degree is to form professional associations of their own in pursuit of self-development. This strategy has potential for high payoff to the extent that evidence accumulates to convince legislators and the laity of the superior effects of peer counseling compared to counseling by persons without disabilities.

Hahn (1985) suggests that little or no progress can be expected in reversing the discrimination built into disability policy and programs in the United States until persons with disabilities are recognized as a minority group, establish themselves as a viable political force with which to be reckoned, and succeed in broadening the focus on "functional impairments" to include "perceptions of a person's appearance." Technology has enabled the creation of "user-friendly" physical environments, but prejudice and discrimination by nondisabled persons remain to be confronted and overcome.

Lest the potential of consumer activism be dismissed as "pie in the sky," consider the possibilities more closely. Perhaps the only way to reduce the increasingly high administrative and overhead costs of the many categorical programs that characterize the American welfare state is to organize consumers with disabilities and their families or family surrogates into cooperatives. Only by eliminating at least some of the middlemen can consumers stretch the value of the available service dollar and at the same time preserve some semblance of acceptable quality (Noble, 1981).

Smith (1979) provides evidence that greater reliance on informal social networks, either in themselves or in conjunction with the formal intervention system, promotes greater independence among persons with disabilities. His study of 950 adults with chronic disabilities living in a metropolitan community found no statistically significant relationship between utilization of rehabilitation services and recovery status. (Recovery status was measured by a four-factor index of independence. Changes toward greater work activity, unrestricted mobility, self-derived income, and not being under a physician's care were deemed indicative of greater independence.) In Smith's view, the evidence suggests:

> that informal social networks play an important role in the rehabilitation of the disabled. Reliance on informal resources is enhanced in the absence of formal rehabilitation intervention, suggesting alternative modes of social support are actively sought and utilized by the disabled. Furthermore, lay-initiative may constitute another effective resource in the process of recovery. (p. 63)

Family, friends, and nonrehabilitation agency sources of help such as unions, employers, and fraternal and religious organizations constitute the informal social network in question. Smith's (1979) study does not stand alone in pointing to the vital role played by family and informal social networks in the face of acute or chronic illness and dysfunction (see, for example, Croog & Levine, 1977; Kaplan, Cassel, & Gore, 1977; Martin, 1978; World Health Organization, 1976).

Persons with disabilities could form cooperatives in order to meet the full range of needs of the membership and could even acquire provider status under a variety of social programs—most notably under the intermediate care facility for the mentally retarded (ICF/MR) authority of Medicaid and the Title XX Social Services Block Grant. Within the constraints of budget afforded by such provider arrangements with state and local governments, persons with disabilities and their families or surrogate families might begin to exercise a greater measure of responsibility for their own lives. They could contract, according to their needs, with a variety of organizations and individuals for whatever goods and services they might require, or they could make purchases on a fee-for-service basis.

The concept of a cooperative for persons with disabilities would differ from that of the Centers for Independent Living, now authorized by Title VII, Part B, of the Rehabilitation Act of 1973, as amended. Persons with disabilities and their families or surrogate families would be provided with something more than a service supplement because of the provider status that the cooperatives would have to obtain. A cooperative would be defined as a nonprofit entity existing for the purpose of providing, on a cooperative basis, goods, services, or facilities primarily for the benefit of its members or voting consumer stockholders. Such status would confer eligibility for loans at below-market rates of interest from the National Consumer Cooperative Bank, as well as eligibility for assistance under the HUD Sections 202, 213, and 265/235 and Home Ownership programs (Schwarzentraub, 1980).

The time is approaching when rehabilitation professionals must take sides—for or against the empowerment of their clients. Available evidence urges support for client aspirations and strivings for a larger measure of control over their lives. Rehabilitation professionals should be actively engaged in community action to give clients more say in the choice of services and the methods of their delivery.

Alternatives to Utilitarianism

The economic model of human resource investment and the prescriptions of benefit-cost analysis that dominate thinking in the field of rehabilitation are grounded in the ethical theory of utilitarianism. In the utilitarian view, actions are right if they produce the greatest happiness for the greatest number of people (Munson, 1983). Translated into client selection criteria, clients are selected or rejected for receipt of rehabilitation services on the basis of their potential to contribute to an optimal yield of benefits from the investment of available resources (Noble, 1977).

Coupled with negative stereotyping about the capacities of persons with severe disabilities and the conclusions reached by some economic studies, the utilitarian ethic has hindered efforts to promote the well-being of people with severe disabilities. The studies (Berkowitz, Fenn, & Lambrinos, 1983; Haveman, 1977; Levitan & Taggart, 1979) conclude that limitations in physical and mental fitness are closely related to diminished ability to produce on the job and/or that employers prefer nondisabled workers, even if disadvantaged, to workers with disabilities. These interpretations of the data ignore the potential of new vocational techniques and careful job placement to enable workers with severe disabilities to engage in substantial employment, as well as the combined and interacting effects of a host of other employment impediments, including age, limited education, work disincentives, and discrimination by employers.

An ethic based on Rawls' theory of justice as "fairness" would be much more sensitive than utilitarianism to the special needs of persons with disabilities. In the Rawlsian scheme, each person has an equal right to the most extensive total system of equal basic liberties compatible with a similar system of liberty for all; social and economic inequalities are arranged so that they create the greatest benefit for the least advantaged. The resultant just society guarantees the worth and self-respect of the individual (Munson, 1983). Unlike utilitarianism, Rawlsian justice will not permit an individual's interests to be sacrificed for the good of the greatest number.

It is recommended that students being educated for the counseling professions be exposed to alternative ethical systems and their tenets. In this way, students can recognize utilitarianism for the influence it exerts on rehabilitation practice, and perhaps acquire the basis for decisions grounded in an alternative ethical system that seeks more just outcomes for persons with disabilities.

Appropriate Technology

There is a need for the exposure of students in the counseling professions to a broader range of theories and practice than they now receive. The focus on theory and practice that seeks to change the individual is much too narrow. Advocacy and community action are grounded in a body of theory and practice that can be taught. Counseling professionals need to know how to be effective advocates and community organizers. To the extent that counseling professionals are expected to help clients to adjust to the environment as a given, but lack knowledge, proficiency, and *motivation* to change the individual's environment for the better, clients will be short-changed in the help they receive.

How much of counseling practice is confined to an office on a 5-day, 9:00 to 5:00 basis? Responsiveness to Smith's (1979) findings would expand that practice considerably, drawing the would-be effective helper into a very different routine—one that encompasses advocacy and community organization activities on behalf of the client. It would probably place much greater emphasis on organizing peer counseling and support groups for individual clients than is now the case in most counseling agencies and practices. And it might even require work on evenings and weekends when the client's family, friends, and other sources of social support are more readily available.

Given the reward structure of the rehabilitation counseling marketplace, advocacy and community action should be directed first to reshaping existing incentives. This is something that requires vision beyond the immediate self-interest of the counseling professions. It is unreasonable to expect counseling professionals to advocate for changes that will be discomforting to their customary work habits and life-styles. Thus, it is necessary to rely on the activism of disgruntled consumers to bring about basic reforms. It would seem that competition from consumers organized to help themselves will be necessary to change the incentives of the rehabilitation counseling marketplace. And that is what the civil rights movement for persons with disabilities is all about.

REFERENCES

Berkeley Planning Associates. (1982). *A study of accommodations provided to handicapped employees by federal contractors* (Vols. 1–2). [Final report for the U.S. Department of Labor, Employment Standards Administration.] Berkeley, CA: Author.

Berkowitz, M., Fenn, P., & Lambrinos, J. (1983). The optimal stock of health with endogenous wages. *Journal of Health Economics, 2,* 139–147.

Croog, S. H., & Levine, S. (1977). *The heart patient recovers.* New York: Human Sciences Press.

Flexner, A. (1910). *Medical education in the United States and Canada.* New York: Carnegie Foundation for the Advancement of Teaching.

Hahn, H. (1985). Disability policy and the problem of discrimination. *American Behavioral Scientist, 28,* 293–318.

Haveman, R. H. (1977). *A benefit-cost and policy analysis of the Netherlands social employment program.* Leiden, Netherlands: University of Leiden.

Kaplan, B. H., Cassel, J. C., & Gore, S. (1977). Social support and health. *Medical Care Supplement, 15,* 47–58.

Levitan, S., & Taggart, R. (1979). *Jobs for the disabled.* Baltimore: Johns Hopkins University Press.

Martin, J. F. (1978). The active patient: A necessary development. *WHO Chronicle, 32,* 51–57.

Munson, R. (1983). *Intervention and reflection: Basic issues in medical ethics.* Belmont, CA: Wadsworth.

National Council on the Handicapped (1986). *Toward independence: A report to the President and to the Congress of the United States.* Washington, DC: U.S. Government Printing Office.

Noble, J. H., Jr. (1977). The limits of cost-benefit analysis as a guide to priority setting in rehabilitation. *Evaluation Quarterly, 1,* 347–380.

Noble, J. H., Jr. (1981). New directions for public policies affecting the mentally disabled. In J. J. Bevilacqua (Ed.), *Changing government policies for the mentally disabled* (pp. 9–37). Cambridge, MA: Ballinger.

Plant, R. (1970). *Social and moral theory in casework.* London: Routledge & Kegan Paul.

Reamer, F. J. (1979). Fundamental ethical issues in social work: An essay review. *Social Service Review, 53,* 229–243.

Rehabilitation International. (1981). *International statements on disability policy.* New York: Author.

Schwarzentraub, K. (1980, June 18). *Cooperatives and their implications to individuals who have special needs.* Sacramento: California Department of Housing and Community Development.

Smith, R. T. (1979). Rehabilitation of the disabled: The role of social networks in the recovery process. *International Rehabilitation Medicine, 1,* 63–72.

Wilensky, H. L., & Lebeaux, C. N. (1958). *Industrial society and social welfare.* New York: Russell Sage Foundation.

World Health Organization. (1976). *Reports on specific technical matters—disability prevention and rehabilitation* (A29/INF.DOC/1). Geneva: Author.

World Health Organization. (1980). *International classification of impairments, disabilities, and handicaps.* Geneva: Author.

2

The Rehabilitation Counselor and the Disabled Client

Is a Partnership of Equals Possible?

Phyllis Rubenfeld

HOW THE COUNSELING relationship between the consumer—the client—and the rehabilitation counselor is defined and structured is examined in this chapter. It is a given that the ideal relationship would allow the consumer to maintain optimal control over the objectives pursued, while remaining open to the benefits to be gained from the substantial contribution of the counselor. Any such discussion must consider that the professional and the consumer enter the counseling relationship from different perspectives, perspectives that often contribute unconsciously to the final shaping of objectives. The counselor usually is not disabled. The consumer is. More often than not, the impact of that fact varies not only from consumer to consumer, but its interpretation also varies from counselor to counselor.

Legislation (Rehabilitation Act of 1973) mandates that all parties involved in counseling agree in writing on ultimate goals, and then concur on a plan of action to implement those goals. Still, the counselor can be perceived as being in control of the decision-making process. Many disabled persons have yet to learn how to take part in decision making. They tend to rely on parents, physicians, nurses, social workers, or physical therapists to make choices for them. The rehabilitation counselor comes to the relationship with a broad professional knowledge of the dynamics of human behavior and a familiarity with disability gained through study and work. This knowledge, if not enriched with the understanding that comes only from listening carefully to what disabled persons experience and envisage for themselves, can result in the counselor's considering only broad social, economic and physical factors—such as accessibility, architectural and communicative barriers, and the likelihood of a welcome by supervisors and peers in the workplace—in assessing the likelihood of the consumer's attaining a specific goal.

It is thus that consumers' aspirations can be undervalued and the resultant counseling short sighted. Such a result can be considered simply inadequate, or can impose severe limitations on the life of the disabled person. It has been the author's experience that such an outcome is characteristic of a hierarchical counseling structure. B. A. Wright (1983) has pointed out "that help frequently connotes an asymmetrical situation in which the one helped occupies a subservient, less powerful position. The helper is the capable one in the situation, whereas the one helped is in a position of dependency" (p. 422). This situation can be somewhat ameliorated through counselor encouragement of active client participation. B. A. Wright (1983) elaborates:

> The specification of active participation becomes clarified when clients are considered to be part of management. It is then that they not only contribute data to their case but also help to evaluate the data and work toward solutions; and finally that they claim veto power as well as voting privileges. The principle of co-management is an apt designation for the kind of relationship advocated. It connotes active participation by both client and specialist. (p. 418)

TOPICS FOR DISCUSSION

In order to delineate the sources of tension in the counseling relationship and suggest some possible ways of reducing them, the following are discussed:

1. The historical characterization of disabled persons as cultural pariahs
2. The presently widespread failure to distinguish between disease and disability
3. The embodiment of this intellectual failure in the medical model of disability which pervades the theory and practice of rehabilitation
4. The resultant emphasis placed by rehabilitation professionals on clients' limitations and their failure to imagine possibilities
5. The effect of self-fulfilling prophecies on counseling outcomes, considered especially in those cases where the rehabilitation counselor does not agree with the consumer's career goals and covertly suggests that other alternative choices will be met with failure
6. The effect of physical, racial, ethnic, and cultural differences between counselors and clients on the selection of vocational programs
7. The effect of counselors' negative, stereotyped attitudes toward disabled persons on both the precise nature of counselor-consumer relationships and the outcomes of counseling

8. The effects on counselors of budgetary pressures, time constraints, and large caseloads
9. Negative attitudes of the consumer
10. The counselor with a disability
11. The co-management alternative

HISTORY

As G. N. Wright (1980) pointed out, "A culture inherits all that has gone before. No civilization has come and gone without leaving some legacy. Rehabilitation, a small element of our culture, is what it is and is becoming as a result of all the variations in human interrelationships to date" (p. 118). While space limitations preclude a review of the entire history of disability, a vast amount of historical research (Obermann, 1967; Rubin & Roessler, 1983; G. N. Wright, 1980) has demonstrated how powerless and how marginal to the rest of society disabled persons have been over the years. In many ancient cultures, disabled children were exposed to the elements and allowed to die for the good of the larger, healthier society.

In various present-day traditional cultures, such as the Chagga of East Africa, disabled persons are viewed as being punished by God or possessed by evil spirits. Conversely, disability is venerated as a transcendent symbol of goodness and suffering by the Dahomeans of West Africa (B. A. Wright, 1983).

The belief that the disabled person is somehow "possessed" is present in contemporary Western society in the fear and hostility that many people feel toward disabled persons. At the very least, disabled persons suffer from the general disregard of the public, to whom they represent an uncomfortable reminder of human vulnerability. For example, at a demonstration meant to impress Joseph Califano, former Secretary of the U.S. Department of Health, Education and Welfare (HEW), with the need to sign the Section 504 regulations, people in the street did not ask the demonstrators what they were doing, and when demonstrators approached people on the street to ask them to sign the petitions, some literally ran away.

The notion of the "transcendent goodness" of the disabled person surfaces today in the thoughtlessly benign image of the understanding and forgiving "cripple," an image that dominates many people's thinking (Obermann, 1967; G. N. Wright, 1980). One could interpret the image of the "patient cripple" as a balm to the conscience of an unheeding public.

Neither of these attitudes has benefitted the disabled person. Both images underlie demands from various *ad hoc* groups to segregate disabled persons, either through institutionalization, through "keeping them at home," or through housing them in someone else's neighborhood. Segregation of disabled persons, like segregation of racial minorities, is really a convenience for the larger society; it sets the disabled population, which can be different or frightening to look at, safely apart from the rest of society; it spares the nondisabled the discomfort of seeing that, through accident or injury, they might become one of "them"; and it effectively conceals from public scrutiny any unfortunate effects of the policy itself. Such a policy assumes, and thus requires, that disabled persons accept their difference and separateness from the "normal" population, forego any expectation of leading normal lives, and accept with gratitude whatever minimal level of care the larger society may deign to offer them.

Whether by segregating disabled persons or by the indifference of condescension, society is not pressed to respond with the initial financial planning that would help to incorporate the disabled population productively into the marketplace. Instead, the appropriation of inadequate funding for programs often results in disabled persons having to remain in institutions, whereas they could be housed in their own apartments with varying degrees of assistance or supervision. Cities lack the funds to change the infrastructure that would make transportation accessible for a person who uses a wheelchair, and the person with disabilities who is on Supplemental Security Income (SSI) lacks the funds to become mobile—to go to a museum or vote in one's district, especially if the polling site is inaccessible. Thus disabled persons are denied self-determination and even basic freedoms. Government, however, loses little of its wealth.

DISEASE – A DESTRUCTIVE SYNONYM FOR DISABILITY

The image of the forbearing and isolated cripple is not confined to sentimental films, Victorian novels, and melodramatic telethons. It is embodied in the U.S. system of maintenance and rehabilitation services today. As Nosek, Narita, Dart, and Dart (1982) noted, disabled persons "live in a therapeutic state, a 'society of the sick,' [where] there is no place for any of the hallmarks of a present or future adult identity; no place for politics, no place for work and sexuality, no place for choice between competing moralities" (p. 9). Even with the best of intentions, the managers of this therapeutic state transform "all political, legal, and ethical issues . . . into questions of disease and health, deviance and normal adjustment, proper and improper management of the disability" (Nosek et al., 1982, p. 9).

Confusion between disability and disease is so widespread that many helping professionals and much of the general public have great difficulty in seeing disabled persons as mature individuals whose pursuits might be affected by more than the usual physical limitations, but whose aspirations are fully shared with the rest of the public. Therapy here operates as a screen, an interpreter. Swimming, for example, is viewed solely in terms of physical therapy for disabled persons rather than for pleasure or for sport. This confusion of illness with physical limitation has led to placing the programs for disabled persons within the medical community, resulting in even further segregation of disabled persons. A more appropriate response would provide for infrastructure design to facilitate independent choice of activity.

THE MEDICAL MODEL OF DISABILITY

Anderson (1975), Glick (1953), and Lowenfeld (1956) have delineated the essential imbalance of the helping relationship. Anderson (1975), for example, pointed out that the relationship itself

> tends to reinforce the attitude that the expert has the answers, or at least should have all the answers. The thought that the answers themselves may frequently require the judgment and decision of the client is quite alien. Instead, it becomes natural for the professional to take over and to receive the credit for successful rehabilitation. The dominance of the expert has been associated with the medical model in contrast to help as a growth-promoting process in which clients co-manage their rehabilitation. (p. 103)

The medical model is, in fact, the clearest expression of this view, and the one that pervades current thinking and policy. The medical model defines disability as

> a medical problem to be treated in the same general way as, for example, a strep infection. Medically certified as ''ill,'' the child becomes a full-time (and often lifelong) patient. Both the child and the parents are expected to accept passively the medical establishment's superior knowledge and therapeutic instructions. The child is defined as having ''something wrong,'' and the goal is to ''get well,'' which of course the child can never do. Indeed, the medical model sometimes suggests that all other activities, including planning for the future, are to be suspended until the child is ''cured.'' (Kenniston, 1980, p. xiii)

Where the medical model dominates the thinking of the rehabilitation counselor, the counselor replaces the role of the all-knowing doctor, identifying the therapeutic issues and ultimately deciding what the client must do to ''get better'' or ''adjust.'' In this scenario, the consumer's role is defined as acceptance of the counselor's superior expertise and judgment. The consumer is even expected to conform to the counselor's timetable. For example, many disabled clients in independent living programs have told the author that their counselors' assessments, and not decisions made jointly by themselves and their counselors, usually determine their career ''choices,'' just as a doctor's diagnosis would determine a course of treatment. Lately one begins to hear from clients who say that their independent living centers (ILCs) have become as bureaucratic and self-protecting as most hospitals, and that the emphasis of the centers is less on helping individual clients to lead self-directed lives than on encouraging all clients to adjust and conform to the administrative routine of the centers. Both the latter emphasis and the medical model of disability place the client in a subordinate position, without a voice.

The authoritarian approach of state rehabilitation agency (office of vocational rehabilitation, or OVR) staff is perhaps better known, so only three examples are cited here from the many the author heard. One disabled young woman decided to enter the field of social work, but her OVR counselor told her that she could not do so because she was "unable to jump." The woman gave this advice the consideration it deserved and went ahead with her plans. She was accepted by many graduate schools of social work and has made a name for herself in the field despite being labeled hostile and aggressive by her counselor. Another example is that of a young man, blind from birth, who wanted to become a lawyer and scored very high on his LSAT exams. His counselor felt that law school would be too much of an academic strain for the young man and that even if he did graduate, it would be difficult for him to build a practice. The counselor labeled him maladjusted when he insisted on entering law school. The young man is now a successful lawyer. The third example is a young man with muscular dystrophy who wanted to attend law school, but his OVR counselor declined his request, stating that he was a "poor risk" and that, since he had a degenerative illness, any money the state invested in him would be "unwisely allocated." After many arguments and the threat of legal action, the OVR office reversed the counselor's decision. Today the young man is a successful lawyer.

Not every disabled person who defies his or her counselor goes on to fame and fortune. However, those who succumb completely to the medical model of disability and do everything the experts tell them, including choosing the job and career the experts select, run the risk of going through life without learning how to defend themselves or how to reach a mature assessment of their own capabilities and limitations. They are often without friends and immaturely dependent on their parents. This might occur in any case, but a system of care that listens last, if at all, to the needs and wishes of the client *as the client understands them* only encourages such a scenario.

EMPHASIS ON CLIENTS' LIMITATIONS

The recent history of rehabilitation has been a glorious one. Rehabilitation has made important theoretical contributions that have been adopted to great advantage by other medical and psychotherapeutic disciplines. Tailoring counseling to the needs of each individual client and involving the client's entire family in the counseling process are only two examples. However, what concerns many disabled persons about the rehabilitation field is something that is difficult to discuss without seeming overly sensitive or perhaps even somewhat hysterical.

Disabled persons simply cannot read much of the literature of rehabilitation without being deeply troubled by its focus on the *limitations* of clients (Bowe, 1980; DeJong, 1984). For example, G. N. Wright (1980) noted that, in general, ''the importance of matching clients' abilities with jobs was recognized'' by rehabilitation professionals, and it ''was advised that care be taken not to place people in jobs that were too demanding physically'' (p. 136). This would seem to be entirely self-evident; no one, surely, would want to give persons with physical disabilities jobs that are beyond their physical capabilities.

It is crucial that every counselor and every client mutually assess the client's level of motivation, expectations, and ability to take risks and accept failure. One of the major complaints voiced by people with disabilities is that OVR counselors seem to see them as primarily incapable, discourage them from taking any risks whatsoever, and would rather place them in jobs that would not tax their bodies or their emotional reserves, but that may be depressing, boring, or intellectually beneath their abilities. Since such placements also protect the counselor from the risk of failure, one may wonder whose interests are really being served. Interviews support this contention. For example, one high school senior who uses a wheelchair wanted to major in biology and minor in art, since she was interested in working as a scientific illustrator for biology textbooks. Although the biology laboratory was architecturally accessible in the college to which she applied, her rehabilitation counselor felt that she would be ''better off majoring in art,'' since she could work out of her home. It was the counselor's idea that she could design cards and sell them from her house. A college sophomore wanted to major in sociology, with the intention of attending a graduate school of social work. She was told by her rehabilitation counselor that because of her disability it would be too physically strenuous, and that therefore she should major in speech pathology, which is essentially ''a desk job.'' It is not within the purview of this chapter to go into the specific details of each situation; however, the rehabilitation counselor in each case minimized the consumer's aspirations and emotional and intellectual capabilities, and in each case, the students, through much drive, accomplished their goals.

THE ROLE OF EXPECTATIONS AND SELF-FULFILLING PROPHECIES

Research (Horney, 1939; Murphy & Salomone, 1983; Rosenthal, 1969; Rubenfeld, 1981; Shearer, 1981) has suggested the importance of service provider expectations and particularly of self-fulfilling prophecies (Rosenthal & Jacobson, 1966) to the outcomes of the clients served. The basic point is that one person's expectations of another person's behavior can, in time, produce or at least greatly encourage the expected behavior. A classic case in point is that of a middle-aged man with cerebral palsy who required assistance to perform most activities of daily living, yet wanted to attend college and live in his own apartment. His rehabilitation counselor was convinced that he could not function in his own apartment, even with a personal care attendant and accommodations made for him at college. The man's parents, who had always taken care of his every need, agreed with the rehabilitation counselor. Upon trying to live independently, this consumer became easily frustrated when things did not work out and finally moved back home. Later, when both of his parents died in an automobile accident, he was placed in a nursing home that he described as "a living hell." Eventually he got in touch with people and groups who helped him get out. Now he has his own apartment and a personal care attendant, attends college, and socializes. He has his share of problems, but expects to learn to live with them. He has come to realize that when little or nothing was expected of him, he fulfilled those expectations.

The beneficial effects of positive expectations also have been demonstrated. Rosenthal and Jacobson (1966) cite an experiment in which a self-fulfilling prophecy brought about academic progress:

> Within each of 18 classrooms, an average of 20% of the children were reported to classroom teachers as showing unusual potential for intellectual gains. Eight months later these "unusual" children (who had actually been selected at random) showed significantly greater gains in IQ than did the remaining children in the control group. These effects of teachers' expectations operated primarily among the young children. (p. 117)

Rehabilitation counselors are not entirely immune to the prejudices and stereotypes about disabled persons that are prevalent in our society. To the degree that their professional training has not counteracted any such pretraining attitudes, they might fail to realize their clients' true vocational potential. If such possible training deficiencies are not seen as equally tragic by both rehabilitation educators and consumers of rehabilitation services, not only does a major problem exist; it is likely to persist.

DIFFERENCES BETWEEN COUNSELORS AND CLIENTS

Clients and counselors are bound to disagree to some extent about the nature and degree of the client's psychological adjustment, vocational needs, and level of ability. These disagreements are often exacerbated by physical, racial, ethnic, or cultural differences between clients and counselors. Many of the disabled persons the author meets cite racial and ethnic compatibility as a major factor in the success of their counseling relationship. In one case, two men, one white and the other black, had the same disability, similar talents and interests, and almost identical career goals. They were close friends and had the same counselor. The white client had little difficulty getting his counselor to agree to his professional plans, but the black client found resistance and doubt every step of the way.

Even when counselor prejudice does not affect the counseling relationship, differences in background can lead to misunderstanding between counselor and client and inappropriate treatment of the client. These differences must be faced directly and discussed with complete openness and the greatest imaginative empathy by both parties.

One of the most significant differences between counselors and clients is that most often the counselor is not disabled.

> Well into the 1960s, disabled applicants to many academic programs for professional training in rehabilitation disciplines were not welcomed by screening committees unless they demonstrated unusual ability to avoid ''identification'' with clients' or patients' problems. Nondisabled professionals feared disabled providers would be unable to separate their own problems (and resulting emotions) from those of their clients, reducing their objectivity and helpfulness. The (largely unrecognized) assumption underlying this prejudice was that a person who is disabled must be so pervasively damaged by it psychologically, that recovery of objectivity and emotional control, when the subject is touched, is virtually impossible. This attitude was tempered first by the increasing realization, within the entire psychosocial/behavioral helping field, that ''identification'' is neither so rare nor so deadly as previously imagined. Second, it was quelled by the rising voice of an increasing political disabled constituency. The ''customers'' began to insist that they could do the job better in some respects, and they demanded the right to try. The ILPs [Individualized Learning Plans] provided a mechanism for them to do so. (Vash, 1981, pp. 211–212)

Another difference between counselors and clients is basic to consumerism,

> . . . which . . . is a distrust of seller or service provider. It is up to the consumer to become informed about product reliability or service adequacy. Consumer sovereignty has always been the hallmark of free market economic theory. In practice, however, it is often the professional who has been sovereign. With the rise of consumer sovereignty, professional dominance in disability policy and rehabilitation is being challenged . . . the Rehabilitation Act of 1973 provides for an ''individualized written rehabilitation plan'' (IWRP) to be drawn up jointly by client and counselor. (DeJong, 1979, pp. 47–48)

COUNSELORS' NEGATIVE ATTITUDES TOWARD DISABLED PERSONS

Wicas and Carluccio (1971) report findings that suggest that in many cases rehabilitation counselors hold negative, stereotyped attitudes toward disabled persons, and that factors other than client needs determine what services are eventually provided. These negative attitudes may be reinforced by many of the factors just discussed—the medical model that casts disabled persons in the sick role, the focus of rehabilitation professionals on clients' limitations, rehabilitation counselor expectations that can limit client options, and counseling relationships in which decision making is significantly dominated by the counselor. At best, such relationships display a severe imbalance resulting in ''a greater tendency for the counselor to fail to note a problem identified by the client than for the client to acknowledge a problem identified by his or her counselor'' (Makas, 1980, p. 235).

NEGATIVE EFFECTS OF EXTERNAL FACTORS

Of course, it is not just the imperfect counselor who stands in the way of realizing an effective counseling relationship; financial pressures, time constraints, and the need to offer rehabilitation services to as many clients as possible also interfere (B. A. Wright, 1983). Clients, especially the newly disabled, often need so much time to adjust to their situations that they may become administrative burdens on busy agencies as well as unrewarding clients for highly motivated counselors. In such cases, the counselor may have to devote special effort to stimulating the client's involvement and cooperation, or risk falling prey to the negative attitudes, mutual distrust, and unsatisfactory counseling relationships outlined in the preceding section.

NEGATIVE ATTITUDES OF THE CONSUMER

Becoming newly disabled more often than not is synonymous with dependency on others. This newly disabled person may have absorbed from society at large the following belief:

> The language of disability indicates that persons with disabilities are usually perceived exclusively in terms of their disabilities, that they are confined to a ''handicapped role'' in which they are seen primarily as recipients of medical treatment, and that this role also includes ascribed traits of helplessness, despondency, abnormality of appearance and mode of functioning, pervasive incapacitation of every aspect of personhood, and ultimately subhumanness. (Longmore, 1985, p. 419)

In the experience of many professionals, a newly disabled person is very angry, frustrated, and does not want to be identified with a group of people that the disabled person did not think much of before anyway. Often anger and lack of motivation characterize the newly disabled person even when one explains and/or shows them how they can continue on with their lives and be happy.

Much time and energy goes into counseling the newly disabled person, whereas those who have been disabled for an extended period of time are usually more familiar with career limitations and possibilities. The newly disabled person can be viewed as an *administrative* ''burden'' simply because of the extra amount of time needed in order to be effective in keeping the client involved in living a life as close to the one he or she did previously. The newly disabled person knows very little about state rehabilitation agencies and the services they have to offer. This client is negative about his or her dependency, usually doesn't believe that he or she can be helped in a significant manner, and indeed may be assigned to a counselor who feels overwhelmed as it is and who thus provides a minimal amount of help. This client does not feel fulfilled nor does he or she know how to appeal for additional services that could make life easier and more satisfying. If the client remains angry, frustrated, and depressed, he or she may have difficulty engendering a satisfactory relationship with his or her counselor.

THE COUNSELOR WITH A DISABILITY

It is extremely helpful to have a counselor with a disability to serve as an example, a role model. Such a counselor probably has encountered many of the same or similar problems the consumer is facing, and is able to set a real-life example that one's life-style can change. This does not mean that a legitimate role does not continue to exist for the nondisabled counselor.

THE CO-MANAGEMENT ALTERNATIVE

Co-management appears to be the strongest viable alternative to the more traditional helping relationship. Where the traditional mode stresses a hierarchical relationship, co-management insists on a team approach. Where the traditional mode tends to view the client as dependent, co-management relies on and nurtures active participation: the client is responsive and responsible. It has been found that an increase in learning potential characterizes the co-management pattern (B. A. Wright, 1983, p. 419). True rehabilitation seeks to build inner strength and self-respect in the client; such values are fostered by a relationship in which the disabled person feels that he or she has an important role in planning his or her life, and that what he or she says and feels are respected.

> Belief in the principle of co-management in a relationship of respect and caring can go far in bringing co-management about. But just because it is easier to subscribe to this in principle than in practice, the professional person must question at all times whether the client is at the helm helping to steer the course of rehabilitation or whether in effect the client is being paternalistically directed as a manipulable charge who is to follow through but not question why. (B. A. Wright, 1983, p. 441)

CONCLUSIONS

Counselors at all levels should examine their attitudes in light of the factors discussed above. Do they see disability and disease as synonymous? Do they subscribe uncritically to the medical model and its total subordination of the disabled client to the clinical expertise of the treating professional? Are they unable to see clients' talents and accomplishments as readily as their limitations? Do they encourage clients to fail through negative expectations and self-fulfilling prophecies? Are they acting out prejudices against disabled persons as such, or as members of racial, ethnic, or cultural groups different from their own? Do they allow their clients to suffer unduly because of the temporal and financial pressures of their jobs? Are they unwilling to accept the burden of equality imposed by co-management?

Only when counselors can answer no to these questions will the field begin to back away from the grim future envisioned by Zola (1983):

> Rehabilitation personnel must change their model of service so that it focuses less on doing something to someone and more on planning and creating service with someone. In short, unless the rehabilitation world frees itself from some of its culture-bound and time-limited standards and philosophy, we may one day find ourselves in the position of Walt Kelly's Pogo, who once exclaimed: "We have met the enemy and he is us." (p. 356)

Rehabilitation counseling should be a collaborative venture; the roles of client and counselor should become more nearly equal. Attitude and behavior change will have to occur in both counselor and consumer, but the greater adjustment will have to be made by the counselor.

> The needs of the helper are also important in role determination. When professionals have a need to assert themselves, flaunt their knowledge, buttress their status, or gain power, the authoritarian role is so satisfying that it is not easily given up. There is also the specialist who does not enjoy or who becomes anxious in real give and take relationships. More impersonal contact with clients in an authoritarian relationship may then be preferred. (B. A. Wright, 1983, p. 423)

Counselors must listen to what their clients are saying without being unduly influenced by common preconceptions and stereotypes about disability, nor about their role as professionals. They should allow their clients to take risks and, perhaps, let them fail. Failure, which can be very instructive, must not be reserved for the nondisabled person.

The best place to begin to affect this adjustment is in the training of rehabilitation counselors. Adjustment here refers primarily to counselors already working in the field, for most have come to their profession with little direct experience with disability and are plunged into fieldwork in traditional settings, such as hospitals, that provide the most extreme model for encouraging dependency in the disabled persons.

In such a setting, a rehabilitation counselor or a colleague from an independent living center with very strong beliefs in client participation should be on the supervisory staff to help change the traditional counselor-client relationship. Why not use independent living centers as preferred field placements? This would allow counseling students to interact with disabled clients in a more positive environment, and to experience disabled persons as fellow staff or even as superiors. Many unconscious prejudices might be recognized and disposed of in the process.

Independent living centers afford more structural flexibility than the traditional approach to rehabilitation, in a climate that fosters a more equal relationship between counselor, client, and the co-management model within their system. What is necessary is that efforts be concentrated toward the adoption of the co-management model within the traditional rehabilitation state agencies. Education is one step toward bringing about this change. It is hoped that the new vision gained through education will change the concepts of role modeling to such an extent that the systems themselves will then reflect that more equal structure.

REFERENCES

Anderson, T. P. (1975). An alternative frame of reference for rehabilitation: The helping process versus the medical model. *Archives of Physical Medicine and Rehabilitation, 56,* 101–104.

Bowe, F. (1980). *Rehabilitating America: Toward independence for disabled and elderly people.* New York: Harper & Row.

DeJong, G. (1979). Independent living: From social movement to analytic paradigm. *Archives of Physical Medicine and Rehabilitation, 60,* 39–63.

DeJong, G. (1984). *Independent living and disability policy in the Netherlands: Three models of residential care and independent living.* New York: World Rehabilitation Fund.

Gleidman, J., & Roth, W. (1980). *The unexpected minority: Handicapped children in America.* New York: Harcourt Brace Jovanovich.

Glick, S. J. (1953). *Vocational, educational, and recreational needs of the cerebral palsied adult.* New York: Springer-Verlag.

Horney, K. (1939). *New ways in psychoanalysis.* New York: Norton.

Keniston, K. (1980). Foreword. In J. Gliedman & W. Roth, *The unexpected minority: Handicapped children in America.* New York: Harcourt Brace Jovanovich.

Longmore, Paul K. (1985). A note on language and the social identity of disabled people. *American Behavioral Scientist, 28,* 419–423.

Lowenfeld, B. (1956). *Our blind children.* Springfield, IL: Charles C Thomas.

Makas, E. (1980). Increasing counselor-client communication. *Rehabilitation Literature, 41,* 235–238.

Marinelli, R. P., & Dell Orto, A. E. (Eds.). (1984). *The psychological and social impact of physical disability* (2nd ed.). New York: Springer-Verlag.

Murphy, S. T., & Salomone, P. R. (1983). Client and counselor expectations of rehabilitation services. *Rehabilitation Counseling Bulletin, 27,* 81–93.

Nosek, P., Narita, Y., Dart, Y., & Dart, J. (1982). *A philosophical foundation for the independent living and disability rights movement.* Houston: Institute for Rehabilitation and Research.

Obermann, C. E. (1967). *A history of vocational rehabilitation in America.* Minneapolis: T. S. Dennison.

Owen, M. J. (1985). A view of disability in current social work literature. *American Behavioral Scientist, 28,* 397–403.

Ratzka, A. D. (1986). *Independent living and attendant care in Sweden: A consumer perspective.* New York: World Rehabilitation Fund.

Rosenthal, R. (1969). Unintended effects of the clinician in clinical interaction: A

taxonomy and a review of clinician expectancy effects. *Australian Journal of Psychology, 21,* 1–20.
Rosenthal, R., & Jacobson, L. (1966). Teachers' expectancies: Determinants of pupils' IQ gains. *Psychological Reports, 19,* 115–118.
Rubenfeld, P. (1981, June). Notes from the bottom of the blackboard. *The Exceptional Parent,* pp. 27–30.
Rubin, S. E., & Roessler, R. T. (1983). *Foundations of the vocational rehabilitation process.* Austin, TX: PRO-ED.
Shearer, A. (1981). *Disability: Whose handicap?* Oxford: Basil Blackwell.
Vash, C. L. (1981). *The psychology of disability.* New York: Springer-Verlag.
Wicas, E. A., & Carluccio, L. W. (1971). Attitudes of counselors toward three handicapped client groups. *Rehabilitation Counseling Bulletin, 15,* 25–34.
Wright, B. A. (1983). *Physical disability: A psychosocial approach* (2nd ed.). New York: Harper & Row.
Wright, G. N. (1980). *Total rehabilitation.* Boston: Little, Brown.
Zola, I. K. (1983). Toward independent living: Goals and dilemmas. In N. M. Crewe & I. K. Zola (Eds.), *Independent living for physically disabled people.* San Francisco: Jossey-Bass.

3

Independent Living and Rehabilitation Counseling

Margaret A. Nosek

The rise of the independent living movement in the early 1970s and the advent of federal funding for the establishment of centers for independent living throughout the country has secured independent living as a permanent part of the rehabilitation discipline and the disability-related service system. The relationship between independent living and rehabilitation on both the systems and professional levels has raised several issues. This chapter presents background information on issues surrounding independent living as a movement, a service, and a profession. It concludes with a discussion of the impact of independent living on the education and job responsibilities of rehabilitation counselors.

OVERVIEW OF INDEPENDENT LIVING

Independent living is defined as control over one's life based on the choice of acceptable options that minimize reliance on others in making decisions and performing everyday activities (Frieden, Richards, Cole, & Bailey, 1979). Living independently in this context includes managing one's affairs, participating in the day-to-day life of the community in a manner of one's own choosing, fulfilling a range of social roles that include productive work, and making decisions that lead to self-determination and the minimization of nonproductive physical and psychological dependence upon others. According to the *National Policy for Persons with Disabilities,*

> the type of independence defined here implies an optimally responsible and productive exercise of the power of choice. It implies that each disabled person,

> regardless of his or her mental or physical ability, should be encouraged and assisted to achieve maximum levels of quality of life, independence and productivity in the least restrictive environment and with due respect for cultural or subcultural affiliation. (National Council on the Handicapped, 1983, p. 20–21)

The philosophy reflected by this definition emerged from the grass-roots civil rights movement of persons with severe disabilities attempting to forge independent life-styles for themselves. The tenets of this philosophy are the individual's right and power to exercise control over his or her life with the greatest degree of self-reliance possible while having acceptable options in the spheres of life judged to be important by that person. It contains a potent advocacy orientation that focuses on changing the environment to suit the individual, rather than molding the individual to fit the expectations and limitations imposed by society (DeJong, 1979; P. Nosek, Narita, Dart, & Dart, 1982; Pflueger, 1977).

Services to support independent living must be tailored to the needs of the individual. Persons with severe physical disabilities usually require assistance with personal care, domestic tasks, transportation, equipment maintenance, and modifications of home and work place for architectural accessibility. Those with sensory disabilities require reader and interpreter assistance with communication and expression. Persons with mental impairments who wish to live independently may require advocates for some assistance with cognitive tasks. All can benefit from information and referral about services and service providers, training in independent living skills, assistance in gaining mobility in the community, and individual advocacy. For those who have extraordinary medical and personal care needs, private and/or public resources are required to help cover such expenses. Those who are not employed usually require income maintenance support and financial assistance with daily living expenses.

Services for independent living include any formal or informal assistance needed by people with disabilities trying to increase control of their life, productivity, and participation in the community. Generally, these services are delivered by community-based organizations that are privately or publicly funded. However, services rendered by residential institutions can also be considered independent living services if they assist residents to achieve maximum control and independence in the least restrictive environment. In this sense, long-term care service providers could provide independent living services if the criteria of assisting residents to exert control over their lives and reach their independent living goals are met.

Almost all persons residing in private and government-operated institutions, regardless of the severity of their disability, could benefit in some way from independent living support services. For a large percentage, it could mean being able to live in the community in a residence and having the life-style of their own choice, as well as the opportunity to realize their potential for productive contribution to society. For those with the most severe disabilities, it could mean receiving life support and enrichment services in a dignified and humane manner that maximizes their quality of life. Independent living services could benefit those who have been rejected by or who have failed in the vocational rehabilitation system. Potential beneficiaries also include the uncounted millions of disabled persons living in rural areas with little access to service providers of any kind, or residing with families or in small group settings that restrict their ability to control their lives and reach their productive potential.

In 1981, an estimated 2,138,970 disabled persons were served in 38,975 residential facilities (including state hospitals, residential facilities for mentally retarded persons, nursing homes, and other long-term care facilities) at a cost to the federal and state government of $22.8 billion (National Study Group on State Medicaid Strategies, 1983; Sirrocco, 1983; Smith, 1984). In 1984, state vocational rehabilitation agencies closed 131,572 cases of clients who had not reached their rehabilitation goals. Out of almost 600,000 applicants, 245,435 were rejected as ineligible. Another 48,372 applicants were placed in the category of extended evaluation; that is, they were not rejected, but were not found to be eligible or ineligible for vocational rehabilitation services (Department of Education, 1985). Although there may be some overlap between these figures and the number of persons in residential facilities, the total number who sought disability-related services and who could extensively use independent living support services probably exceeds 2.5 million (M. A. Nosek, 1986).

THE GENESIS AND STATUS OF INDEPENDENT LIVING SERVICES

Prior to the independent living movement, traditional services for persons with severe disabilities emphasized medical recovery and employability as the major indicators of success. This narrow focus relegated a large percentage of persons with disabilities to the limited life options of institutional placement or extensive dependence on family care. The potential for recovery or employment and the ability to live independently in the community were either underestimated or unrecognized by the rehabilitation and social service systems. The independent living movement was initiated about 15 years ago, primarily by young adults with physical disabilities who sought to broaden the approaches and services available to them for acquiring the necessary knowledge, skills, confidence, and assistance to participate more fully in society. Their efforts to develop the necessary support services for maintaining their own independence were expanded and formalized in the establishment of what are now called centers for independent living.

DeJong (1979, p. 34) set out three major propositions that underlie the philosophical context of the community-based independent living movement:

1. *Consumer sovereignty* Disabled persons, the actual consumers of the services, not professionals, are the best judges of their own interests. They should ultimately determine how services should be organized on their behalf.
2. *Self-reliance* Disabled persons must rely primarily on their own resources and ingenuity to acquire the rights and benefits to which they are entitled.
3. *Political and economic rights* Disabled persons are entitled to participate fully and freely in the political and economic life of the community.

The practice of delivering independent living support services to disabled persons by disabled persons, combined with advocacy for community accessibility, had its start in Berkeley in the early 1970s. The Berkeley Center for Independent Living (Zukas, 1975) and the Boston Center for Independent Living, which was developed soon after (Fay, Bartels, Corcoran, & McHugh, 1977), became service delivery models. It is upon the Berkeley model that independent living legislation is based. This model, a community-based, nonprofit, nonresidential program controlled by the disabled consumers it serves, provides directly, or coordinates indirectly through referral, those services that assist severely disabled individuals to increase personal self-determination and to minimize unnecessary dependence upon others (Frieden et al., 1979). The minimum services provided by an independent living center include housing assistance; referral of attendants, readers, and/or interpreters; peer counseling; financial and legal advocacy; and community awareness and barrier removal programs. Other services either provided or coordinated by independent living centers include transportation provision or registry, peer counseling, advocacy or political action, independent living skills training, equipment maintenance and repair, and social-recreational services.

Examples of other approaches to the independent living concept include cooperative living (Stock & Cole, 1977); ''New Options'' (Institute for Information Studies, 1979); and programs in Illinois (Jeffers, 1978), New England (Driscoll, Marquis, Corcoran, & Fay, 1978), Massachusetts (Bartels, 1978), California (Brown, 1978), and Houston (Frieden, 1978). The various program models are described by Frieden et al. (1979).

Conceptually, the term *independent living program* is generic—the most broadly defined term relating to organizations that work with disabled individuals who wish to live independently. Several different kinds of independent living programs exist. They differ from one another in at least six primary ways:

1. *The service setting* may range from residential to nonresidential.
2. *The service delivery method* may range from direct to indirect, or a combination of both.
3. *The service delivery style* may range from professional to consumer.
4. *The vocational emphasis* may range from primary to incidental.
5. *The goal orientation* may range from transitional to ongoing.
6. *The disability type* served may range from single to many.

The features of the independent living program are determined by the needs of the consumers served, the availability of existing community resources, the physical and social makeup of the community, and the goals of the program itself. Custodial care facilities and primary medical care facilities are specifically excluded from the definition of an independent living program (Frieden et al., 1979).

In 1978, Congress authorized direct support of independent living programs as part of the discretionary programs of the Rehabilitation Services Administration (RSA). The Rehabilitation Act of 1973 was amended to add Title VII—Comprehensive Services for Independent Living. As expressed in the legislation, Title VII was intended to assist in development of community-based service centers to provide information and referral, transportation, attendant care, peer counseling, skills training, and other services. The goal was to facilitate the integration of severely disabled adults into the mainstream of community social and economic life; that is, to decrease their dependence and increase their self-determination and ability to be productive, contributing members of society.

Title VII authorization was based upon the program development experience of early independent living centers and led to the substantial growth of independent living centers across the country. Using an approach that philosophically and operationally differs from more traditional service systems, independent living centers actively developed and implemented needed programs to facilitate increased independence for the people they sought to serve.

In short, the impetus and strength of the independent living movement resulted in a viable service alternative that: 1) emphasized consumer sovereignty, self-reliance, and economic and political rights; 2) resisted approaches that put the onus of the problem on the consumer and left decisions about service in the hands of the professional; and 3) resisted the use of assessment systems that were experienced as paternalistic. The hallmark of the independent living movement is advocacy for change, on both individual and community levels.

As a policy issue, independent living has only recently been examined (Dalrymple & Richards, 1983; Galvin, 1980; M. A. Nosek, 1986; Siegman, 1980). In 1983, the concepts of independent living were incorporated into the *National Policy for Persons with Disabilities* by the National Council on the Handicapped. This was the first policy document to apply actively the concepts of independent living to all disability groups and call for an independent living orientation in the provision of all human services. It was followed by specific recommendations by the council to Congress for legislative changes which would promote community-based programs for independent living (National Council on the Handicapped, 1986).

LEGISLATION

Since 1920, a federal-state rehabilitation program has existed to provide services to disabled people who could demonstrate immediately achievable vocational goals (PL 66-236). The program was amended in 1965 to authorize an extended vocational evaluation period of up to 18 months. As a result of this extended evaluation clause, many previously excluded disabled people were able to obtain services from vocational rehabilitation that enhanced their abilities to live independently; however, if they were not vocationally ready at the end of the evaluation period, they were dropped from the rehabilitation program (Dalrymple & Richards, 1983).

Proponents of the independent living movement—including disabled individuals, family members, rehabilitation professionals, health professionals, policy makers, and other advocates—lobbied for changes in the federal-state rehabilitation program. In particular, they urged changes in two respects: 1) elimination of the requirement of vocational potential, and 2) inclusion of disabled people to a greater degree in developing policy for the program (Lorenz, 1982).

In 1972, a bill authorizing provision of independent living services without requiring a vocational goal was passed by Congress but vetoed by President Nixon (Rubin & Roessler, 1983). However, in the following year funds for a comprehensive needs study were authorized by Congress to establish five research and demonstration projects to provide independent living services. Finally, in 1978, independent living legislation was passed that did not require vocational potential as a requirement for participation. This took the form of a separate title of the act, however, rather than as an amendment that could have changed the focus of the entire vocational rehabilitation program, as independent living supporters had hoped.

This independent living entitlement, Title VII of the Rehabilitation Act, contains three sections. The following is a summary of these sections and an assessment of the extent to which each section has been fulfilled to date.

Part A. Comprehensive Services

Part A authorized grants to assist states in providing comprehensive services for independent living designed to meet the current and future needs of individuals with severe disabilities who presently lack the potential for employment, but who may benefit from vocational rehabilitation services enabling them to live and function independently (*Rehabilitation Act,* 1984). States are thus authorized to provide comprehensive independent living services, including traditional services such as vocational counseling, physical rehabilitation, orthotics and prosthetics; and nontraditional services, such as health maintenance, recreational activities, services for children, and housing modification. The scope of service provision appears to be from birth to death. An especially notable requirement of Part A is that disabled consumers have a substantial role in developing the state's plan of service. As of 1986, $5 million had been appropriated by Congress to implement Part A.

Versions of the Part A program (independent living services without vocational requirements) are presently being operated by state agencies for mentally disabled people, visually disabled people, and hearing-impaired people. State mental health and mental retardation agencies nationwide have been given authority and substantial funding to carry out community programs to facilitate independent living for mentally retarded and mentally ill people. Some programs for this disability group have been developed by combining Housing and Urban Development loan/subsidy housing programs with operating funds from combined state funds and federal income support sources such as Social Security Disability Insurance and Supplemental Security Income. In addition, community mental health centers provide a wide range of services for mentally disabled persons, including counseling, day programs, and, frequently, housing and supportive services. One missing element, though, appears to be an extensive, goal-oriented case management coordination system like the one found within vocational rehabilitation agencies.

Many state agencies for blind individuals have independent living programs that include independent living coordinators along with mobility and homemaker specialists. More states are beginning to establish councils for people with hearing impairments. While these programs do not limit service advocacy and provision to those people with vocational goals, they are frequently small programs with limited staffing and few direct services.

Physically disabled people without apparent vocational potential, however, are still ineligible to receive federally funded services from state vocational rehabilitation agencies. Recently, a few state legislatures have authorized the use of state funds to provide certain independent living services, including equipment purchase, attendant care, peer counseling, independent living skills training, and others. Among these states are Texas, California, New York, Massachusetts, Maine, North Carolina, Ohio, Minnesota, and Wisconsin (Dalrymple & Richards, 1983).

Part B. Centers for Independent Living

Part B authorizes grants to establish independent living programs and requires substantial involvement of disabled people in policy direction, management, and employment within the independent living program. The general intent of Part B is the provision of services that are multiple and comprehensive, such as intake counseling, advocacy, independent living skills training, housing and transportation referral and assistance, health maintenance, peer counseling, education and training, recreation, and attendant care.

In fiscal year 1979, $2 million was appropriated for Part B, funding only 10 grants. Subsequent appropriations were $15 million for fiscal year 1980, $18 million for fiscal year 1981, and $17.28 million for the fiscal year ending September 1983, expanded to $19.4 million by continuing resolution and maintained at that level for 1984. Appropriations for fiscal year 1985 were $22 million. Altogether, over 160 programs are being at least partially supported by these funds.

For the most part, the grant awards made to state vocational rehabilitation agencies were subcontracted with community-based organizations that had boards largely composed of disabled persons. There are some variations on this pattern. For instance, a small number of grant awards were made to local organizations when state agencies chose not to apply. Also, in a few instances, state agencies chose to operate independent living programs themselves, fulfilling the requirement of substantial consumer involvement in policy direction by setting up advisory boards of disabled persons (Dalrymple & Richards, 1983).

The most comprehensive analysis to date of the full range of independent living programs has been done by the Independent Living Research Utilization Project. This project has identified 281 programs which deliver independent living support services (Independent Living Research Utilization, 1985). Of the 157 programs responding to a 1983 survey, 63% met the criteria for an independent living center, including being consumer controlled and community based (Independent Living Research Utilization, 1984; Veerkamp, 1984). The average program budget funding was 79% federal and state, 4% local, 8% private agency or foundation, and 9% program generated (fees, memberships, etc.). While 70% of the programs served only persons in the immediate community, 15% provided services in rural areas, and 13% served those in other cities around the state. The most prevalent disability types served were spinal cord injury (18%), blindness (16%), mental retardation (12%), and cerebral palsy (10%).

In the 1984 amendments to the Rehabilitation Act, Congress mandated comprehensive evaluation of all programs receiving funding under Title VII. This evaluation study (Berkeley Planning Associates, 1986) revealed that of 156 centers receiving this funding, 79% subcontracted to the state vocational rehabilitation agency, 10% were located and operated within the agency itself, and 21% of the centers received funds directly from the federal government. One hundred twenty-one of the centers reported delivering independent living services to 48,000 counsumers, 75% of whom had severe disabilities, and to 14,000 nondisabled individuals (such as family members), with 56,000 additional persons receiving only information and referral assistance. Centers receiving Title VII funding primarily served persons with orthopaedic impairments (48%), followed by those with hearing impairments (17%), visual impairments (12%), and other disabilities (15%). Mental illness and mental retardation were the categories least frequently served by this type of independent living program, constituting 8% of the consumer population.

Part C. Independent Living Services for Older Blind Individuals

Part C authorizes grants to states to provide independent living services to persons 55 years of age or older whose visual impairment makes employment difficult to attain, but for whom independent living goals are possible. No appropriations have been made for Part C. For the 1986 budget, the House has recommended a funding level of $5 million.

INDEPENDENT LIVING PROFESSIONALS

A new profession within the discipline of rehabilitation is being born: the independent living service provider. The critical element that distinguishes an independent living specialist from traditional rehabilitation professionals is a heightened awareness of and commitment to advocating for the rights of the individual.

Although some traditional professions specialize in one component of independent living, such as occupational or physical therapists teaching independent living skills, psychologists with disabilities offering peer counseling, or persons with a legal background serving as individual advocates, the independent living specialist is usually a generalist. Such persons have competencies, either through formal training or personal experience, in the psychological and social aspects of disability, barriers to the integration of persons with disabilities into society, case management, and the array of services available in the local community to assist persons with disabilities. Independent living program managers or center directors have additional abilities in personnel management, project planning, fund raising, and other skills required of administrators.

There are many different settings in which independent living services can be provided and professionals can be employed: community-based centers for independent living, comprehensive medical rehabilitation facilities, public and private residential facilities, public school systems, vocational rehabilitation agencies, private rehabilitation counseling organizations, and any setting in which persons with disabilities receive services to increase their abilities and quality of life.

As in other generalist fields, many different paths in formal training can lead to a profession in independent living service provision. In the community-based center for independent living setting, while some level of postsecondary education is usually prerequisite, personal experience is the most valuable source of information. In the rehabilitation facility or agency setting, rehabilitation counseling is one of the most appropriate backgrounds due to certification and other educational requirements that hold together traditional salary and promotional hierarchies. The filling of such positions is made difficult by the fact that only a few educational institutions have course offerings specifically in independent living. At this writing, there are no standardized criteria for independent living specialists or any movement toward establishing such.

INDEPENDENT LIVING AND REHABILITATION COUNSELING

The inclusion of independent living services among the responsibilities of rehabilitation counselors was initiated with the implementation of Title VII of the Rehabilitation Act. When monies became available through Part B to establish centers for independent living, state rehabilitation agencies were given the right to refuse the targeted funds, in which case such funds were then made available to the field through a competitive application process. All but a few states accepted the funding and appointed an administrator to identify appropriate community organizations as potential recipients, worked with them to develop proposals, and monitored grants subsequently awarded to establish and operate centers for independent living. In some states, such as Illinois and Massachusetts, the state agency hired a former director of a center for independent living to administer this program.

Under Part A, only 20% of the funds are required to be designated for fee-for-service or contract arrangements with centers for independent living. The remainder is to be used by the state rehabilitation agency to deliver what is called ''independent living rehabilitation services'' to clients who could not otherwise be served by the state rehabilitation agency. Designated, if not all, counselors within the agency must be familiar with independent living, understand how it relates to vocational rehabilitation, and be able to identify and obtain access to available goods and services that can be purchased with these funds.

Although independent living services have formally existed since funding started flowing through Title VII, the profession of rehabilitation counseling has been very slow to incorporate it. There are many reasons for this. First and foremost, there remains strong concern that adding independent living counseling and services dilutes the vocational focus of traditional rehabilitation counseling. There is resistance to the notion that independent living is a holistic construct that includes productivity (in terms of increasing both financial gain and quality of life) as one of its components (P. Nosek et al., 1982).

Second, the law has provided a convenient rationale for the belief that independent living services dilute traditional rehabilitation counseling by its declaration that Title VII services are for those without immediate vocational potential. There is much confusion and contradiction over this point in various parts of the law and its regulations. In many state rehabilitation agencies, counselors are able to refer clients judged not to have vocational potential, but found to have independent living needs, to other counselors or service divisions within the agency and thus feel little responsibility to become more familiar with this area. They fail to realize that clients judged to have vocational potential and accepted for Title I services may also have independent living needs. Many of these needs could be met by a properly trained rehabilitation counselor.

Third, the concept and process of closure is fundamentally inappropriate for many independent living services. Independent living service needs are often long term and cannot be subjected to the outcome assessment currently used in the closure system of state rehabilitation agencies. An individual cannot be said to have achieved independence until all the support services needed to maintain independence are financed by a stable and continuous source. A state agency, for example, could conceivably purchase a wheelchair for a client to allow more mobility around the home and then "close" the case as having achieved an independent living goal. Such action, however, would be premature and short sighted for individuals with more extensive independent living needs and with potential still to be explored. To achieve true independence according to independent living philosophy, the client would probably also require attendant services, transportation, housekeeping assistance, and other ongoing services to reach his or her potential for independence. Nor can independence be judged attained and the case closed if state financing for these services is offered for a trial period but then terminated after 90 days of "successful placement" without ensuring the presence of similar benefits (Rice & Roessler, 1980). Individuals' independent living needs change as life circumstances change and as opportunities arise. The need for assistance in acquiring independent living support services and finding new resources for financing them can extend throughout the lifetime.

Fourth, there are several conflicts between the rehabilitation paradigm and the independent living paradigm reflected in the daily job activities of rehabilitation counselors and independent living specialists. The rehabilitation paradigm places the locus of the problem in the individual while the independent living paradigm places it in the environment (DeJong, 1979). Most of the activities of rehabilitationists are designed to assist the individual to change in order to meet the demands of society. While independent living directs considerable attention to assisting individuals to improve their ability to function and interact productively with others, there is also a strong focus on changing society to meet the needs of the individual and to allow that individual the freedom to participate equally. It can be difficult for a professional to adopt both philosophies and engage in concurrent activities from both camps.

The relationship between professional and consumer is sometimes a barrier to the acceptance of independent living concepts by rehabilitation counselors. The tradition of maintaining professional detachment from the people one serves directly contradicts the model of peer counseling that underlies the independent living philosophy. The independent living movement believes that effectively assisting a person with a disability toward greater independence often requires more than just referrals or delivering support services. While acknowledging the important role played by nondisabled counselors with facilitative attitudes, the movement believes that independent living counselors should be living examples of the goal; to have faced the barriers, overcome them, and established an independent life-style for themselves and to be able to call upon these experiences in giving the consumer information that is relevant to real life. Given that independent living services are becoming a larger part of the rehabilitation counselor's responsibilities, the movement believes that persons with disabilities will best be served when a significant proportion of rehabilitation counselor positions are occupied by counselors with disabilities.

Independent living philosophy also requires a commitment to disability issues that extends beyond the work day; that is, advocacy expressed through involvement in organizations and activities that seek to remove the societal barriers to independent living, often alongside persons one is currently serving as clients. This type of involvement can occupy evenings and weekends and can consume personal financial resources, but it demonstrates one's dedication to independent living philosophy. While tradition does not recognize this type of involvement as professional behavior, it is this author's belief that independent living services cannot be effectively delivered without it.

This list is in no way inclusive. Additional issues have been articulated by Rice and Roessler (1980) and Rice, Roessler, Greenwood, and Frieden (1983). The demands and influences on rehabilitation counselors are complex and many. Independent living is a new concept still undergoing refinement as a service area. Interaction between the two professions will probably be subjected to analysis for several years before they are comfortably intermixed and a productive partnership is established. One critical area remains to be discussed: what the rehabilitation system is doing to prepare counselors to meet the independent living needs of persons with disabilities.

INDEPENDENT LIVING IN REHABILITATION COUNSELOR EDUCATION

One gauge of the future of independent living in the profession of rehabilitation counseling is the degree to which it is taught in university counselor education programs. A survey of these programs was conducted in 1986 by the Independent Living Research Utilization (LRU) Research and Training Center in Independent Living at the Institute for Rehabilitation and Research in Houston, at the request of the board of the American Rehabilitation Counseling Association. The study investigated Council on Rehabilitation Education (CORE) standards and Council on Rehabilitation Counselor Certification (CRCC) requirements to determine adequacy in the area of independent living, and gathered data on the status of instruction in independent living in rehabilitation counselor education programs.

Seventy of the 83 programs were surveyed in a telephone interview. Only 20 currently offer courses in independent living, 8 of which require that it be taken for the rehabilitation counseling degree. Sixty-five offer independent living as a subject in other courses that are usually introductory in nature. Sixty-two offer practica and/or internships in independent living programs. Sixty-four bring in panels of persons with disabilities for discussion at least once in the semester the course is taught. Only three programs showed significant involvement of a person with a disability in instruction on independent living, and two of these persons were staff of a center for independent living who were serving as instructors of a course.

These findings suggest that while there seems to be some exposure to concepts and techniques of independent living in the training of rehabilitation counselors, it is minimal. Although most programs discuss the topic of independent living in coursework, this discussion is generally only introductory. Exposure to persons with disabilities from an independent living perspective is totally inadequate. The significant involvement of persons with disabilities in the education of rehabilitation counselors is practically nonexistent.

CORE standards were examined and found to allow the inclusion of concepts and techniques of independent living under many provisions. There is, however, no requirement to offer instruction in this subject. Similarly, CRCC requires an understanding of several areas essential to independent living services, such as community services and psychological and social aspects of disability. However, coverage of barriers to independence, principles of independent living counseling (as discussed earlier related to self-determination, life options, and self-reliance), self-advocacy, and other areas key to the delivery of independent living services are inadequate.

After a student graduates from a rehabilitation counselor education program, opportunities for continuing education are available in independent living services through Regional Rehabilitation Continuing Education Programs (RRCEPs), agency in-service training programs, and conferences of professional organizations such as the American Rehabilitation Counseling Association and the National Rehabilitation Association. There is a need to survey RRCEPs, agencies, and organizations to determine the frequency of such opportunities. The evaluations of one training session offered by the Region VI RRCEP indicated that while participating rehabilitation counselors generally appreciated the information, there was ambivalence about how useful it would be in their jobs. Several comments reflected a disinterest in independent living history and philosophy, and called for more specific information on how to deliver independent living services to their clients. Interviews with miscellaneous rehabilitation counselors revealed an interest and curiosity in independent living and a sincere desire to be better able to serve clients with severe disabilities, but also confusion about exactly how this need related to the responsibilities of a counselor in a vocational rehabilitation system. A survey of 69 rehabilitation professionals and paraprofessionals corroborated these observations by identifying significant gaps in service delivery. An extensive list was developed of concepts and techniques that professionals found important for independent living. However, results indicated that there was a significant difference between ratings of importance and the level at which these techniques were used in the field (Walton, Schwab, Cassatt-Dunn, & Wright, 1980).

Conclusions from the study of rehabilitation counselor education programs indicate that current and newly graduating rehabilitation counselors are generally unprepared to deal with the independent living needs of their clients. In view of the establishment of independent living as a permanent part of the disability-related service system and the recommendations of the National Council on the Handicapped to Congress (1986) regarding full funding and implementation of Title VII, Part A, entitled "Services for Independent Living," this deficit in the education of rehabilitation counselors will have serious ramifications in the near future.

SUMMARY

The independent living movement is changing the face of rehabilitation. In addition to being instrumental in establishing a new component of the disability-related service delivery system accompanied by a new set of techniques, it has presented a new philosophy of how services should be delivered to persons with disabilities that has been well received by policy makers at the highest levels. The movement has also given rise to a new profession: the independent living specialist. The future is rich in possible settings in which such a professional could function to assist persons with disabilities increase their level of independence. Barriers to breaking down the artificial distinctions between independent living and rehabilitation counseling on both the professional and the systems level are many. The challenge to persons who have an interest in lessening the negative effects of disability on the quality of life is to affirm an unwavering commitment to the development of cooperative and productive relationships that focus on the enhancement of human potential, and to support this affirmation with personal action.

REFERENCES

Bartels, E. C. (1978). IL in Massachusetts. *American Rehabilitation, 3*(6), 22,33.

Berkeley Planning Associates. (1986). *Comprehensive evaluation of the Title VII, Part B Centers for Independent Living Program.* Berkeley, CA: Author.

Brown, B. M. (1978). Second generation: West coast. *American Rehabilitation, 3*(6), 23–30.

Dalrymple, J., & Richards, L. (1983). *Independent living and policy changes: Reflections on a decade's progress.* Houston: Independent Living Research Utilization.

DeJong, G. (1979). *Report of the national conference on independent living service regulations per PL 95-602.* Boston: Tufts University Medical Rehabilitation Research and Training Center.

Department of Education. (1985). *Caseload statistics, state vocational rehabilitation agencies, fiscal year 1984.* Washington, DC: Office of Special Education and Rehabilitation Services, Rehabilitation Services Administration.

Driscoll, J. V., Marquis, B., Corcoran, P. J., & Fay, F. A. (1978). Second generation: New England. *American Rehabilitation, 3*(6), 17–21.

Fay, F., Bartels, E. C., Corcoran, P., & McHugh R. (1977). In P. Reich (Ed.), *The BCIL Report.* Boston: Tufts University Regional Medical Rehabilitation Research and Training Center No. 7.

Frieden, L. (1978). IL: Movement and programs. *American Rehabilitation, 3*(6), 6–9.

Frieden, L., Richards, L., Cole, J., & Bailey, D. (1979). *ILRU sourcebook: A technical assistance manual on independent living.* Houston: The Institute for Rehabilitation and Research.

Galvin, D. E. (1980). *Policy issues in independent living rehabilitation.* East Lansing: Michigan State University, University Center for International Rehabilitation.

Independent Living Research Utilization. (1984). *ILP registry: An annotated directory of independent living programs.* Houston: Author.

Independent Living Research Utilization. (1985). *Directory of independent living programs.* Houston: Author.

Institute for Information Studies. (1979). *New life options: Independent living and you.* Falls Church, VA: Author.

Jeffers, J. S. (1978). The Illinois approach. *American Rehabilitation, 3*(6), 16–33.

Lorenz, J. R. (1982). Part III: ''Practice.'' Introduction to issues: Independent living and public rehabilitation. *Journal of Rehabilitation Administration, 6*(1), 24–28.

National Council on the Handicapped. (1983). *National policy for persons with disabilities.* Washington, DC: Author.

National Council on the Handicapped. (1986). *Toward independence: An assessment of federal laws and programs affecting persons with disabilities—with legislative recommendations; Appendix.* Washington, DC: U.S. Government Printing Office.

National Study Group on State Medicaid Strategies. (1983). *Restructuring Medicaid: An agenda for change: Background papers.* Washington, DC: Author.

Nosek, M. A. (1986). Community-based services for independent living. In National Council on the Handicapped. *Toward independence: An assessment of federal laws and programs affecting persons with disabilities—with legislative recommendations; Appendix.* (pp. G1–49). Washington, DC: U.S. Government Printing Office.

Nosek, P., Narita, Y., Dart, Y., & Dart, J. (1982). *A philosophical foundation for the independent living and disability rights movements* (Occasional Paper No. 1). Houston: The Institute for Rehabilitation and Research.

Pflueger, S. S. (1977). *Independent living. Emerging issues in rehabilitation.* Washington, DC: Institute for Research Utilization.

PL 66-236. An act to provide for the promotion of vocational rehabilitation of persons disabled in industry or otherwise and their return to civil employment. 66th Congress, Session 2, Chapter 219, 735–737. U.S. Statutes at Large, V. 41, Part 1 Public Laws, 1920.

Rehabilitation Act of 1973 as amended through February 22, 1984 by Public Law 98-221. (1984). Washington, DC: U.S. Government Printing Office.

Rice, B. D., & Roessler, R. T. (1980). *Introduction to independent living rehabilitation services.* Fayetteville: Arkansas Rehabilitation Research and Training Center, University of Arkansas, Arkansas Rehabilitation Services.

Rice, B. D., Roessler, R. T., Greenwood, R., & Frieden, L. (1983). *Independent living rehabilitation program development, management and evaluation.* Fayetteville: Arkansas Rehabilitation Research and Training Center, University of Arkansas, Arkansas Rehabilitation Services, The Institute for Rehabilitation and Research.

Rubin, S. E., & Roessler, R. T. (1983). *Foundations of the vocational rehabilitation process* (2nd ed.). Baltimore: University Park Press.

Siegman, S. J. (1980). *Policy planning and development in independent living: Proceedings of a Region V workshop.* East Lansing: Michigan State University, University Center for International Rehabilitation.

Sirrocco, A. (1983). An overview of the 1980 national master facility inventory survey of nursing and related care homes. *NCHS Advancedata, 91.*

Smith, M. F. (1984). *S. 2053 and the transfer of mentally retarded persons from large institutions to small community living arrangements.* Washington, DC: The Library of Congress, Congressional Research Service.

Stock, D. D., & Cole, J. (1977). *Cooperative living.* Houston: The Institute for Rehabilitation and Research.

Veerkamp, E. (1984). *A national profile of independent living programs for people with disabilities.* Houston: Independent Living Research Utilization.

Walton, K. M., Schwab, L. O., Cassatt-Dunn, M. A., & Wright, V. A. (1980). Techniques and concepts: Independent living perceptions by professionals in rehabilitation. *Journal of Rehabilitation, 6*(3), 57–63.

Zukas, H. (1975). *CIL history: Report of the state of the art conference, Center for Independent Living.* Berkeley, CA: Center for Independent Living.

4

Life-threatening Disabilities

Barriers to Rehabilitation

Harry A. Allen, John D. Dolan, Doreen Miller, and Richard Millard

ALLEN AND JAET (1982) defined the term *life-threatening condition* as "any illness, disease or physical condition which is likely to cause an untimely death" (p. 18). This broad definition accommodates such disabilities as acquired immune deficiency syndrome (AIDS), amyotrophic lateral sclerosis (ALS), cancer, coronary heart disease, cystic fibrosis, Duchenne muscular dystrophy, end-stage renal disease, sickle cell anemia, and stroke, which are also the major causes of death in America today.

Heart and blood vessel disease is the leading cause of death in the United States. The American Heart Association (1986) estimates that there will be over 63 million persons with some form of cardiovascular disorder in 1986, with an overall cost to the public exceeding $78 billion. Included in this figure is $13 billion in lost output due to disability. In 1983, heart attacks were associated with 347,100 deaths and strokes with 156,400 deaths. In 1986, it was estimated that 4,740,000 persons were presently living with some history of heart attack, angina pectoris, or both. In addition, in 1986 there were 1,930,000 survivors of stroke and 1,500,000 individuals had heart attacks (only 530,000 of whom died). Based on the Farmingham Heart study, 5% of all heart attacks occur before the age of 40, and 45% occur in individuals under the age of 65 (American Heart Association, 1986). Thus a large number of these individuals fall well within the age range of persons who should receive rehabilitation services.

The second leading cause of death and disablement in this country is neoplastic disease. The American Cancer Society estimated that 910,000 people were diagnosed as having cancer in 1985. All told, over 5 million persons are alive today in the U.S. with a history of cancer. Three million of these individuals are considered to be cured and to have the same life expectancy as persons who have not had the disease. Indeed, the "relative" survival rate of the newly diagnosed cancer patient is about 49% (American Cancer Society, 1985).

When considering the incidence and/or prevalence of some other forms of life-threatening diseases, the magnitude of the problem can be better understood. Amyotrophic lateral sclerosis has an incidence of 5 cases per 100,000 population (Corcoran, 1981) and a prevalence of 5,000–10,000 cases at any given point in time (Bender, Schumacher, & Allen, 1976). The incidence of cystic fibrosis varies between 1 in 1,500 to 1 in 2,600 live births and has a prevalence of 13,000–30,000 persons (Goldberg, Shwachman, & Isralsky, 1980). Duchenne muscular dystrophy affects only males, and has an incidence of 4 out of every 100,000 persons (Corcoran, 1981). Parrish (1981) notes that in 1976, 25,000 patients were undergoing dialysis, and estimated that the number was growing by 5,000–10,000 per year. Further, 1 out of every 500 black children has at least one of the sickle cell diseases (Johnson, 1981).

Considering these diseases in combination with cancer and coronary heart disease, it appears that 11–12 million persons could benefit from some form of vocational or independent living rehabilitation services. Yet when the state-federal rehabilitation closures for 1980 (N=914,729) were investigated, persons with the conditions noted constituted less than 3% of all case closures (D. Harrison, personal communication, November 12, 1985). These figures confirm what several researchers (Allesberry et al., 1977; Dietz, 1981; Goldberg, 1977; Goldberg et al., 1980) have suggested, namely that many persons with life-threatening disabilities are not receiving the rehabilitation services for which they are eligible under the 1973 Rehabilitation Act and its subsequent amendments. When considering the financial loss to society as well as the loss of human potential, the cost is phenomenal.

The purpose of this chapter is twofold. Current barriers to rehabilitation for individuals with life-threatening disabilities are reviewed, and recommendations for overcoming some of these barriers made. The barriers examined are associated with the individual's physical condition, state-federal agency policy, employer attitudes, the person's psychosocial adjustment to the condition, and the competence and training of the rehabilitation professional.

THE PERSON'S PHYSICAL CONDITION

The first, and perhaps deceptively obvious, barrier to rehabilitation is the individual's physical condition. This barrier is deceptive because of confusion between the concept of diagnosis and that of physical condition. While persons with the same diagnosed condition often share similar symptomatology, it is a critical mistake to make broad assumptions based exclusively on diagnosis. For example, Janiszewski, Caroscio, and Wisham (1983) note that because the cause and cure of ALS is unknown, the diagnosis has been regarded as a death sentence. The data suggest, however, that while the majority of persons have a life expectance of 3–4 years after onset of ALS, some individuals remain active for 10 or more years with periods of apparent arrest from the disease (ALS Association, undated).

The idiosyncratic response of each person to disease and its treatment must be dealt with on an individual basis. It is important to realize that in all disease the symptomatology may at times show remission, arrest, and even reversal. A clear and accurate medical evaluation is mandated and often a psychological and/or vocational evaluation is helpful. The basic rule with any high-risk population is to evaluate the individual's specific strengths and weaknesses, rather than to make assumptions based upon the diagnosis alone. While a number of persons will be so limited by their physical condition that vocational or independent living rehabilitation may not be achievable, research suggests that there are many persons with the above physical conditions that can benefit from rehabilitation services (Allen & Falvo, 1983; Goldenson, Dunham, & Dunham, 1978; Stolov & Clowers, 1981).

STATE-FEDERAL AGENCY POLICY

The state-federal rehabilitation system varies from state to state and region to region. Agency policy can affect services to persons with life-threatening disabilities through acceptance criteria or by more subtle barriers. Addressing the feasibility for employment criteria as a policy barrier, Goldberg et al. (1980) made the following observation in regard to the availability of vocational rehabilitation services to persons diagnosed as having cystic fibrosis:

> At present the vocational rehabilitation system has turned its back on patients with cystic fibrosis because it has used the third criterion of eligibility—that is, reasonable expectation that the client may enter employment by provision of rehabilitation services—as a means of denying services to persons with potentially fatal disease. Under the Rehabilitation Act of 1973 and the Rehabilitation Amendments of 1978 cystic fibrosis is listed as a severe disability eligible for assistance under the Federal Rehabilitation Act, but few states provide these patients with counseling, training and job placement. (p. 224)

Goldberg suggested that restrictive federal-state rehabilitation agency policy may negatively affect the vocational rehabilitation of the cancer patient (Goldberg, 1977; Goldberg & Habeck, 1982). This is supported by a national study on the economic impact of cancer that concluded that the Vocational Rehabilitation Act of 1973 had not had substantial impact on the rehabilitation of cancer patients (Mayo Comprehensive Cancer Center, 1977).

A subtle way agency policy may affect the successful rehabilitation of persons with potential terminal conditions is related to the individual's time of entry in the rehabilitation process. For example, Dietz (1981) noted:

> Historically, in disabilities associated with other diseases early rehabilitation has been more readily encouraged and arranged. However, it is still often delayed or withheld from the patient who has had cancer strictly on the basis of "cancer" without consideration of the patient's prognosis or rehabilitation potential. (p. 164)

Early intervention by rehabilitation specialists has been suggested to be beneficial for persons with coronary heart disease (Brammell, McDaniel, Niccoli, Darnell, & Roberson, 1979; Hansen, 1978; Thoreson & Ackerman, 1981); cancer (Dietz, 1981; Goldberg, 1977; McCollum, Powell, & Gaiser, 1978); cystic fibrosis (Goldberg et al., 1980); and sickle cell anemia (Allesberry et al., 1977). Despite evidence suggesting the positive impact of early intervention, it has not been a widespread practice in the state-federal rehabilitation system. The practice appears to be limited to the rare demonstration project.

A final example of how agency policy may influence the rehabilitation of persons with life-threatening disabilities is the degree of aggressiveness with which agencies seek referrals. The Mayo Comprehensive Cancer Center (1977) found that only 15% of their sample of 940 cancer patients who were eligible for vocational rehabilitation services were receiving services. Allesberry et al. (1977) suggested that lack of an aggressive case-finding policy may lead to inadequate rehabilitation service provision for persons with sickle cell anemia. Whether the lack of active recruitment of individuals with life-threatening disabilities is an overt attempt to deny services to persons who may be eligible is open to question. Whether an act of commission or omission, however, the result is the same. The individual is not served.

This does not imply that all state agencies create barriers to persons with life-threatening disabilities. Rather, the data reflect an imbalance in regard to the nature of the disability groups served. One explanation for this imbalance may be agency policy. Should this be the case, it is suggested that rehabilitation professionals have a responsibility to rectify this situation.

EMPLOYER ATTITUDE

A third barrier facing persons with life-threatening disabilities is employer attitude. Communities will often isolate persons with catastrophic illness out of fear, ignorance, or perhaps feelings of inadequacy (Blumberg, Flaherty, & Lewis, 1980). Employers reflect the attitudes of their communities (Wright, 1980). Thus the very label, such as *cancer*, may elicit fear and apprehension in the employer's mind (Vash, 1981). The prejudice effect associated with this labeling phenomenon may be linked with other employer concerns, such as the work potential or potential absenteeism of the disabled person. These are important concerns that must be addressed by the rehabilitation profession.

Fear of the Disease

We all have idiosyncratic perceptions and fears of the effects of life-threatening diseases. These are often projected upon the person who has the disease (Blumberg et al., 1980; Ehrle, 1969; Miller, 1985). These preconceived notions may lead to feelings of prejudice, hostility, avoidance, and anxiety toward an employee or co-worker with a life-threatening disability.

The rehabilitation professional may need to serve as both an advocate and educator in the work place. For example, several studies suggest that recovering cancer patients may require assistance dealing with co-workers' hostility and suspicion (Blumberg et al., 1980). This would seem a valid role for the rehabilitation professional.

Employment Potential

The evidence suggests that the employment potential is very high for many persons with life-threatening disabilities. Shwachman, Kowalski, and Shaw (1977) report findings on 70 outpatients with cystic fibrosis. They found 67 of the patients working successfully in a wide range of occupations varying from medical doctor to truck driver. Dimsdale, Hackett, Hutter, and Block (1982) report 53% of their sample of myocardial infarction patients were satisfactorily performing their premorbid job or had obtained a better job 1 year following the heart attack.

Research conducted by the Metropolitan Life Insurance Company (Wheatley, Cunnick, Wright, & Van Kueren, 1974) and Bell Telephone System (Bond, 1977; Stone, 1975) support the positive nature of vocational potential for persons diagnosed as having cancer. Wheatley et al. (1974) explored the work performance of 74 persons with known cancer histories employed by Metropolitan between 1959 and 1971. The company's policy was to accept applications of persons who had a history but showed no evidence of disease since treatment. Indeed, over 50% of those persons in the study had been hired within 5 years of treatment. When results were reported, 55% of the 74 employees were still working, 3% were on disability, and the remaining 42% had been "discontinued." Members of the latter group were considered by the company to have left their jobs voluntarily. When comparing this turnover rate with other "noncancer history" employees, the company found the rates comparable and thus not significantly associated with cancer. In addition, the work performance for the majority of the sample was found to be satisfactory. The absenteeism rate for the majority of the group was found to be comparable with other employees. The study concluded that the appropriate hiring of persons with cancer and the placement of them in positions for which they are physically qualified was a sound policy.

Stone (1975) reported on 800,000 employees of the Bell Telephone System. Of the 1346 employees treated for cancer in 1972, 77% returned to work after absences averaging 106 days. The majority of these employees had been employed by the Bell Systems for longer than 5 years and were older (i.e., 40 years and older in age). In general, Stone found that older experienced employees were more readily rehired than young employees with less experience. Thus it appears that the value of the employee to the company, in terms of experience, was the major factor affecting post disability employment rather than the disabling condition. Bond (1977) studied this same population at a later time and confirmed Stone's findings. Both Stone's and Bond's findings suggest that persons able to return to work presented no unusual problems for the employer.

Goldberg (1975) reported on the vocational rehabilitation of persons who had had laryngectomies resulting from cancer. He explored the home, social, and work adjustment of these persons. His findings indicated that the best predictors of vocational and social adjustment after laryngectomy were motivation and realism in rehabilitation outlook, vocational plans, education, and speech acquisition. Of his sample of 62 persons, 41% returned to the competitive labor market. Severity of laryngeal cancer was not significantly related to employment or degree of social activities after laryngectomy.

Thus, the literature suggests that many persons with life-threatening disabilities are satisfactory and productive workers. The literature also indicates that factors other than disability, such as employer attitudes and company medical policy, especially in the case of coronary disease and cancer, may be associated with the hiring or rehiring of these persons. The research does not imply, nor do the authors mean to suggest, that vocational rehabilitation of persons with life-threatening conditions is without challenge. Indeed, there are environmental and work considerations that must be considered and managed. For example, persons with cystic fibrosis should not consider occupations that would expose them to heat, dust, and fumes (Goldberg et al., 1980). The client with sickle cell disease needs to avoid exposure to hot, humid environments because of the extra stress it places upon the heart. Further, while follow-up studies suggest that 70%–90% of all persons who survive a heart attack are able to return to work, 33% require some modification of job task in order to return to their previous occupation (Brammell et al., 1979, p. 99). The literature indicates that many challenges are faced by the counselor, client, and employer. However, it appears that when the problems are confronted, the outcomes are rewarding for all involved.

Absenteeism

Employer concerns about absenteeism seem very legitimate. However, the validity of such concerns cannot be strictly determined from the label of the person's disability. Still, the research does suggest that certain conditions may present greater problems than others in regard to health management. Brammel et al. (1979) noted that coronary patients when compared with noncardiac employees were absent more often and had more days lost per incidence. In terms of sickle cell anemia, Allesberry et al. (1977) stated:

> Two characteristics of sickle cell disease appeared to be most problematic to the successful vocational rehabilitation of individuals. First was the occurrence of crisis which has at least a disrupting effect upon an individual's performance on the job and possibly the consequence of causing an individual to lose his job. Secondly was the fluidity of the disease . . . not only was sickle cell anemia capable of affecting virtually every body system it was also capable of being manifest in many different forms within the individual. (p. 60)

Shwachman, Kowalski, and Shaw's (1977) findings in regard to cystic fibrosis patients suggest that while virtually none of their patients were so incapacitated that they could not work, the number and frequency of crises and hospitalizations varied from patient to patient. Parrish (1981) stated that the patient with end-stage renal disease is typically involved in dialysis two to three times a week, each session lasting 3–6 hours. He also noted that at any one point in time 10%–12% of hemodialysis patients are hospitalized.

Thus, the evidence suggests that for several of these high-risk disability groups there may be a legitimate concern about absence from work. Unfortunately there appear to be few if any well-controlled studies that specify the reasons for absence or the impact absences may have upon the person's future employment. For the rehabilitation counselor this suggests that postplacement follow-up may be a vital ingredient of successful rehabilitation. Job restructuring and modification needs to be studied in addition to wellness and health promotion strategies. Such interventions may prove helpful to disabled as well as nondisabled employees.

THE PERSON'S PSYCHOSOCIAL ADJUSTMENT TO THE DISABILITY

A fourth major barrier to rehabilitation of persons with life-threatening disabilities is the person's psychosocial adjustment to the disability. Medical technology has extended the functional life of persons who would have been thought of as "hopeless cases" 20 years ago. This functional life extension has forced many into a new life phase identified by Pattison (1977) as a living-dying interval. This interval is the period of time that exists between the point in time when the person is diagnosed as terminal and the time of death. The nature of the living-dying interval differs for each individual in terms of both duration and psychosocial adjustment. For some, this interval occurs during the early developmental years (e.g., Duchenne muscular dystrophy, cystic fibrosis, sickle cell anemia), while for others it is more likely to occur later in life (e.g., ALS, stroke). The time of occurrence certainly has an impact both upon the individual and the family. For example, the family with a son born with Duchenne muscular dystrophy (DMD) will normally know the diagnosis before the child's fifth birthday, and the child will probably require a wheelchair for mobility by the age of 10 (Corcoran, 1981). While the life expectancies of individuals with DMD may vary, death usually occurs between the ages of 20 and 30 from either respiratory infection or cardiac arrest (Madorsky, Radford, & Neumann, 1984). When family reactions to this disease were studied, Buchanan, La Barbera, Roelofs, and Olsen (1979) found that 76% of the families identified psychological problems rather than physical problems as the major concern. The child with this progressive life-threatening disease will experience the living-dying interval differently than a young mother diagnosed at the age of 28 as having breast cancer that has metastasized, who has a 70% chance of surviving for 5 years. These two persons will differ from the 45-year-old black male who survived a myocardial infarction but who now experiences angina pectoris with any emotional excitement or unusual physical exertion. Thus, this living-dying interval is filled with many idiosyncratic changes and symptoms (Barton, 1977). Anxiety, anger, denial, pain, weakness, guilt, depression, fatigue, grief, weight change, changes in sleeping patterns, changes in eating and bowel patterns, changes in mobility, recurring acute episodes, negative response to medical intervention, and other physical and emotional responses are all powerful reminders of the presence of illness and progressive changes in the individual (Allen & Sawyer, 1984).

Pattison (1977) identified fear of: 1) loneliness, 2) sorrow, 3) loss of family and friends, 4) loss of body, 5) loss of self-control, 6) suffering and pain, 7) loss of identity, and 8) regression as experiences of the living-dying interval. He assumed these fears have an impact on the individual with a life-threatening disability as well as on family members, and may vary in degree and intensity throughout the living-dying interval. Carey (1976) suggested that persons with a life-threatening illness will experience four major areas of anxiety: 1) fear of pain, 2) fear of being separated from loved ones, 3) fear of being a burden on loved ones, and 4) concern about how the loved ones will care for themselves. Abram (1969) expanded the list by adding the fear of mutilation and loss of sexuality. Stewart and Sheilds (1985) called attention to grief as a common component in chronic illness that can and frequently does impede the rehabilitation process. Gelfman and Wilson (1972) suggested that the individual may be caught in a double bind. This bind involves a true fear of living with the life-threatening disability and all the changes, potential pain, and suffering it may bring, while at the same time being equally afraid of dying. For some individuals, facing death may be easier than facing life with a serious disability (Kubler-Ross, 1974). Allen and Sawyer (1984) suggest that while the dynamics of the living-dying interval are not well understood, with the advancement of medical technology this interval is likely to increase for a number of persons with life-threatening disabilities.

The research, in general, suggests that the emotions people experience during this phase can dramatically affect their personal, interpersonal, spiritual, social, and vocational life. For example, a fair amount of research on the vocational stability of post-myocardial infarction patients suggests that they are greatly affected by their emotional response to the disability. Dimsdale et al. (1982) cited research that suggested that 40%–60% of males surviving their first myocardial infarction did not return to work for 6 months after infarction, although they were physically capable of doing so. They argued that the low return to work rate may be due to depression, lack of understanding of their disease, employer discrimination, and secondary gains for insurance benefits. Ell, Guzman, and Haywood (1983) suggest that depression, anxiety and other stress factors are important in regard to the functional recovery of the post-myocardial infarction patient. Stern, Pascale, and McLoone (1976) found that over 75% of their subjects did return to work, yet the ''poor rehabilitation'' group (13% of the sample) were not working and demonstrated marked signs of depression and significant levels of anxiety. These studies reflect only a portion of the data suggesting that for persons who have survived a heart attack, emotional factors may play as great a role as physical factors in successful rehabilitation.

For hemodialysis patients, the psychosocial adjustment to disability may play not only an important role in vocational rehabilitation but in life continuation itself. It is estimated that at any given time 10%–12% of hemodialysis patients are known to be hospitalized. The evidence in general shows that well-motivated persons do fairly well. However, for those who appear to lack motivation and who are noncompliant in regard to medication and diet, life expectancy is severely shortened (Parrish, 1981). Gonsalves-Ebrahim, Gulledge, and Miga (1982) suggested that there are a number of factors that influence the success of the peritoneal dialysis patient. They list, as important psychological factors related to survival, the person's mood and ability to test reality, cognitive function, previous ability to handle crisis, personality structure, and the support and acceptance of treatment by family members (Gonsalves-Ebrahim et al., 1982, p. 945). Other researchers have also stressed the importance of goals, interests, and values as factors in satisfactory adjustment to the disability (Goldberg, 1975).

Evidence overwhelmingly suggests that the individual's psychosocial adjustment to his or her disability is a major factor in rehabilitation and the quality of life experienced by the individual. When adjustment is poor, rehabilitation is impeded, if not completely thwarted. Thus, the counselor working with such persons must attend to personal aspects of counseling crucial to the individual's psychosocial adjustment.

THE REHABILITATION COUNSELOR

The final barrier discussed is the level and appropriateness of training of rehabilitation counselors who are serving persons with life-threatening disabilities. Due to the complexities and demands of serving these high-risk groups, adequate training is vital, and the lack of such training is a substantial barrier (Brickner, 1979; Bugen, 1979; Kalish, 1976; Krieger, 1978; Miller, 1985).

The available data (Allen & Jaet, 1982; Allen & Miller, 1986; Bascue, Lawrence, & Sessions, 1977; Boerema, 1981; Rauzi, 1985) suggest that rehabilitation counselors who have little or no training in serving this high-risk group are serving clients with life-threatening conditions. Bascue et al. (1977) found that 46% of their sample of vocational rehabilitation counselors served persons with terminal illness, and 61% could recall a client's death. Allen and Jaet (1982) found that 73% of their sample of counselors employed by the Illinois Department of Rehabilitation Services recalled working with persons who had a life-threatening disability, and 77% of them had experienced one or more client deaths over a 3-year period. Their results indicated that the death of a client affected the counselor both emotionally and existentially. Only 15% of the counselors reported having had any form of training in working with persons who were terminally ill, and 24% had no preparation for death and bereavement issues. When queried about their needs, 70% saw a need for training to work with persons having life-threatening disabilities, and 59% felt that training in death and bereavement issues was needed.

In a more broadly based study, Allen and Miller (1986) surveyed randomly selected certified rehabilitation counselors from a national list in an effort to investigate counselors' experiences in serving persons with life-threatening disabilities, and in dealing with clients' deaths. Of direct care providers, 61% experienced the death of one or more clients on their caseload between the years of 1982 and 1985. It was also found that 40% of the direct service providers served persons with life-threatening conditions (e.g., cancer, coronary heart disease, diabetes). The data also indicated that 71% of the sample had no training in serving persons with life-threatening conditions, and that 91% of the respondents felt more advanced training was needed.

The impact of this lack of training for the rehabilitation counselor is unknown. Judging from the nursing and health provider literature, such lack of preparation is harmful for both the patient and the care provider (Barton, 1977; Bugen, 1979; Kalish, 1976; Maslach, 1979; Pearlman, Stotsky, & Dominick, 1969; Vachon, Lyall, & Freeman, 1978). Intuitively, one might suspect that it serves as a barrier to rehabilitation service delivery and may be associated with counselor burnout (Allen & Jaet, 1982; Miller, 1985).

If the rehabilitation professional's values reflect the society's values as a whole (Scofield, Pape, McCracken, & Maki, 1980), and if a lack of information causes society to respond in a prejudicial way toward persons with a life-threatening disability, it would be reasonable to assume then that rehabilitation professionals will respond in a similar manner. Brickner (1979) stated that:

> I find the primary reasons for low level of cancer patient involvement in vocational rehabilitation are: 1) the lack of updated information on the care, treatment, and prognosis of the disease on the part of those engaged in vocational rehabilitation; 2) the lack of an aggressive and consistent educational program directed toward the health care and rehabilitation professions on the rehabilitation potential of persons whose cancer has been cured or contained; and 3) the lack of consideration of rehabilitative and vocational goals early in the treatment planning for the individual. (p. 2)

Brickner's statement could be made in terms of each condition traditionally assumed to be terminal. If the term *cancer* or *cystic fibrosis* signals the concept of hopelessness in the counselor's mind, then rehabilitation is severely hampered if not totally blocked. Without accurate information, people respond from personal and/or social biases that may not reflect the true facts of a given condition or situation. Ignorance walks hand in hand with prejudice, and these two form greater barriers than have ever been caused by architecture or legislation.

SUMMARY, RECOMMENDATIONS, AND CONCLUSIONS

Several barriers to the rehabilitation of persons with life-threatening disabilities have been discussed. They are: 1) the person's physical condition, 2) the policy of the state-federal rehabilitation system, 3) the attitudes of employers, 4) the person's psychosocial adjustment to the disability, and 5) factors associated with the rehabilitation counselor's preparation and training. These barriers may serve to prevent the disabled person from entering or reentering the world of work, as well as exacerbate the degree of isolation from the community experienced. If effective rehabilitation is to be accomplished, these barriers must be overcome.

The research and literature in the field suggest that policy changes are needed. Specifically, the state-federal rehabilitation system should reevaluate the use of the third criterion—"reasonable expectation of employment"—and other restrictive agency policies if persons with life-threatening disabilities are to be served effectively. Since the 1973 Rehabilitation Act and the 1978 amendments mandate that priority service be given to these high-risk groups, there appears to be a legal as well as a moral responsibility to serve such individuals. If the spirit of these laws is to be implemented, it is suggested that the state and federal systems need to serve as advocates for these high-risk populations. This implies that state agency personnel need to be aggressive in their case-finding efforts, and that field counselors need further training that focuses on serving these clients. Attitudinal barriers that confront persons with life-threatening disabilities are so ingrained in society that they influence all areas of culture. Often subtle and veiled as humanitarian, such attitudes serve to limit human potential and dignity. Judging from the work of several investigators (Allesberry et al., 1977; Blumberg, et al., 1979; Goldberg et al., 1980), these attitudinal barriers may exist within state agency policy. Thus, agency policy review and examination appears warranted.

The literature also suggests that if these high-risk populations are to be served, educational preparation of service providers and administrators must be strengthened. Available research strongly suggests that both service providers and administrators have not been adequately prepared to serve persons with life-threatening conditions (Allen & Miller, 1986). This problem may also extend to rehabilitation educators, though there are no data to support this contention. Rehabilitation educators may not have stressed this area of training because of their own lack of training in the area.

Education focusing on life-threatening disabilities must be demanded in both professional preparation training programs as well as in-service training. This should include the basic biomedical nature of the condition, the psychosocial correlates of the condition, and the consideration of the issues of death, dying, and bereavement. Furthermore, trainees must examine their own values, beliefs, and attitudes toward life-threatening illnesses, suffering, and death, and their attitudes about serving persons with life-threatening conditions. They must examine the personal and social factors that block effective communication with these clients. They must also develop an awareness of the tangible and intangible needs of persons with life-threatening illness (e.g., tangible—living arrangements, occupation, food, transportation; intangible—emotionally coping with the fear of dying, of suffering, of further physical incapacitation). Understanding the person's needs also requires that the service provider become aware of the client's family dynamics and ways of successfully interacting with these. Life-threatening disabilities normally occur within a family constellation. The person requires a great deal of support and attention from family members. Family units serve to either enhance or thwart the person's efforts at rehabilitation. Understanding the complex web of interpersonal interactions in the context of the disability is extremely important to the successful rehabilitation of the individual (Power & Dell Orto, 1980).

Beyond the education and training of the service provider, there is a need for public education to overcome the barriers presented by negative employer attitudes. It is suggested that the federal-state rehabilitation service system could help correct these attitudes by increasing their own public relations efforts. Offering employers current factual information about the specific disability may serve to reduce both fear and prejudice (Wright, 1980). Service providers might also encourage their clients to act on their own behalf, agitating for "additional enforceable legal proscriptions to combat the discrimination they face" (Eisenberg, 1982, p. 10). The efforts to overcome prejudice, isolation, and fear will require creativity and courage on the part of the disabled client and the service provider.

Finally, further research and demonstration projects must be undertaken to provide a systematic body of knowledge regarding the rehabilitation of persons with life-threatening illnesses. As Allen and Falvo (1983) have noted regarding coronary disease, neoplastic disease, and end-stage renal disease, much of the present research is fragmented, nonsystematic, atheoretical and poorly designed. While there is evidence that rehabilitation efforts have been successful when persons with life-threatening disabilities have received special attention (Allensberry et al., 1971; Brammel et al., 1979; DeNour, 1982; Goldberg & Habeck, 1982; Isralsky, Goldberg, & Schwachman, 1979), overall there is an apparent lack of information regarding effective service delivery to persons with such disabilities. There also seems to be a lack of comprehensive understanding of the characteristics and needs of this high-risk population. While, as noted in this chapter and others in this book, pockets of data do exist, they are often shallow and of limited generalizability.

A growing recognition that the majority of Americans will personally encounter a long-term, life-threatening disability (Allen & Sawyer, 1984) points to the importance of this issue. The vast majority of U.S. families are affected at some time by these groups of disabling conditions (American Cancer Society, 1985; American Heart Association, 1986). The rehabilitation professional can play a major role in improving the quality of life of these disabled individuals and their families.

REFERENCES

Abram, H. S. (1969). The psychiatrist, the treatment of chronic renal failure, and the prolongation of life. *American Journal of Psychiatry, 12*, 1351–1358.

Allen, H. A., & Falvo, D. (1983). *The principles and practices of vocational rehabilitation with persons with hidden disabilities.* Washington, DC: National Rehabilitation Information Center.

Allen, H. A., & Jaet, D. (1982). Rehabilitation counselor's response to a client's death. *Journal of Applied Rehabilitation Counseling, 12*(2), 17–21.

Allen, H. A., & Miller, D. (1986). *Client death: A national survey of Certified Rehabilitation Counselors' experience.* Manuscript submitted for publication.

Allen, H. A., & Sawyer, H. W. (1984). Individuals with life-threatening disabilities: A rehabilitation counseling approach. *Rehabilitation Literature, 15*(2), 26–37.

Allesberry, D., Bonner, O. J., Jenkins, W. W., Parks, B. W., Fairly, H. D., & Driver, A. L. (1977). *Assessment of vocational potential of sickle cell anemics*

(Federal Innovation and Expansion Grant #25-P-15471/3-01, State Clearinghouse #74-05-2-076).

Amyotrophic Lateral Sclerosis Association. (Undated). *What is amyotrophic lateral sclerosis?* (Available from the ALS Association, 158 Madison Avenue, New York, NY 10016.)

American Cancer Society. (1985). *1985 cancer facts and figures*. New York: Author.

American Heart Association. (1986). *1986 heart facts*. Dallas: Author.

Barton, O. (1977). *Dying and death: A clinical guide for caregivers*. Baltimore: Williams & Wilkins.

Bascue, L. O., Lawrence, R. E., & Sessions, J. (1977). Counselor experience with client death concerns. *Rehabilitation Counseling Bulletin, 1,* 36–38.

Bender, E., Schumacher, B., & Allen, H. A. (1976). *Medical aspects of disability*. Minneapolis: MRC, Inc.

Blumberg, B., Flaherty, M., & Lewis, J. (Eds.). (1980). *Coping with cancer* (NIH Publication No. 80-2080). Washington, DC: National Institutes of Health.

Boerema, R. N. (1981). *The role of the rehabilitation counselor in serving the terminally ill, bereaved, and suicidal*. Unpublished master's research report, Southern Illinois University, Carbondale.

Bond, M. (1977). Employability of cancer patients. *Rocky Mountain Medical Journal, 74,* 153–156.

Brammell, H. L., McDaniel, J., Niccoli, S. A., Darnell, R., & Roberson, D. R. (1979). *Cardiac rehabilitation*. Denver, CO: Webb-Warring Lung.

Brickner, A. (1979). Cancer: Action for reducing to employment and community participation. In L. G. Perlman (Ed.), *The role of vocational rehabilitation in the 1980s serving those with invisible handicaps. A report of the third Mary E. Switzer Memorial Seminar*. Washington, DC: National Rehabilitation Association.

Buchanan, D. C., La Barbera, C. J., Roelofs, R., & Olsen, W. (1979). Reactions of families to children with Duchenne muscular dystrophy. *General Hospital Psychiatry, 1,* 262–268.

Bugen, L. A. (1979). Emotions: Their presence and impact upon the helping role. In C. A. Garfield (Ed.), *Stress and survival: The emotional realities of life-threatening illness* (pp. 138–145). St. Louis: C. V. Mosby.

Carey, R. G. (1976). Counseling the terminally ill. *Personnel and Guidance Journal, 55,* 124–126.

Corcoran, P. J. (1981). Neuromuscular diseases. In W. C. Stolov & M. R. Clowers (Eds.), *Handbook of severe disability* (pp. 329–340). Washington, DC: Department of Education, Rehabilitation Services Administration.

Cystic Fibrosis Foundation. (undated). *Questions and facts about cystic fibrosis*. (Available from Cystic Fibrosis Foundation, 6000 Executive Boulevard, Suite 309, Rockville, MD 20852.)

DeNour, K. (1982). Psychosocial adjustment to illness scale (PAIS): A study of chronic hemodialysis patients. *Journal of Psychosomatic Research, 26*(1), 11–22.

Dietz, H. J. (1981). *Rehabilitation oncology*. New York: John Wiley & Sons.

Dimsdale, J. F., Hackett, T. P., Hutter, A. M., & Block, P. C. (1982). The association of clinical, psychological, and angiographic variables with work status in patients with coronary artery disease. *Journal of Psychosomatic Research, 26*(2), 215–221.

Ehrle, R. A. (1969). Mutilation, death and the rehabilitation counseling student. *Rehabilitation Counseling Bulletin, 13,* 197–202.

Eisenberg, M. G. (1982). Disability as stigma. In M. Eisenberg, C. Griggins, & R. J.

Duval (Eds.), *Disabled people as second class citizens.* New York: Springer-Verlag.

Eissler, K. R. (1955). *The psychiatrist and the dying patient.* New York: International University Press.

Ell, K. O., Guzman, M. O., & Haywood, L. J. (1983). Stressful life events: A predictor in recovery from heart attacks. *Health and Social Work, 8,* 133–142.

Falvo, D., Allen, H., & Maki, D. (1982). Psychosocial aspects of invisible disability. *Rehabilitation Literature, 43*(1–2), 2–6.

Gelfman, M., & Wilson, E. G. (1972). Emotional reactions in a renal unit. *Comprehensive Psychiatry, 13,* 283–290.

Goldberg, R. T. (1975). Vocational and social adjustment after laryngectomy. *Scandanavian Journal of Rehabilitation Medicine, 7,* 1–8.

Goldberg, R. T. (1977). Vocational rehabilitation: Outlook for persons with cancer. *Rehabilitation Literature, 38,* 310–321.

Goldberg, R. T., & Habeck, R. (1982). Vocational rehabilitation of cancer clients: Review and implications for the future. *Rehabilitation Counseling Bulletin, 26,* 18–28.

Goldberg, R. T., Shwachman, H., & Isralsky, M. (1980). Rehabilitation with cystic fibrosis: From utopia to reality. *Rehabilitation Literature, 41,* 218–228.

Goldenson, R. M., Dunham, J. R., & Dunham, C. S. (Eds.). (1978). *Disability and rehabilitation handbook.* New York: McGraw-Hill.

Gonsalves-Ebrahim, L., Gulledge, A. D., & Miga, S. (1982). Continuous ambulatory peritoneal dialysis and psychological factors. *Psychosomatics, 23,* 944–949.

Grouscth, E., Martison, J., Kersey, J., & Nesbit, M. (1981). Support systems of health professionals as observed in the project of home care for the child concerned. *Death Education, 5,* 37–50.

Hansen, M. C. (1978). In L. G. Perlman (Ed.), *The role of vocational rehabilitation in the 1980s serving those with invisible handicaps. A report of the third Mary E. Switzer Memorial Seminar:* Washington, DC: National Rehabilitation Association.

Isralsky, M., Goldberg, R. T., & Shwachman, H. (1979). Vocational rehabilitation of the person with cystic fibrosis. *Rehabilitation Counseling Bulletin, 23,* 114–119.

Janiszewski, D. W., Caroscio, J. J., & Wisham, L. H. (1983). Amyotrophic lateral sclerosis: A comprehensive rehabilitation approach. *Archives of Physical Rehabilitation, 64,* 304–307.

Johnson, C. S. (1981). Sickle cell disease. In W. C. Stolov & M. R. Clowers (Eds.), *Handbook of severe disability* (pp. 349–362). Washington, DC: Department of Education, Rehabilitation Services Administration.

Kalish, R. A. (1976). A little myth is a dangerous thing: Research in the service of the dying. In C. A. Garfield (Ed.), *Psychosocial care of the dying patient.* San Francisco: University of California School of Medicine.

Krieger, G. W. (1978). Loss and grief in rehabilitation counseling of the severely traumatically disabled. *Journal of Applied Rehabilitation Counseling, 7,* 223–228.

Kubler-Ross, E. (1974). *Questions and answers on death and dying.* New York: Macmillan.

Madorsky, J. G., Radford, L. M., & Neumann, E. M. (1984). Psychosocial aspects of death and dying in Duchenne muscular dystrophy. *Archives of Physical Medicine Rehabilitation, 65,* 79–82.

Martin, R. (1975). *Legal challenges to behavior modifications: Trends in schools, corrections, and mental health.* Champaign, IL: Research Press.

Maslach, C. (1979). The burn-out syndrome and patient care. In C. A. Garfield (Ed.),

Stress and survival: The emotional realities of life threatening illness (pp. 111–120). St. Louis: C. V. Mosby.

Mayo Comprehensive Cancer Center, Cancer Rehabilitation Program. (1977). *A study of discrimination toward cancer patients by insurers, employers and vocational rehabilitation agencies* (National Cancer Institute Contract No. CN 45120-F). Rochester, MN: Mayo Clinic.

McCollum, P. S., Powell, R., & Gaiser, R. (1978). The state rehabilitation agency and the cancer patient: Receptivity and service delivery. *Rehabilitation Counseling Bulletin, 21,* 224–229.

Miller, D. (1985). *The impact of client death upon rehabilitation counselors.* Unpublished doctoral dissertation, Southern Illinois University, Carbondale.

Parrish, A. E. (1981). End-stage renal disease. In W. C. Stolov & M. R. Clowers (Eds.), *Handbook of severe disability* (pp. 329–340). Washington, DC: Department of Education, Rehabilitation Service Administration.

Pattison, E. M. (1977). *The experience of dying.* Englewood Cliffs, NJ: Prentice-Hall.

Pearlman, J., Stotsky, B., & Dominick, J. (1969). Attitudes toward death among nursing home personnel. *The Journal of Genetic Psychology, 114,* 63–75.

Pickert, L. M. (1981). *Terminal illness, dying, and death: Training of caregivers.* Unpublished doctoral dissertation, University of Pittsburgh.

Power, P., & Dell Orto, A. (1980). *Role of the family in the rehabilitation of the physically disabled.* Baltimore: University Park Press.

Rauzi, R. G. (1985). *Minnesota D.V.R. counselors' experience, perceptions, and needs regarding client death and dying.* Unpublished master's thesis, Mankato State University, Mankato, MN.

Scofield, M., Pape, D., McCracken, N., & Maki D. (1980). An ecological model for promoting acceptance of disability. *Journal of Applied Rehabilitation Counseling, 11,* 183–187.

Shwachman, H., Kowalski, M., & Shaw, K. T. (1977). Cystic fibrosis: A new outlook. *Medicine, 56*(2), 129–150.

Stern, M. J., Pascale, L., & McLoone, J. B. (1976). Psychosocial adaption following an acute myocardial infarction. *Journal of Chronic Disability, 29,* 513–526.

Stewart, T., & Sheilds, C. R. (1985). Grief in chronic illness: Assessment and management. *Archives of Physical Medicine Rehabilitation, 66,* 447–450.

Stolov, W. C., & Clowers, M. R. (Eds.). (1981). *Handbook of severe disability.* Washington, DC: U.S. Department of Education, Rehabilitation Service Administration.

Stone, R. W. (1975). Employing the recovered cancer patient. *Cancer, 36*(1), 285–286.

Thoreson, R. W., & Ackerman, M. (1981). Cardiac rehabilitation: Basic principles and psychosocial factors. *Rehabilitation Counseling Bulletin, 24,* 223–255.

Vachon, M., Lyall, W., & Freeman, S. (1978). Measurement and management of stress in health professionals working with advanced cancer patients. *Death Education, 1,* 365–375.

Vash, C. L. (1981). *The psychology of disability.* New York: Springer-Verlag.

Wheatley, G. M., Cunnick, W., Wright, B., & Van Kueren, D. (1974). The employment of persons with a history of treatment for cancer. *Cancer, 33,* 441–445.

Wright, G. N. (1980). *Total rehabilitation.* Boston: Little, Brown.

5

The Role of the Rehabilitation Counselor in the Provision of Transition and Supported Employment Programs

Marvin L. Tooman, W. Grant Revell, Jr., and Richard P. Melia

THE REHABILITATION COUNSELOR has been, and continues to be, a key player in the provision of services to persons with disabilities. Over the years, the rehabilitation counselor has been charged with the responsibility of meeting with individuals who are disabled, and with interpreting the services and resources available for their entry or reentry into the mainstream of life.

Recent developments within the rehabilitation profession suggest that transition and supported employment will be recognized as rehabilitation service components within the Rehabilitation Act of 1986. As these service components become part of the traditional service delivery system, special staff competencies may be required. A study commissioned by the National Institute for Handicapped Research (NIHR), performed by Harold Russell Associates (HRA), addressed transition and supported employment (Cohen, Patton, & Melia, 1986). Within these service components, a new job role

The opinions expressed are those of the authors and do not necessarily reflect the views of the department or agency for which they work.

entitled "employment training specialist" has been suggested. The relationship between the rehabilitation counselor and the employment training specialist, and other roles within transition and supported employment (i.e., job coaches, job developers, vocational trainers) raises questions about the role of the rehabilitation counselor.

The purpose of this chapter is to define the role of the rehabilitation counselor within transition and supported employment services. Recognizing that these employment programs are currently being written into law, this discussion is prescriptive in nature. After the reauthorization of the Rehabilitation Act, the development of these programs will be greatly accelerated. In addition, this chapter discusses the future beyond transition and supported employment from the perspective of the rehabilitation counselor.

TRANSITION AND SUPPORTED EMPLOYMENT DEFINED

The development of any new service program may foster confusion and misunderstanding as the meaning of particular terms, usages, and program goals are discussed. To further a new and developing service program, participants need a common understanding of these terms, usages, and goals.

Webster's Dictionary defines transition as "the passage from one state, stage, or place to another, or change." Transition employment focuses on the passage or movement of youth with disabilities from school to working life. Rather than a particular state or condition, transition more accurately represents a process encompassing a variety of activities that enable a youth with a disability to move from childhood to an adult life in which employment represents a vocational outcome.

The process of transition occurs during a period of time that includes high school, the point of graduation, additional post-secondary education or adult services, and the initial years of employment (Will, 1984). This process may be thought of as a bridge between the security and structure offered by the school and the opportunities and risks of adult life.

Whereas the defining of transition employment may be more abstract, in reference to the services available to youth with disabilities, supported employment can be more directly defined and described. However, the definition of supported employment may be viewed from either a legal or an operational perspective. Legally, the definition of supported employment may be established through the reauthorization of the Rehabilitation Act of 1986, Section 103(f):

> Competitive work in integrated work settings for individuals with severe handicaps for whom competitive employment has not traditionally occurred, or for individuals for whom competitive employment has been interrupted or intermittent as a result of a severe disability and for individuals who, because of their handicap, need ongoing support services to perform such work. (Duncan, 1986)

The operational definition of supported employment enhances and extends the legal definition. Recently, a meeting of personnel from 10 states conducting supported employment demonstration projects discussed the definition and minimum standards for supported employment. Their operational definition of supported employment is:

> Paid employment which:
> a. is for persons with severe disabilities for whom competitive employment at or above minimum wage is unlikely, and who, because of their disabilities, need intensive ongoing support to perform in a work setting;
> b. is conducted in a variety of settings, particularly worksites in which persons without disabilities are employed; and
> c. is supported by an activity needed to sustain paid work by persons with disabilities, including supervision, training, and transportation. (RSA State Demonstration Projects, 1985, p. 3)

Their criteria for supported employment are:

> Paid employment:
> a. in groups of eight or less persons with disabilities;
> b. at least 20 hours of work each week; and
> c. with ongoing support funded and provided. (RSA State Demonstration Projects, 1985, p. 3)

Drawing from the previous definitions, supported employment can be one of the vocational outcomes resulting from the process of transition. For rehabilitation counselors, supported employment represents one alternative to the traditional rehabilitation closures and employment settings that were categorized as competitive, sheltered, or homebound. Due to the potential of this new vocational outcome, rehabilitation counselors who use supported employment will find that they will be working with clients having a broader range of severity of disabilities. Individuals who traditionally were not thought of as rehabilitation clients, due to the severity of their disabilities, will become eligible.

Supported Employment Models

The definition of supported employment can be brought into finer focus through a brief discussion of the activities that establish supported employment's uniqueness when compared to other rehabilitation modalities. Job placement services for persons with severe disabilities traditionally come after a long and sometimes arduous series of service programs that focus on such things as work adjustment, prevocational training, and behavior modification training. Severely disabled clients that successfully demonstrate their capabilities through these preplacement activities are asked to "generalize" their previous learning in a new work environment. Unfortunately, on a national scope, few persons with severe disabilities complete this process (M. Hill, Hill, et al., 1985). In contrast to the train-and-place approach to employment, supported employment emphasizes the place-and-train method. There are four program components that distinguish supported employment from other approaches to job placement (Wehman & Kregel, 1985).

Program Component I: Job Placement Supported employment techniques emphasize initial client assessment concurrent with job development. Nonwork-related factors such as transportation, Social Security, and housing are dealt with as a part of the initial placement effort.

Program Component II: Job Site Training and Advocacy Generally an employer is the party responsible for training an individual on the job. In contrast, supported employment programs provide job site training and advocacy services to promote a client's initial adjustment to the work environment and long-term job retention.

Program Component III: Ongoing Monitoring Ongoing monitoring activities include the collection and analysis of subjective information obtained from employers, clients, and parents/caregivers. There is a need to gauge employer perception of the worker's performance. Problems require immediate intervention strategies.

Program Component IV: Job Retention and Follow-Up The supported employment approach views follow-up services as long-term activities that are provided over a period of years. A change in the job may require the supported employment staff person to initiate retraining of the client.

Summary

Supported employment is designed to serve persons with severe disabilities for whom employment in an integrated setting (i.e., with nondisabled persons) has not been traditionally feasible. Placement, training, and support services for these persons occur in the community versus in a controlled and segregated environment. Ongoing monitoring and support is provided to maintain the individual in productive and profitable employment. Support services may be necessary throughout a person's adult life.

IDENTIFICATION OF ROLES IN SUPPORTED EMPLOYMENT

Supported employment requires teamwork. The members of the team can be identified in many ways—profession, function, or perhaps setting. The team membership will vary depending on individual needs, program characteristics, and job availability. Since supported employment is an adult lifecycle activity that involves ongoing support in job preparation, initiation, and enhancement, some team members may have long-term involvement with the process, while others may have responsibilities that are episodic. In the discussion that follows, a range of roles are identified without pigeonholing team members into a rigid classification system. A discussion of relationships among the players is presented, followed by a more detailed description of the role of case management and the provision of job site services in a supported employment program.

Participants in a Supported Employment Program

There are a variety of participants in a supported employment program. From the perspective of a rehabilitation counselor and utilizing a marketing approach (Corthell & Boone, 1982), these participants could be divided into two groups—consumers and service providers. While there may be a number of consumers of a supported employment program, this chapter primarily focuses on three groups of consumers: the parents of a supported employee, the supported employee, and the employer involved. Service providers whose roles in supported employment are discussed include:

Rehabilitation counselor
Residential coordinator
Community advocates
Special educators
Evaluators
Work adjustment specialists
Employment training specialists
Co-workers
Job coach

They represent an array of advocates and professional service providers who are ideally linked together to provide a continuum of services. The purpose of such a linkage is to place and sustain an individual with a severe disability in productive and profitable employment in a community-based setting.

Consumers The employer's role goes beyond the obvious acceptance of labor and payment of wages in return. A primary consumer of supported employment services, the employer must be aware of how his or her human resource needs can be appropriately satisfied by a person with a severe disability through supported employment. Employers of persons in need of supported employment should clearly understand the potential and limitations of the disabled employee and the nature and terms of the assistance available from employment training specialists, parents/advocates, educators, rehabilitation staff, and others assisting in the provision of support at the job site, such as co-workers or supervisors.

Parents of a supported employee often know that person best. However, while having had extensive experience with child-oriented services, they may lack knowledge of adult services. Parents may have significant concerns as to whether "their child" can "make it" in employment. They need to know the contributions that "their child" can make through supported employment.

The supported employee will obviously be the key consumer in the provision of rehabilitation services. The matching of employer human resource needs and the skills and talents of a potential supported employee requires an individualized service delivery program. Supported employment services are intended for persons who traditionally have not entered the labor force, and who often are presumed ineligible for rehabilitation benefits due to the severity of their disabilities. The supported employee, and his or her parents where appropriate, must be active participants in the selection of an appropriate vocational goal. Further, disabled workers in supported employment will need to understand and appreciate the support services available at a job site and be fully informed of the effect that a job may have on any benefits for which they are eligible.

Service Providers Rehabilitation counselors assist individuals who are eligible for vocational rehabilitation in entry to and continued participation in supported employment programs. In some instances, rehabilitation counselors provide some of the direct employment services in place-and-train settings. However, rehabilitation counselors involved in most supported employment settings usually purchase or assist in arrangement of supported employment through a specialized place-and-train provider.

Community advocates and residential support staff are important team participants for supported employees who live in group homes or other supported living arrangements. Resident staff teach independent living skills, assist disabled individuals with consumer affairs, and help to integrate the disabled individual into the community through social and recreational interaction. Adjustments made by supported employees to their living arrangements often are a crucial component in determining continued vocational success. Residential support staff are in a key position to provide other supported employment service providers with information that may have an impact on a supported employee's ultimate job success. The residential support staff or community advocate can, through daily contact with the supported employee, provide vital reinforcement of work-related social skills, assist in promoting independent mobility to and from the job, and provide vital early warning of off-the-job factors that may influence job performance.

Teachers and other instructional personnel, through daily classroom contact, will ideally be the first to introduce disabled pupils who require substantial support in employment to the world of work and the promise of the future. Working with parents, instructors can create opportunities for the student to obtain knowledge about workers, including some who are severely disabled, through experiential learning in the community. They also teach the mobility, self-care, and communication skills vital to success in the work environment (Snell & Browder, 1986).

Usually the roles of evaluators and vocational adjustment specialists are de-emphasized in supported employment. Instead of predictive measures of potential or "readiness" for work, supported employment emphasizes place-and-train methods in which employee productivity is assessed as the client performs typical tasks in the actual settings in which the job will be done (Schalock & Karan, 1979). Yet every student, every applicant for income benefits, every candidate for supported employment faces some psychometric testing and similar assessments. Applied negatively or inappropriately, such "diagnostics" and "labeling" can have detrimental consequences, and can become part of the process of discouraging the individual from participating in supported employment. It is important for those administering evaluations as well as for those using results from such assessments to be aware of such potential outcomes.

Employment training specialists or job coaches are a hallmark of supported employment and other place-and-train approaches. They provide individualized training and support in the actual job to be performed at the job site. Their specific activities may involve individualized task analysis, work accommodation, job modeling, monitoring or "shadowing," and other direct assistance to increase worker accuracy and productivity. Assistance is provided in as unobtrusive a manner as possible. A key aspect of intensive direct employment assistance is withdrawal of support as the learning curve builds. Reducing direct support is desirable for it can increase the independence of the disabled worker as he or she assumes more and more responsibility for job performance. Such "fading out" of staff assistance also "frees up" staff to take on new supported employment clients and reduces the cost of long-term support. Support is usually completely withdrawn from persons in transitional employment programs, but in supported employment, maintenance levels of ongoing assistance remain available. At this point, a paraprofessional may be used to provide ongoing contact with the supported employee and employer.

Sometimes co-workers provide key support. In any case, social integration into the world of work is an essential element of supported employment. Strategies to integrate disabled workers into the regular work force and normal work activities at the job site should include natural approaches to co-workers. Labor unions and employee associations should be available to supported employees in the same way any worker would participate in such organizations.

Relationship of the Roles of Participants

With so many relationships involved, supported employment requires continued attention by all parties to the fostering of positive teamwork. Among the major tasks, the following should be addressed by participants seeking to establish a supported employment program: 1) role identification, including lead responsibilities, for existing needs; 2) role amendments/transitions within existing programs; 3) definition of responsibilities for newly emerging needs; and 4) identification of new roles/positions, if necessary.

Lead responsibilities can be designated in formal documents, such as individualized written rehabilitation programs (IWRPs), individualized education programs (IEPs), cooperative agreements, vendor agreements, and eligibility statements. A good rule of thumb would be to assign lead responsibility on a functional basis by asking the question: "Who is most involved in this activity?" But practical considerations have to be followed as well. Communication methods such as conferences, written progress reports, and scheduled "keep-in-touch" phone calls are important. Planned decision points can assure that persons with responsibility for accountability (such as a rehabilitation counselor) receive timely information on the client's progress. Three primary consumers—the employee, the employer, and the employee's parent or advocate—must always know who the primary contact person is for direct supported employment needs.

Role changes will inevitably occur over the life-cycle of employees in supported employment. Agencies and employers will change staff. Agreements and purchase arrangements will be renegotiated. Supported employees will experience major changes in their families, advocates, and living arrangements. Each change of employer, job enhancement, job reduction, or termination will be reflected in role changes for those assisting the supported employee. Many role changes should be viewed as probable and should be planned in advance. For example, a planned event requiring a change in direct employment support services could be reassignment of the supported employee to new duties. Specifically, at the time of the reassignment, the employee could be receiving monitoring of work performance by a community social services specialist employed by the local agency that serves persons with mental retardation. Upon identifying the need for a significant vocational service, the social services specialist would notify the rehabilitation counselor, who would then arrange for employee retraining using post-employment services provided by the employment training specialist. When the supported employee reaches full productivity in the new job, the social services specialist would resume ongoing monitoring responsibility.

Research as well as innovation in practice will lead to new role relationships. One area of probable change involves investigation of the importance of direct staff roles at the job site. New forms of supported employment, as well as new jobs for supported employees to perform, will lead to role changes. Research (Southwest Business, Industry, and Rehabilitation Association, in press) is currently studying the use of employee assistance programs to provide support to developmentally disabled workers. Further research may suggest ways of franchising supported employment and ways of providing supported employment to nondisabled as well as developmentally disabled persons (Berkeley Planning Associates, Inc., in press). Studies are underway to develop measures of supported employment outcomes, including wages, personal satisfaction, integration, impact on benefits and related indicators (Berkeley Planning Associates, Inc., 1986). The more known about the variables that determine positive supported employment outcomes, the more role responsibilities will be defined or redefined to address these factors. A key example might be relationships with employers and co-workers. Studies looking at the use of advocates or mentors in the workplace might result in enhanced roles for co-workers and employers in providing support now provided by employment training specialists or community advocates (Shafer, 1986). If such practices become common, co-worker and employer responsibilities will play an expanded role within the definition of supported work.

There are many other areas where more research is needed. The substantial expansion of supported employment projected through the current Rehabilitation Services Administration ''state-change'' demonstration projects will increase the knowledge base but will also lead to new questions. Supported employment studies to date have largely described model programs in isolation from one another. There have been few evaluations of outcomes over multiple sites where similar approaches have been used with similar clients. The growth of new programs and the expansion of existing programs is resulting in increased numbers of published studies, and in research efforts that compare results and practices across settings with substantial numbers of disabled workers (Wehman & Kregel, 1985).

New supported employment roles likely to gain widespread professional recognition are employment training specialists and special vocational educators. Not all individuals employed in these emerging professional roles will work in supported employment, but those who do will have key responsibilities.

Employment training specialists are direct service trainers who work with severely disabled individuals at the job site, providing the behavioral and vocational assistance needed to meet the job requirements. Sometimes called ''job coaches,'' employment training specialists have up to now been trained largely by the innovators of the supported employment concept. Just as supported employees learn on the job, so too have their trainers and coaches. The professional development of these new staff roles has largely been within the demonstrations and projects that have pioneered supported employment. In turn, the persons trained have gone on to jobs where small groups (usually eight or less) of supported employees work under guidance of the trainer or coach in an enclave, work crew, manufacturing, or dispersed job setting. This managerial/organizational approach has led to less hierarchy, less overhead, and less supervision for employment trainers than is experienced by many other rehabilitation professionals. A current issue in supported employment focuses on how future employment training specialists will be trained (*Federal Register,* 1986a, 1986b), and the extent to which traditional long-term training programs, such as those in rehabilitation counseling, will incorporate components of the employment training specialist training.

Special vocational educators and vocational resource educators are professionals who have special education skills applicable in vocational education or employment settings, or as preparation for such settings (U.S. Department of Education, 1985a). These educators provide the foundation for the high school student who may later have a career that is built with the aid of supported employment. Through their efforts during the secondary school years, students learn in much the same way that they will later learn to perform a meaningful, integrated, paid job. Often it is a volunteer or summer work experience program that provides the vocational dimension (U.S. Department of Education, 1985b), but the support assistance provided has many elements in common with adult supported employment. Personnel preparation programs and professional education associations are currently studying the emergence of these new roles.

ROLE OF THE REHABILITATION COUNSELOR

The previous section of this chapter identified a variety of participants, including a multidisciplinary group of professionals, who may potentially be involved in a supported employment program. For the rehabilitation counselor, primary reference is to responsibilities related to case management. The rehabilitation counselor who carries a caseload can also potentially provide job site training and follow-along services in support of the employment training specialist. Well-timed case management and effective job site services are both integral parts of a successful supported employment program. The description that follows discusses the role of the rehabilitation counselor both as a case manager and as a provider of employment services within a supported employment program.

The rehabilitation counselor working within the public vocational rehabilitation program will probably approach supported employment with a time limit in mind. Vocational rehabilitation participation in representative supported employment demonstration efforts frequently involves ongoing case management and funding participation by other agencies and organizations that are involved in adult long-term work services (M. Hill, Hill, et al., 1985; M. Hill, Revell, et al., 1985). The components of the counselor role discussed here mainly focus on the initial phase of a program of supported employment that heavily involves the vocational rehabilitation program. Recognition is given to the ongoing nature of supported employment and the importance of maintaining case management and job site follow-along services.

CASE MANAGEMENT

Provision and coordination of effective services require attention to a number of case management services. A representative sample of required case management activities are:

Select Appropriate Clients

Supported employment programs are for clients who require an intense level of training and follow-along to successfully enter and retain employment. Functional characteristics of potentially appropriate clients are: repeated failures to maintain employment without support; failure or inability to generalize skills from preemployment training programs, or problems acquiring skills; significant communication problems where job site advocacy would help social integration with co-workers and supervisors; and the need for extended training support to develop production rates (M. Hill, Hill, et al., 1985). The functional need for the service is not limited to specific disability groups. Clients currently participating in segregated, center-based day or work services are primary candidates for supported employment programs.

Assure Client/Family Readiness

Many potential clients for supported employment programs are unemployed or underemployed. Frequently, their work experience and work expectations have not prepared them or their families for the demands of work in regular industry. A change in job status might necessitate a change in personal or family routine. The family unit requires preplacement preparations and post-placement support to reduce the risk for conflict and misunderstanding regarding the responsibilities and experiences involved in moving into community-based integrated employment.

Recognize the Impact of Preplacement Experience

The supported employment approach is a movement away from an emphasis on extended periods of preemployment readiness training. Where preplacement training has taken place, demonstration efforts in supported employment indicate that work experience through enclaves, crews, or actual employment can contribute to successful employment (J. Hill, Banks, Wehman, & Hill, 1986). Case planning involving clients, such as public school special education students, who have supported employment as a probable goal, should emphasize participation in regular work opportunities whenever possible.

Define a Point of Case Closure by the Vocational Rehabilitation (VR) Program

Case closure can occur when a participant in a supported employment program reaches the point of job stabilization. Specific indicators of job stability are:

Employer satisfaction
Completion of the training, adjustment, and fading activities of the job coach
An average intervention by the job coach of less than 20% of the client's working hours over a 2-week period (Virginia Department of Rehabilitation Services, 1986)

For example, a client working 32 hours a week, who can be maintained in that job by intervention at the job site by a job coach at no more than 6.4 hours per week (20% of 32 hours), would be considered potentially stable in employment. The final determination of job stability would require employer satisfaction with the client's performance and at least a 2-week demonstration that the intervention schedule of under 6.4 hours is adequate to maintain the job (Virginia Department of Rehabilitation Services, 1986). It is at the point of job stability and resulting VR case closure that funding from an ongoing support agency or resource must be initiated.

Assure Commitment to Ongoing Support

Case management responsibilities include ensuring that the training time needed and the ongoing support that constitute a supported employment program are available prior to committing long-term job site services to an employer and a client. Coordination is needed with the provider agency and long-term adult service agencies. Supported employment programs potentially involve the blending of support from a variety of funding agencies.

Rehabilitation counselors have historically, as a part of case management activities, screened clients, planned preplacement training on the basis of decisions about eventual goals, and worked with families (Muthard & Salomone, 1969; Rubin & Puckett, 1984). Supported employment does not require a complete redefinition of the case management role of the counselor. Successful client participation in supported employment programs does require that the counselor extend the case management role beyond the normal confines of case closure while continuing to recognize the importance of coordination in case planning, service provision, and funding.

EMPLOYMENT SERVICES

The provision of specific employment services involves substantial job development, job site training and support, and extended follow-along activities.

The role of the rehabilitation counselor, either as an employment service specialist or as a backup to that specialist, includes:

Job Development

During job development the counselor works intensively with both the client and the potential employers. To increase the chances for proper match, counselors frequently complete a job analysis of each job. Areas analyzed include: salary and benefits, hours and days of work, task description, physical requirements, cognitive requirements, motivational factors, social requirements, and working conditions (Moon, Goodall, Barcus, & Brooke, 1985). The job analysis can help structure the task of matching client strengths to job requirements.

After completing the analysis and matching the potential job to the client, the counselor then describes the services that will be provided to help assure that the job will be done acceptably. This description includes information on the Targeted Job Tax Credit program (as available) and the on-site training and support provided by the counselor after placement. During job development, the counselor must accurately inform the employer of the abilities and needs of the client to minimize misunderstandings that might jeopardize the placement. The counselor must also resolve problems relating to the disincentives to employment that are a part of the disability income system. Finally, parent/family reaction to the anticipated job must be clarified and a transportation or travel training plan must be initiated.

Job Site Training and Assistance

The role of the counselor during the training period that follows placement focuses on a number of areas:

Providing on-site training to familiarize the client with the specific job demands

Assisting the client to develop a standard of production acceptable to the employer

Further refining work-related behaviors in the areas of mobility to and from work, timeliness, following work schedules, and personal appearance

Assisting the client to develop positive relationships with co-workers and resolving those rare situations where abuse of the client by co-workers occurs

Serving as a source of awareness to supervisors and co-workers on the many productive and positive qualities of persons who are disabled

Assisting the client and family in properly managing the money earned working in competitive industry

The counselor is responsible for seeing that the job is done properly and, during the initial period of employment, the counselor can actually help the client complete required tasks. As the client develops required skills and productivity, the counselor attends to relationships with co-workers and to helping the client become a member of the work force. The counselor also monitors the relationship between the client and the supervisor to assure that effective methods of giving directions and changing routines are understood. The counselor, during the training and adjustment period, concentrates on integrating the client into the work force as an individual who can contribute productively and personally to the job environment.

Follow-Along and Job Maintenance

When the client is first placed on the job, the counselor might spend up to a full 8 hours a day at the job site. Once the client is established on the job, the counselor will reduce the time spent on the job site, for example, to 1–2 hours per week or less. To make this transition, the counselor must establish a number of conditions in the areas of client performance and independence, co-worker acceptance and awareness, and family commitment to maintaining the work schedule. Frequently problems that affect job stability are not related specifically to the job. During periods of reduced performance by the client or in crisis intervention situations, the counselor might temporarily increase the time spent with the client until job performance returns to levels acceptable to the employer. If relocation to a new job becomes necessary, the job development and training process is reinitiated.

Of necessity, the responsibilities of the rehabilitation counselor within supported employment encompass those of the previously discussed employment training specialist. The services of job development, job site training and assistance, follow-along, and job maintenance may be assumed by either of these two service providers. However, if an employment training specialist or any other provider with similar duties is not available, the rehabilitation counselor has the ultimate responsibility to see that the services associated with supported employment are satisfactorily provided.

SUMMARY

The supported employment initiative is an effort to make integrated paid work opportunities available to persons with severe disabilities who historically have not had the support necessary for them to successfully enter and remain in the competitive labor force. Our knowledge to date about supported employment and our concept of the role of rehabilitation counseling in this area comes largely from experience with demonstration efforts. With the September, 1985, funding by the federal Rehabilitation Services Administration (RSA) of 10 states to develop state programs of supported employment, there is now progress toward formal efforts to make supported employment a work option more readily available to those workers with severe disabilities who require ongoing job site support to remain successfully in the competitive labor force. Successful large-scale development of those work opportunities will require full participation by the rehabilitation counselors and their professional associations in the system development activities currently being initiated.

This chapter has discussed the variety of roles that are potentially a part of a successful supported employment program. Coordination of these roles into a focused effort understood by the service consumer and valued by the employer is central to a successful program. The rehabilitation counselor is in the best position to understand the importance of these various roles.

REFERENCES

Berkeley Planning Associates. (1986). *Development of supported employment performance measures* (Contract #300-85-0138 from the National Institute of Handicapped Research). Berkeley, CA: Author.

Berkeley Planning Associates. (in press). *Development of small business innovation for promoting supported work opportunities* (Contract #NIE-R-85-006 from the U.S. Department of Education's Small Business Innovative Research [SBIR]. Berkeley, CA: Author.

Cohen, D., Patton, S., & Melia, R. (1986). Staffing supported and transitional employment programs. *American Rehabilitation, 12,* 20–24.

Corthell, D. W., & Boone, L. (Eds.). (1982). *Marketing: An approach to placement.* Menomonie: University of Wisconsin–Stout Research and Training Center, Stout Vocational Rehabilitation Institute.

Duncan, J. (1986). Weicker introduces Senate version of Rehabilitation Act extension. *Washington Update* (L-86-9). Washington, DC: National Rehabilitation Association.

Federal Register. (1986a). Application notice for grants under long-term training in rehabilitation counseling (CFDA Number 84-129B).

Federal Register. (1986b). Rehabilitation workshop and facility personnel training announcement (CFDA Number 84-129X).

Hill, J., Banks, P. D., Wehman, P., & Hill, M. (1986). *Individual characteristics and environmental experiences related to competitive employment success of persons with mental retardation.* Richmond: Virginia Commonwealth University Rehabilitation Research and Training Center.

Hill, M., Hill, J., Wehman, P., Revell, G., Dickerson, A., & Noble, J. (1985). Time limited training and supported employment: A model for redistributing existing resources for persons with severe disabilities. In P. Wehman & J. Hill (Eds.), *Competitive employment for persons with mental retardation: From research to practice* (p. 134). Richmond: Virginia Commonwealth University Rehabilitation Research and Training Center.

Hill, M., Revell, G., Chernish, W., Morrell, J. E., White, J., & McCarthy, P. (1985). Social service agency options for modifying existing systems to include transitional and supported work services for persons with severe disabilities. In P. McCarthy, J. Everson, S. Noon, & M. Barcus (Eds.), *School-to-work transition for youth with severe disabilities* (p. 195). Richmond: Virginia Commonwealth University Rehabilitation Research and Training Center.

Moon, S., Goodall, P., Barcus, M., & Brooke, V. (Eds.). (1985). *The supported work model for competitive employment for citizens with severe handicaps: A guide for job trainers*. Richmond: Virginia Commonwealth University Rehabilitation Research and Training Center.

Muthard, J. E., & Salomone, P. R. (1969). The roles and functions of the rehabilitation counselor. *Rehabilitation Counseling Bulletin, 13*(1).

RSA State Demonstration Projects. (1985). *Summary of meeting Nov. 14–15*. Washington, DC: Office of Special Education and Rehabilitation Services.

Rubin, S., & Puckett, F. (1984). The changing role and function of the rehabilitation counselor. *Rehabilitation Counseling Bulletin, 27*(4), 225–231.

Schalock, R., & Karan, O. (1979). Relevant assessment: the interaction between evaluation and training. In G. T. Bellamy, G. O'Connor, & O. C. Karan (Eds.), *Vocational rehabilitation of severely handicapped persons* (pp. 33–54). Baltimore: University Park Press.

Shafer, M. S. (1986). Utilizing coworkers as change agents. In F. Rusch (Ed.), *Competitive employment issues and strategies* (pp. 215–224). Baltimore: Paul H. Brookes Publishing Co.

Snell, M., & Browder, D. (1986). Community referenced instruction: Research and issues. *The Journal of the Association for Persons with Severe Handicaps, 11*, 1–11.

Southwest Business, Industry, and Rehabilitation Association. (in press). *Industry-based employee assistance program model to increase the job retention rate of developmentally disabled persons* (Contract #G-008535141 from the National Institute for Handicapped Research).

U.S. Department of Education, Office of Special Education and Rehabilitation Services, and the National Institute of Handicapped Research. (1985a). *Cooperative programs for transition from school to work* (pp. 12–14). Washington, DC: U.S. Government Printing Office.

U.S. Department of Education, Office of Special Education and Rehabilitation Services, and the National Institute of Handicapped Research. (1985b). *Cooperative programs for transition from school to work* (pp. 117–125). Washington, DC: U.S. Government Printing Office.

Virginia Department of Rehabilitation Services. (1986). *Interim guidelines for use in the review and approval of vendor applications to DRS for transitional employment services within a supported employment program*. Richmond: Author.

Wehman, P., Hill, M., Hill, J., Brooke, V., Pendleton, P., & Britt, C. (1985). Competitive employment for persons with mental retardation: A follow-up six years later. *Mental Retardation, 23*, 274–281.

Wehman, P., & Kregel, J. (1985). A supported work approach to competitive employment of individuals with moderate and severe handicaps. *The Journal of the Association for Persons With Severe Handicaps, 10*, 3–11.

Will, M. (1984). *OSERS programming for the transition of youth with disabilities*. Washington, DC: Department of Education, Office of Special Education and Rehabilitation Services.

6

Transition from School to Work for Individuals with Learning Disabilities

A Comprehensive Model

Patricia Schmitt, Bruce Growick, and Michael Klein

THE TRANSITION FROM school to work for individuals with disabilities is an issue that has recently received wide public attention. Transition involves more than just finding suitable employment. Rather, it is a complex process, occurring simultaneously with the transition from adolescence to adulthood, and involves a broad spectrum of life issues related to separating from the family, facing new challenges, learning decision-making and problem-solving techniques, and preparing for the many pressures of adult life (Davis, Anderson, Linkowski, Berger, & Feinstein, 1985).

Transition is also not a one-step process. It requires communication and action among school personnel, parents, and adult service providers in a coordinated effort to move the adolescent through school instruction, planning for the transition process, and placement and continuance in employment. Recent research indicates that learning disabled individuals experience particular difficulty in making this transition due to functional limitations and learning disability—related problems such as organizational and prob-

The Ohio State University recently has been awarded a 3-year federal demonstration grant to implement and evaluate the efficacy of the treatment approach that is described in this chapter.

lem-solving deficits and inadequate life-planning skills (Hallahan, Gajar, Cohen, & Tarver, 1978; Schmitt & Hall, 1986; Schumaker, Hazel, Sherman, & Sheldon, 1982; Tollefson, Tracy, Johnsen, Buenning, & Farmer, 1981). These problems tend to be pervasive and persistent unless actions are taken, not only to remediate the academic deficits of the learning disability, but also to address the functional and vocational consequences. In this way, the limitations of a learning disability are minimized while adjustment and transition from school to work are maximized.

HISTORICAL DEVELOPMENTS RELATED TO LEARNING DISABILITY

Many events have taken place over the last several years that have focused attention on the transitional problems of persons who are learning disabled, the least of which have been legislative initiatives. When Public Law 94-142, the Education for All Handicapped Children Act of 1975, was established as a national policy that extended education to all handicapped children, individuals with learning disabilities were included within this mandate. Accordingly, the number of children identified as learning disabled and receiving special education services in the nation's public schools grew from 800,000 in 1976–1977 to 2,000,000 in 1983–1984 (*Seventh Annual Report to Congress on the Implementation of PL 94-142*). This led to an awareness of the prevalence of learning disability in our schools (which should increase as the process of diagnosis becomes more refined) and highlighted the need for this population to receive rehabilitative services upon graduation. The person who is learning disabled, as with many persons who have disabling conditions, finds it very difficult to make the transition from school to work.

Interestingly enough, as PL 94-142 was being planned, the Rehabilitation Act of 1973 (PL 93-112) was enacted to further develop and implement comprehensive programs of vocational rehabilitation and independent living for all handicapped persons. As part of the 1981 amendments to PL 93-112, ''specific learning disabilities'' was established as a separate disability category. The eligibility requirements for vocational rehabilitation services help to serve as guidelines in developing a plan for transition from school to work for learning disabled individuals. The definition of learning disability that follows is consistent with the definition used in PL 94-142 and is used here to describe the disability:

> A specific learning disability is a disorder in one or more of the central nervous system processes involved in perceiving, understanding and/or using concepts through verbal (spoken or written) language or nonverbal means. This disorder manifests itself with a deficit in one or more of the following areas: attention, reasoning, processing, memory, communication, reading, writing, spelling, calculation, coordination, social competence and emotional maturity.

> Individuals who manifest these characteristics would be eligible to receive vocational rehabilitation services if they satisfy the following criteria:
>
> The disorder is diagnosed by a licensed physician and/or a licensed or certified psychologist who is skilled in the diagnosis and treatment of such disorders;
>
> The disorder results in a substantial handicap to employment for the individual; and
>
> There is a reasonable expectation that vocational rehabilitation services may benefit the individual in terms of employability. (Amendments to PL 93-112)

In response to these legislative mandates and documented transitional impediments, many schools and rehabilitation agencies have joined forces to help alleviate the problems faced by learning disabled students. This chapter focuses not only on some proposed guidelines that can bridge the gap from school to work for learning disabled individuals, but also describes the role that rehabilitation can play in this process.

UNIQUE PROBLEMS OF THE LEARNING DISABLED ADOLESCENT THAT AFFECT VOCATIONAL OUTCOME

Individuals with a learning disability often face a poor prognosis for vocational success (Marsh, Gearheart, & Gearheart, 1978). They are frequently unemployed or underemployed (i.e., they find themselves in jobs that offer less than competitive pay, lower status, and diminished career potential and advancement). A number of factors contribute to this poor prognosis, particularly a poor self-concept, inappropriate or unacquired social and interpersonal skills, and vocational immaturity.

For the adolescent with a learning disability, this time of transition can be a very difficult and frustrating period, leading to confusion, alienation, and drifting. Because a learning disability is an invisible disability, families, peers, teachers, and employers often expect the adolescent to "grow out" of the problems associated with the learning disability (President's Committee on the Employment of the Handicapped, 1985). The limitations of a learning disability do not occur only in the classroom. A learning disability does not improve or disappear with age. Limitations often become markedly worse upon entry into the world of work (Cruickshank, Morse, & Johns, 1980).

Due to the incongruity between society's expectations based on physical growth and chronological age, and the psychosocial characteristics of the disability, which can retard the maturation process, tremendous confusion in the search for a personal identity may result. Learning disabled individuals struggle to develop an identity, though they may have no positive or clear self-concept, especially if they have not accepted the disability. Repeated failure in school, denial and concealment of the disability, and familial reinforcement of negative experiences can combine to create tremendous anxiety and confusion. Psychologically, this ambiguous search for an identity leads to marked variations in mood, reduced frustration tolerance, extreme restlessness, poorer appraisal of reality, and impaired ability in organizing abstract attitudes. These lead to problems with the acquisition of appropriate interpersonal skills.

A learning disability is also a disorganizing factor in a family (Farnham-Diggory, 1978). It can create problems among siblings, who may feel a learning disabled brother or sister receives inordinate time and attention, which is probably the case. Parental anxiety about the ability of the learning disabled child to acquire appropriate social skills that will lead to independent decision making and living often overlay the adolescent's same fears and anxieties.

Much ambiguity surrounds learning disability. Many people, including teachers, view it as an inability to learn, rather than a different orientation for receiving and processing information. Although learning disabled students typically possess average or above average intelligence, they are frequently not directed toward the same future opportunities as their peers. Again, this is a problem that results from a lack of understanding about the limitations caused by the learning disability, and the accommodations that can be made to minimize these limitations.

Time and energy spent in denying the disability can leave little, if any, time for working through the normal problems of adolescence and the acquisition of appropriate social skills. This results in reduced motivation and an inability to identify personal and vocational goals as well as to develop a commitment to a plan of action for achieving those goals. Learning disabled clients bring with them to the rehabilitation process these obstacles to vocational planning and growth. Failure to solve the developmental issues of adolescence guarantees the loss of a strong foundation for sound vocational decision making and life planning (Marsh et al., 1978; Szymanski & Danek, 1985). Like their nondisabled peers, learning disabled youth face major decisions about their futures. But they face these decisions with fewer available options. They need not only special support, but also special services for the school to work transition.

FOUNDATIONS OF A COMPREHENSIVE SERVICE DELIVERY MODEL

A comprehensive array of special services is needed to address the basic personal, social, and vocational deficiencies of learning disabled individuals. A detailed description of a service delivery model follows below (see Table 1).

Development of an Individualized Transition Plan (ITP)

Current findings suggest that standardized test results, which are now being used, may be of little value for predicting vocational success (McCue, 1984). Although there is a paucity of information available in this area, especially

Table 1. Comprehensive service delivery model for transition from school to work

1. *Development of an individualized transition plan*—based upon a comprehensive assessment of vocational, academic, and interpersonal functioning that yields an individualized transition plan (ITP).
2. *Learning styles evaluation*—identification of appropriate individualized learning style that will result in maximum use of program information and facilitate planning and delivery of services. Learning style preference is adapted to worker style preference.
3. *Vocational exploration and career education*—individually planned career exploration, counseling, utilizing computer interactive programs and planning services based upon ITP assessment.
4. *Employability skills training*—development of vocational, social, and emotional skills necessary to enter the placement phase of the program.
   a. Interpersonal—skill development in basic listening, problem exploration, goal setting, and problem-solving and decision-making skills. Includes social skills, assertiveness, and conflict management training.
   b. Intrapersonal—development of a variety of behavioral, cognitive, and cognitive-behavioral skills. Includes self-instruction, cognitive restructuring, cognitive rehearsal, cognitive modeling, imagery, and stress inoculation experiences.
   c. Extrapersonal—development of skills to gain access to and effectively utilize community resources.
5. *Supported job search/placement/follow-up*—program includes job-seeking skills, job clubs, and business- and industry-based community linkages.
6. *Parent and agency cooperation and involvement*—active, structured involvement and participation of parents and schools, agencies, and business and industry.

regarding the kinds of measurement that will yield the most useful treatment planning data, a diagnostic battery that can be used for generating vocationally relevant information for the development of the ITP is clearly needed.

This assessment battery should ideally be designed to assess vocational interests, aptitudes and achievement levels, career maturity, and work readiness. Such a battery could be administered individually as well as in a group and could comprise the following diagnostic tools: The APTICOM, the Career Maturity Inventory (CMI), and the Work Readiness Inventory.

APTICOM The APTICOM is a computerized program designed to assess interest, aptitude, and achievement, and to relate these to specific U.S. Department of Labor levels. It summarizes and integrates the results into a written narrative that lists job titles that correspond to the *Dictionary of Occupational Titles (D.O.T.)*, in which the student will encounter the greatest likelihood of success.

The Career Maturity Inventory (CMI) The CMI measures six characteristics shown to be important indices of career maturity in adolescence. Five cognitive tests examine the appropriateness of different career actions based on a description of the person's attributes, matching occupations with descriptions, selecting an occupation based on one's attributes and experiences, recognizing steps necessary to realize career goals, and solving career problems stemming from external impediments or conflicts.

Work Readiness Inventory The Work Readiness Inventory is a computerized assessment of 344 skills related to getting and keeping a job. The skills cover such areas as personal work behaviors, the use of tools, participation in a job interview, and using a time clock. Standards for mastery of skills are clearly stated, including three broad areas of evaluation: prevocational, vocational, and work/community adjustment skills.

An individualized transition plan can be formulated from the diagnostic information provided by the school and/or referring agency, and further developed by the rehabilitation team through the above battery. The ITP contains the following information:

1. A summary of the vocational evaluation and assessment, detailing the student's present level of academic, interpersonal, and vocational functioning
2. Identification of learning style preference to facilitate an understanding of the treatment phases and how they transfer to the work site
3. A statement of short- and long-term goals, and services to be provided to meet those goals
4. Appropriate consent and permission forms for participation in clinic services
5. Appropriate objective criteria and evaluation procedures for determining whether goals are being met

Learning Styles Identification

A learning styles assessment is a relatively new concept in the area of vocational evaluation and adjustment. Its usefulness lies in its ability to help individuals understand the optimal conditions under which learning occurs. The counselor can use the information garnered from a learning styles assessment to select a learning strategy that will compensate for learning weaknesses (Swiercinsky, 1985). Such variables as environmental, emotional, sociological, physical, and psychological stimuli are among the categories of personal preference that are assessed. Upon identification of an individual's learning style, this information can be translated and adapted to develop an individual's worker preference style; that is, newly acquired learning strategies that minimize the functional limitations caused by the learning disability can be adopted for use on the work site to provide the requisite training and orientation for a job in a mode of presentation, or learning style, that is most suitable to the individual.

Vocational Exploration and Career Education

Vocational exploration and career education are designed to provide an examination of job options and to assist in the selection of vocational goals appropriate for individuals with learning disabilities. This component can be used to gain an understanding of the individual's level of work orientation and vocational maturity. Many resources are available to assist in the career counseling and vocational placement of learning disabled individuals, including a broad range of psychological assessment tools, vocational evaluation programs, and computer career development and job search systems.

Computer-assisted career exploration and guidance systems are designed to help individuals understand themselves and the world of work, and to develop decision-making skills in the career selection process (Sampson, McMahon, & Burkhead, 1985; Schmitt & Growick, 1985). Computer-assisted career education has been demonstrated to be efficacious in serving individuals with learning disabilities. Through interactive computer programs, the individual can learn to integrate self-knowledge and occupational knowledge, to relate work from broad occupational classifications to specific clusters of jobs, and to appreciate the demands and working environments of a variety of jobs. There are many computer-assisted guidance systems available to facilitate this phase of counseling, among them *DISCOVER* (American College Testing, Inc.) and the *Career Planning System* (Conover Company).

DISCOVER The DISCOVER system is a career guidance program that provides individuals with vocationally related self-knowledge in order to help them make satisfying vocational choices. After identification of self-interests, abilities, and values, DISCOVER displays a "World of Work Map" to provide students with a sense of direction for career exploration. The world of work map is based on job analysis data for the 12,099 occupations in the fourth edition of the *D.O.T.* and on interest scores for 421 educational and occupational groups.

Career Planning System (CPS) The CPS is an interactive program specifically designed for individuals with limited reading ability. Students progress through the exploration experiences on the basis of personal, individual interests and reactions. They complete the CPS experience by making individual education plans in order to synthesize the career knowledge and self-awareness gained through exploring occupations in the interest areas, and plan specific activities for the continued investigation of favored occupations.

Other Computer-Assisted Programs Additionally, individuals can use the information obtained from these programs in combination with statewide computer occupational information systems that provide data on national and state occupations, employment trends and markets, 2- and 4-year colleges, the military, and sources of scholarships and financial aid, as well as other career-related answers to the world of work.

Selection of a computerized program and progress through one depend, of course, on the specific learning style of the individual. Adaptations can be made, such as having a counselor/tutor assisting the individual to read and understand system instructions.

Employability Skills Training

The purpose of the employability skills phase of the total program is to assist the individual in the development of prevocational, social, and emotional skills that are prerequisites to the job placement phase of the program. Prevocational skills are basic work attitudes and habits. Emotional skills include coping skills focusing on stress management, anxiety reduction, and skills needed as prerequisites to entering the job placement phase of the program. Three major components of training and learning addressed in employability skills training are interpersonal (interaction between individuals), intrapersonal (within the individual), and extrapersonal (dealing with outside agencies, bureaucracies, the community, etc.). Several examples might contribute to a better understanding of why this program needs to be individually tailored to meet the learning style and entry-level skills of each client with learning disabilities. An individualized approach is needed in the design and implementation of an employability skills program beyond what may be used in more traditional rehabilitation settings.

The delivery of training to persons with learning disabilities must be dictated by learning style preferences. Table 1 demonstrates how individual learning style characteristics can be linked to specific techniques to deliver specific program content. For example, the use of self-instructional training to teach an individual one method of coping with an overly demanding employer or a distractive co-worker involves auditory perception, emotional responsibility, self/group sociological preference, and analytic learning style characteristics.

The interpersonal skill development component requires that the individual develop specific competencies for seeking and maintaining gainful employment. This includes extensive training in basic communication skills, assertiveness, and conflict management training. Basic interpersonal skills training, which serves as the foundation for much of the employability and placement phases, includes empathetic listening, problem exploration, goal setting, and problem-solving and decision-making skills, with emphasis on the transfer of these skills to the work setting. Effective job seeking is essentially the marketing of oneself to potential employers. Employable individuals acquire the assertiveness skills in their behavioral repertoire to deal effectively with job-seeking and maintenance situations (Bolles, 1985). Learning basic interpersonal skills will require a wide range of activities depending on the learning needs of the learning disabled client. A client with severe reading deficits will need to have experiences that include visual, auditory preference, visual perception, reflective, memory skill, and analytic learning style activities. Conflict management skills are needed by an individual to address employment as well as personal conflict situations that may affect the individual's ability to maintain employment. This training will draw upon the conflict management model developed by Klein and Scofield (1984). Helping the client deal with potentially emotional interpersonal conflicts with co-workers, supervisors, and/or the members of the community is emphasized, utilizing a variety of interpersonal and behavioral strategies.

The interpersonal phase of the employability skills program focuses on the development of a variety of behavioral and cognitive skills to assist the client in dealing with the difficulties and stress of the employment search and job acquisition process. A comprehensive behavioral programming process is utilized to facilitate the objectives of this phase. The growth of the employee assistance movement attests to the inability or unwillingness of individuals to resolve these problems without intervention. Many employers feel that there is a significant need at the workplace to deal with issues such as stress management, interpersonal problems, and the effects of physical disability (Klein & Kelz, 1986).

This model focuses on the intrapersonal needs of clients by the provision of three major areas of service. First, clients need to be taught methods to deal effectively with the physiological effects of stress, anxiety, and anger that may accompany employment. This can be accomplished by teaching progressive relaxation techniques (Jacobsen, 1938), and other techniques to manage stress in a variety of work-related situations. Second, using the self-instructional training models of Meichenbaum (1977), and Burns and Beck (1980), trainees can learn to deal with maladaptive thought patterns that lead to dysfunctional anger, fear, anxiety, and depression. By using these cognitive behavioral methods, dysfunctional cognitive distortions and patterns that may often interfere with employment seeking, occupational adjustment, and placement can be proactively addressed. Finally, ongoing individual and group counseling should be available to assist the individual in the transition process, as well as to deal with issues of self-esteem and self-concept.

Instructional modes must again be determined by the learning style of the client. A learning disabled student with reading skills may be encouraged to read program manuals on coping skills, complete logs of behavioral and cognitive activity, and read written materials related to self-control. Other individuals with reading and perceptual difficulties may require an approach that utilizes lectures, the development of audiotapes of these curricular phases, and the keeping of verbal logs on audiotape. A student who needs to work on anger management, for example, may be taught relaxation through modeling and the use of audiotapes between classes. Cognitive self-control can be taught using lecture and the modeling of self-instruction designed to reduce anger and physiological arousal.

The extrapersonal component of the employability section of the program is designed to assist the individual in obtaining access to community resources. The model operates on the premise that strong community linkages and support networks need to be established to assure a successful school-to-work transition. Trainees should learn about the state-federal agency and its services, such as placement and postclosure services required for finding and maintaining employment. Within the model programs, if clients are not already linked to the local vocational rehabilitation agency, such a referral should be made, if appropriate, for consideration for eligibility and placement services. The client needs to become aware of and utilize other community support and advocacy groups and service agencies. Parent awareness meetings can be held during the employability skills program as well as during the placement phase to assure active involvement in all phases of the program.

Supported Job Search/Placement/Follow-up

The purpose of this phase is to deliver a program in job-seeking skills, job clubs, and business and industry linkages to prepare severely learning disabled clients for entry into the workforce. Alternative modes of obtaining job leads, information, and job interviews should be highlighted (Bolles, 1985).

Training in these areas can be accomplished by the use of live and filmed models performing the desired employment-seeking behavior (Bandura, 1969, 1971). Another key element in the job-seeking skills program is the use of live and cognitive rehearsal. This program effectively overlaps other segments in the employability skills sequence. For example, the inexperienced job seeker may profit from a combination of coping skills (relaxation and self-instruction) and an opportunity to learn skills in a graduated manner with the least difficult skills first, followed by increasingly more challenging activities. This stress inoculation approach has been found to be effective in teaching a variety of behavioral skills to individuals handicapped by excessive emotionality (Klein & Scofield, 1984; Meichenbaum, 1977; Meichenbaum & Turk, 1978).

Another essential element in this comprehensive behavioral approach to the placement process is the introduction of a job club program modeled after the Azrin and Besalel (1980) program. This behaviorally oriented group experience provides a supportive atmosphere with structured exercises demonstrated to have a positive effect on the placement process.

Finally, perhaps the most essential element in the transition model is the development of active linkages with local business and industry. On-site industrial tours enhance career exploration, make students more aware of the requirements of the local labor market, and establish contacts for possible future employment. In addition to the industrial site visits, informational interviews can be arranged with cooperating business personnel, thus giving the student an opportunity to apply what was learned in earlier phases of the program.

Shadowing experiences can be an important aspect of the business and industry segment. Students can be matched with workers in business and industry, spending full work days observing employees complete work tasks.

Summer work experiences planned with cooperating industry for supervised work experience are a valuable step in the transition process. By paying careful attention to student interests and aptitudes as well as to labor market realities, a carefully planned placement can be the culmination of the transition process. This may be accomplished through financial support by the business, the school district, the state-federal agency, or a combination.

Involvement of the project staff is essential to the success of this part of the program. Student readiness must be assessed prior to assignment to outside industrial experiences. Some severely learning disabled individuals have great difficulty in finding their way around a rehabilitation facility. A counselor often needs to help the client develop appropriate maps (cognitive and real) and rehearse movement throughout the facility. This one-to-one interaction is essential in this phase of the program. It is important that the client not be sent to the worksite, site tour, or shadowing experience unprepared, for this can result in an extremely anxious, traumatic, and confusing experience for the client. Throughout the program, the local business and industry consortium should be actively involved through consultation, classroom lectures, and discussions. The state rehabilitation agency should also be involved in the event that its expertise and support is needed to implement the final phases of the transition plan, and also to provide follow-up services to the client and employer.

Parent and Agency Cooperation and Involvement

Appropriately preparing handicapped individuals with the necessary academic, social, emotional, and vocational skills to function in society is a complex process. To achieve even modest goals requires input and cooperation from all those involved in the individual's growth and development. Next to the client, the most important and often the least consulted entity in this process is the parent. Only in the last decade has significant national attention been focused on a parent-professional partnership based on mutual respect and decision making (Turnbull, Turnbull, & Strickland, 1986). While this particular component of the model appears last in the authors' discussion, parent cooperation and involvement is necessary throughout the provision of services. The multidisciplinary approach to the development of the individualized transition plan requires the input of referring agencies, schools, parents, and clients, as well as the maintenance of their participation throughout the supported job search and job placement.

It is essential that the parents be aware of what to expect from a transition program, the scope and nature of the individual program components, the program's standards and provisions, and the program's expectations of the parents. Parents must learn to: 1) deal with student management problems in the home, 2) transfer skills learned in the program to the home environment, and 3) anticipate future needs for vocational and social development.

Throughout this service delivery model, large and small parent group meetings as well as individual conferences to review the goals and progress of the individualized transition plan are conducted.

Agency cooperation is important for the identification of both community resources and rehabilitative services, and also as part of the linkage with the business and industry community for job development and placement. The model described in this chapter represents a fluid process of service delivery. The components of the model are not static or separate entities. The success of this delivery plan is dependent upon the active participation and involvement of the student, parents, schools, agencies, and business and industry linkages.

A CASE STUDY

A case study of a client seen at the Rehabilitation Clinic at the Ohio State University illustrates the unique problems of learning disabled individuals as well as the application of treatment suggestions for effectively dealing with these problems.

The Case of EJ

EJ is a learning disabled young adult referred to the clinic by a family member who works at the university. He was seen in the clinic for 9 months for extensive vocational, individual, and family counseling. EJ presented a fairly typical profile of a learning disabled client in terms of problems at school, at home, and in the community.

EJ graduated from high school at age 19 with a general diploma, and began counseling 3 months later. He was diagnosed by a family physician, private psychologist, and school psychologist as having "severe dyslexia with attention deficit." Medication, in the form of Ritalin, was prescribed for the hyperactivity; he had taken this medication daily throughout elementary and middle school. His first acknowledgment of his learning disability was during the first grade when he was initially diagnosed. He described it as, "Everything was really slow and seemed to happen later for me than everyone else. It got worse all along and I might as well as have been totally blind in school."

EJ's parents were divorced during his first year of school. His father moved from the Midwest to Colorado 2 years after the divorce, and his mother found full-time employment to try to manage financially. The father was often negligent or tardy about child support and ignored requests from the mother for financial help for special services, such as after-school tutoring, for their son.

At the beginning of the 10th grade, EJ developed serious problems with truancy and was often in trouble for minor offenses at school, such as smoking on school premises. With the exception of shop and an auto body course in the school career center, his academic performance was very poor. A month before the end of the school year, the family had a fire in their home and was forced to vacate to a small apartment for about 6 months. Due to this event, EJ's problems at school, and financial stresses, he was sent to live with his father.

He started school in Colorado at the beginning of a summer session. Although he did not have enough credits, his father persuaded the school to admit him to regular classes in the 11th grade. His father, embarrassed by the learning disability, would not acknowledge it to anyone, including the school. His father and stepmother traveled to Europe during the winter of this year and left EJ home alone for over 2 months. During this time, he was frequently truant, held drinking parties for his friends, wrecked the family car, and held a number of short-term jobs, such as housepainter and busboy. Upon his return from Europe, EJ's father severely beat EJ for the damages that occurred during his absence, and EJ ran away from home. The police located him within 2 weeks and he begged to return home to live with his mother, which he did.

He found part-time employment during the summer and worked two jobs (as a busboy and custodian) to pay for damages done to the father's car. He started 12th grade, returning to the school he had attended in the 10th grade, and tried to establish a social network as well as complete school. Due to the extraordinary circumstances surrounding EJ's educational history, the high school thought he was "beyond" intensive academic remediation and concentrated its efforts on "getting him out." He had a tutor, took tests orally, and graduated with severely limited reading ability. When EJ came to the clinic, he was working two part-time jobs, as an autobody trainee and busboy, both at minimum wage. Neither employer knew EJ was dyslexic, as he had convinced his employers that he possessed normal academic ability. However, his dyslexia was so severe that he could not read a job application.

EJ also tried to hide his disability from his friends, as he thought they would consider him "mentally retarded" if they knew he could not read. His dating relationships involved a great deal of creativity in trying to find things to do that would not require reading (e.g., he avoided going to a restaurant and reading a menu, or looking up a movie time and location in the newspaper). EJ repeatedly got traffic violations and amassed a great debt in fines and late payments because he could not read his tickets. Moreover, he was embarrassed by being served notices at work to appear in court for unpaid fines.

Treatment with this young man at the clinic was designed to accommodate his severe dyslexia. Vocational evaluation and career exploration was conducted orally and auditorily (i.e., both tape-recorded and oral administration of instruments) to maximize his learning style preferences. Individual counseling focused on resolving family issues, building his self-esteem and confidence, getting him to accept his disability, and moving him toward the problem-solving and decision-making skills needed for independent living and life planning. Family counseling was conducted with EJ's mother to work through some of the serious home problems so that mother and son could develop some trust, honesty, and means of communication.

EJ's vocational interests in mechanical work were reflected in self-report and results on orally administered vocational interest inventories such as the Kuder and California Assessment Inventory. Specific job titles and information (corresponding to *D.O.T.* titles) were searched in the area of mechanical work on the Ohio Career Information System (OCIS), a computer-based system that provides detailed information on national and state occupations. Titles such as automobile mechanic helper (*D.O.T.* 620.684-014), service mechanic helper (*D.O.T.* 630.664-018), and tractor mechanic helper (*D.O.T.* 620.683-030) were searched on the system to provide information such as job title (*D.O.T.* code), job description, occupational outlook, number of such jobs nationally and locally (within the state), salary range, and appropriate training required for the job.

Based on this information, EJ was able to progress through the Career Planning System (CPS) to seek additional information about jobs in this interest area. The CPS is geared toward handicapped clients with limited or low reading ability. Individuals advance through the program at their own rate. This interactive program addresses the user by name and provides helpful hints and positive reinforcement when difficulty is experienced in responding to questions. The programs on the CPS are written and graphic in presentation. Completion of an occupational area of interest provides information on specific job titles (again using *D.O.T.* classifications). EJ's progress through this program was slow, though he was able to spend as much time as needed to complete the sequence. His results correlated with information from the other instruments.

Several counseling sessions were devoted entirely to teaching EJ how to read, comprehend, and complete a job application. Role-play interviews were conducted, with the counselor using the job application as a starting point. EJ was taught to elaborate on application information and to talk knowledgeably about himself. The most significant aspect of this part of treatment focused on getting him to reveal and explain his severe dyslexia to a potential employer and discuss accommodations that could be made (e.g., watching another worker perform job responsibilities) for his own orientation to the job.

EJ was very verbal and personable, and he obviously built on these personality assets as he quickly moved through the employability skills training. After 6 months, he applied for a full-time job with an auto parts company. He went to the personnel office, requested an application, filled it out by himself, and interviewed with the company. He told his prospective employer about his learning disability and also about the therapy he was receiving at the clinic to assist him in planning his vocational future and finding suitable employment. He got the job and is continuing to work at present.

Though EJ could still benefit significantly from extensive academic remediation, he was able to find appropriate and suitable employment with the opportunity for salary increases and full-time benefits. His self-confidence was greatly bolstered by this accomplishment and the family relationships improved. He talks about saving money from his current job and going to a technical training institute to learn advanced skills.

At the time of treatment with EJ, the clinic was not equipped to administer a learning styles inventory. It was through research efforts to identify the necessary components for a model treatment program that it was decided to include it as part of the overall strategy in serving clients with learning disabilities.

Upon a review of learning styles instruments, an instrument such as the Productivity Environmental Preference Survey by Dunn, Dunn, and Price (Price Systems, Incorporated) was found to be very useful. This survey is a 100-item, paper-pencil Likert scale inventory that measures the following environmental factors related to educational or occupational activities: immediate environment (sound, temperature, light, and design), emotionality (motivation, responsibility, persistence, and structure), sociological needs (self-, peer-, authority-oriented, or combined), and physical needs (perceptual preferences, time of day, intake, and mobility). Respondents indicate whether they agree or disagree with each of the 100 statements about ways people like to study or work.

CONCLUSIONS

This model is based upon the authors' work with learning disabled individuals seen at The Ohio State University's Rehabilitation Clinic, which is within the Department of Human Services Education. Through the disciplines of special education, school psychology, and rehabilitation services, the clinic is designed to help individuals with learning problems, using a multiplicity of services, from comprehensive psychoeducational assessment to academic remediation to support services. The rehabilitative services component of the clinic was established to provide services for learning disabled individuals age 16–30. As described in the model, services are individualized to address the specific academic, vocational, and psychosocial adjustment needs of the individual.

Based upon experience in serving this population in a clinical laboratory setting designed for research and instruction as well as for direct service, a comprehensive treatment plan was developed. This developmental model assists individuals with severe learning disabilities in making the transition from school to work with the intention of finding and maintaining gainful employment. Programs that attempt to facilitate such a transition using a more unidimensional approach are frequently less likely to be as effective in either the short term or the long term. What is unique about this approach is its comprehensiveness, focusing on the holistic needs of the individual, and utilizing a combination of modalities that have themselves been tested in experimental and field research.

Research is needed to evaluate program implementation in a variety of settings and treatment variations. Rigorous field trials are encouraged to test the efficacy of the program on a variety of program variables. Ultimately, the primary goal of the program should be directed toward job placement and job retention. Studies should be initiated to test the hypotheses that this comprehensive approach is the most effective strategy in both facilitating and implementing the transition process. Thus, evaluations that test the relative efficacy of the individual program components are needed.

This program is most unique in applying multiple educational and psychological approaches in a comprehensive treatment plan. At the same time, the model is adapted and tailored to the individual through the identification and implementation of the individualized transition plan. Cooperation among students, parents, community resources, rehabilitation agencies and professionals, as well as involvement of the private sector, is a key strength of the program.

While traditional approaches to vocational rehabilitation for individuals with severe learning disabilities have demonstrated some success, new creative approaches need to be developed and evaluated. Although a facility such as the Rehabilitation Clinic may not be available to all learning disabled youth, parents, teachers, and adult service providers must combine their efforts to gain access to resources in the community that will help meet the unique needs of the learning disabled person. The model has also sought to recognize and incorporate the advances in clinical and counseling psychology that have occurred over the last decade. Many of the innovative techniques described within this chapter can be implemented with the realization that such a holistic approach, which has always been a hallmark of rehabilitation, can offer greater opportunities to assist learning disabled individuals in achieving a successful, lasting, and personally rewarding transition from school to work.

REFERENCES

Azrin, N., & Besalel V. (1980). *Job club counselor's manual.* Baltimore: University Park Press.

Bandura, A. (1969). *Principles of behavior modification.* New York: Holt, Rinehart and Winston.

Bandura, A. (1971). Psychotherapy based upon modeling principles. In A. E. Bergin & S. L. Gorfield (Eds.), *Handbook of psychotherapy and behavior change: An empirical analysis* (pp. 653–708). New York: John Wiley & Sons.

Bolles, R. (1985). *What color is your parachute?* Berkeley, CA: TenSpeed Press.

Burns, D., & Beck, A. (1980). Cognitive-behavior modification of mood disorders. In J. Foreyt & D. Rathejan (Eds.), *Cognitive behavior therapy: Research and application*. New York: Plenum Press.

Cruickshank, W., Morse, W., & Johns, J. (1980). *Learning disabilities: The struggle from adolescence to adulthood.* New York: Syracuse University Press.

Davis, S., Anderson, D., Linkowski, D., Berger, K., & Feinstein, C. (1985). Developmental tasks and transitions of adolescents with chronic illnesses and disabilities. *Rehabilitation Counseling Bulletin, 29*(2), 69–80.

Farnham-Diggory, S. (1978). *Learning disabilities: A psychological perspective.* Cambridge, MA: Harvard University Press.

Hallahan, D., Gajar, A., Cohen, S., & Tarver, S. (1978). Selective attention and locus of control in learning disabled and normal children. *Journal of Learning Disabilities, 11*(4), 47–52.

Jacobsen, E. (1938). *Progressive relaxation.* Chicago: University of Chicago Press.

Klein, M., and Kelz, J. (1986). *Counseling in business and industry: A survey of major corporations.* Manuscript submitted for publication.

Klein, M., & Scofield, M. (1984). The development of rehabilitation counselor competence in conflict management: The need for an experiential training approach. *Rehabilitation Counseling Bulletin, 27,* 303–311.

Marsh, G., Gearheart, C., & Gearheart, B. (1978). *The learning disabled adolescent: Program alternatives in the secondary school.* St. Louis: C. V. Mosby.

McCue, M. (1984). Assessment and rehabilitation of learning disabled adults. *Rehabilitation Counseling Bulletin, 27,* 287–290.

Meichenbaum, D. (1977). *Cognitive behavior modification: An integrative approach.* New York: Plenum Press.

Meichenbaum, D., & Turk, D. (1978). Cognitive behavioral management of anxiety, anger and pain. In P. Davidson (Ed.), *The behavioral management of anxiety, depression and pain.* New York: Plenum Press.

President's Committee on the Employment of the Handicapped. (1985). *Supervising adults with learning disabilities.* Washington, DC: U.S. Government Printing Office.

Sampson, J., McMahon, B., & Burkhead, J. (1985). Using computers for career exploration and decision making in vocational rehabilitation. *Rehabilitation Counseling Bulletin, 28*(4), 242–261.

Schmitt, P., & Growick, B. (1985). Computer technology in rehabilitation counseling. *Rehabilitation Counseling Bulletin, 28*(4), 233–241.

Schmitt, P., & Hall, R. (1986). About the unique vocational adjustment needs of students with learning disabilities. *The Directive Teacher, 8*(1), 7–8.

Schumaker, J., Hazel, J., Sherman, J. & Sheldon, J. (1982). Social skill performances of learning disabled, non-learning disabled, and delinquent adolescents. *Learning Disability Quarterly, 5,* 388–397.

Swiercinsky, D. (1985). *Testing adults: A reference guide for special psychodiagnostic assessments.* Lawrence, KS: Test Corporation of America.

Szymanski, E., & Danek, M. (1985). School to work transition for students with disabilities: Historical, current and conceptual issues. *Rehabilitation Counseling Bulletin, 29*(2), 81–89.

Tollefson, N., Tracy, D., Johnsen, E., Buenning, M., & Farmer, A. (1981). *Implementing goal setting activities with LD adolescents.* (Research Report No. 48). Lawrence: University of Kansas Institute for Research in Learning Disabilities.

Turnbull, A., Turnbull, H., & Strickland, B. (1986). *Families, professionals and exceptionality: A spatial relationship.* Columbus, OH: Charles E. Merrill.

7

Rehabilitation Counseling in Supported Employment

A Conceptual Model for Service Delivery and Personnel Preparation

Edna Mora Szymanski, Jay Buckley, Wendy S. Parent, Randall M. Parker, and John D. Westbrook

In the past decade, questions have arisen about the adequacy of the traditional rehabilitation service system for persons with developmental disabilities (Bernstein & Karan, 1979; Gold, 1975; Pomerantz & Margolin, 1980). Sheltered workshops and day activity programs, while growing in number, have been questioned with respect to their methods and results (Buckley & Bellamy, 1986; Wehman, 1986; Will, 1984b). Whitehead (1979) found that each year only 7% of individuals in activity centers and 12% of those in workshops move into competitive employment. Bellamy, Rhodes, Bourbeau, and Mank (1986) found that approximately 75% of those individuals who move from workshops into competitive employment do so within the first 3 months and only 3% of those remaining in workshops for more than 2 years are placed into competitive jobs.

Supported employment has emerged as an alternative to the traditional system for persons with severe disabilities (Bellamy, Rhodes, & Albin, 1986; Conley, Noble, & Elder, 1986; Rusch, Mithaug, & Flexer, 1986; Wehman,

1981). It has afforded new options in both service delivery and employment (Lagomarcino, 1986; Revell, Wehman, & Arnold, 1984; Twelfth Institute on Rehabilitation Issues, 1985). The evolution of employment as a goal of education for students with severe disabilities has provided added impetus to the development of supported employment opportunities (Stainback, Stainback, Nietupski, & Hamre-Nietupski, 1986; Wehman, Kregel, Barcus, & Schalock, 1986; Will, 1984a).

Supported employment is a relatively new service option. As its terminology and technology have evolved, some confusion of terms and concepts has occurred. For the purposes of this chapter, supported employment is defined as paid employment for persons with severe disabilities who require ongoing (long-term) support to sustain employment, offered in settings that provide integration with persons without disabilities who are not paid caregivers (*Rehabilitation Research and Training Center Newsletter,* 1985; Twelfth Institute on Rehabilitation Issues, 1985).

This chapter explores supported employment service delivery and personnel preparation issues from a rehabilitation counseling frame of reference. A conceptual model for service delivery is presented that illustrates the different phases or steps of supported employment service delivery. Potential rehabilitation counselor activities are described by phase. These activities, along with supported employment outcomes, are used to examine preservice and in-service rehabilitation counselor training. Suggestions are made for incorporating competencies related to supported employment into existing rehabilitation counseling preservice and in-service training programs.

DIFFERENCES BETWEEN SUPPORTED EMPLOYMENT AND TRADITIONAL REHABILITATION SERVICE DELIVERY

Major differences in philosophical orientation and service delivery provide a stark contrast between the traditional and supported employment models. Table 1 compares the two approaches in the employment preparation of persons with developmental disabilities. It has been argued that some variations of the traditional model contain characteristics of the supported employment approach and vice versa. Table 1 is not intended to define absolute differences, but rather to highlight contrasts between the two approaches.

Cornerstones of the supported employment approach are behavioral training techniques and emphasis on training in the actual work environment. According to the supported employment approach, it is critical for persons with severe disabilities to receive training and other interventions under the circumstances and in the environment where performance is ultimately required (Bellamy, Rhodes, & Albin, 1986). Individuals with mental retardation often have difficulty transferring the job skills and work-related behaviors learned in one environment to a new job site. Supported employment pro-

Table 1. Employment preparation for persons with developmental disabilities: Contrasts between traditional and supported employment approaches

Characteristics of model/approach	Traditional (train/place)	Supported employment (place/train)
Assumptions	Behaviors learned in one setting can transfer to another setting	Behaviors best taught in settings and under circumstances where they are eventually expected to be performed; is extremely difficult for many developmentally disabled individuals to generalize behaviors learned in one setting to another setting
Types of interventions	Therapeutic day activities; prevocational training; life skills training	Task analysis; individual job-specific training; training in actual work environment
Level of support, instruction, supervision	Relatively constant; amount determined more by program size and regulation rather than by individual need	Intensive initially, decreasing over time; flexible, amount determined by individual needs; support faded as performance stabilizes
Evaluation/assessment	Traditional, measuring prior learning and traits; occurs before development of vocational goal and initiating of training	Contemporary assessment of applied performance in the context in which the performance is expected; used throughout service delivery to adjust programmatic support according to current abilities
Typical program types	Medicaid-funded day activities and day treatment; prevocational training; sheltered workshop (without community job-site training)	Sheltered workshop with community employment opportunities; supported employment program; transitional employment program (support in actual work setting); on-the-job training; entrepreneurial ventures that provide work opportunities for persons with disabilities (e.g., enclave, mobile crew, benchwork model)
Opportunities for integration with nondisabled individuals	Usually limited	Emphasized; available in varying degrees according to specific program
Nonvocational skills	Frequently considered prerequisite to vocational skills	Emphasized and taught along with vocational skills on the job
Wage opportunities	Nonexistent in Medicaid-funded day treatment programs; limited, usually piece rate, in other programs	Frequently competitive; if not competitive, substantially higher than more traditional programs; outcomes are wage oriented

grams utilize initial client assessment and detailed job analyses to determine the most appropriate job/client match (Wehman & Kregel, 1985). Individualized training by a trained job coach or employment training specialist is provided on the job site from the first day of paid employment. Behavioral training strategies are used to teach the job skills and work-related behaviors, such as social skills, in the community where they actually occur (Snell, 1983). As skills are acquired and job tasks performed to the employer's standards, the trainer's time on the job site is gradually reduced or faded.

In contrast, the traditional rehabilitation approach has emphasized training clients to be "job ready" before placement into competitive employment. Clients are evaluated, trained, and then placed into employment. Individuals who are deemed not ready for competitive employment may be placed in prevocational or sheltered workshop programs for extended employment or continued training.

The particular characteristics of individuals with developmental disabilities have caused some questions regarding the efficacy of the traditional approach. Since individuals with developmental disabilities may lack many of the skills being evaluated and have difficulty transferring skills learned in one environment to another, traditional evaluations and training programs are often not adequate to predict future work performance (Schalock & Karan, 1979; Stokes & Baer, 1977). In addition, in many cases sheltered workshops use subcontracts requiring assembly or other skills not representative of real jobs in the community, and therefore not valid predictors of successful community employment (Moon, Orelove, & Beale, 1985; Revell et al., 1984).

The traditional and supported employment approaches can also differ in regard to the sequencing of services for the client. In the traditional approach, a city resident who could not sign a time sheet, or who lacked the independent travel skills to take a bus, might not be placed in a competitive job if those skills were considered requisite for employment. With the supported employment approach, however, that same person might be placed in a selected job. Job skills and job-related skills, like signing a time sheet and taking a bus, would then be taught by a job coach or employment training specialist at the job site or the bus stop and in the context of the individual's job.

A CONCEPTUAL MODEL FOR SUPPORTED EMPLOYMENT SERVICE DELIVERY

Different types of supported employment options exist, each offering a variety of benefits depending on individual and community needs and resources (O'Neill & Associates, 1985; Mank, Rhodes, & Bellamy, 1986). Common supported employment options include: individual supported competitive employment (job coach/employment support), mobile crews, supported jobs, enclaves, benchwork, and the entreprenurial model. All supported employment options share the following features: 1) employment as the desired outcome, 2) ongoing support (or follow-up), 3) paid jobs as a primary focus rather than services for job preparation, 4) a basic assumption that all persons regardless of severity of disability (including those with multiple or profound disabilities) have the capacity to work if they receive appropriate ongoing support, 5) an emphasis on social integration with nondisabled persons who are not paid caregivers, and 6) variety and flexibility of job and support possibilities (*Rehabilitation Research and Training Center Newsletter,* 1985). Three of the more common supported work options are described below (Mank et al., 1986; O'Neill & Associates, 1985; Smith, 1986).

The *individual supported competitive employment (ISCE)* option is also referred to as job coach/employment support and independent placement. A person with a disability is placed in a regular job within an area business or industry. Training and support are provided by a job trainer or employment training specialist to help the individual learn job skills and work-related behaviors consistent with the employer's standards. When competitive performance on job tasks and behaviors is reached, support is faded at a rate determined by individual needs. Individuals in this option earn minimum wage or higher from the first day of employment. A variation of this model is the supported jobs model in which individuals may earn less than minimum wage and may work shorter shifts. This variation of the ISCE approach involves a higher level of ongoing support and is designed as an option for persons with more severe disabilities.

An *enclave* involves a small group of individuals with disabilities working in a community-based industry with full integration with nondisabled workers. Generally, six to eight workers will be supervised by a trained specialist employed initially by the supported employment program. Back-up supervision is provided by the host industry, which may later put the employment training specialist on its staff. Because workers are paid at the same rate per work quantity as the other workers in the industry, actual wages may be above or below the minimum wage depending on individual production rate and established piece rates (Rhodes & Valenta, 1985).

The *mobile crew* is a versatile arrangement especially suited for communities where other work opportunities may not be readily available. A small group of individuals with disabilities responds to such employment needs of the area as janitorial services and groundskeeping. A nonprofit company provides the training, supervision, and equipment. Wages vary depending on the program. There is an emphasis on integration with nondisabled individuals in the community, either through service provision or break times.

The different supported employment options offer an array of service delivery and employment options for individuals with severe disabilities. While all of the supported employment alternatives have common features, the method of service delivery and levels of support vary among the models.

Flexibility, in types of support services and job opportunities, allows for variations in individual choice, community resources, and job mobility. Periodic assessment and ongoing support provide the opportunity to evaluate individual abilities for movement to less restrictive employment options. Because supported employment is a new concept that can be implemented in a variety of options, it is helpful to place it in the context of a conceptual model.

The conceptual model must have each of the following attributes. First, it must account for all the different supported employment options. Second, it must show the possible relationship of these options to traditional rehabilitation service delivery. Third, it must be sufficiently general to allow for a wide variety of service delivery applications. The conceptual model presented in Figure 1 describes a broad, general, approach that covers existing supported employment options within the context of traditional rehabilitation service delivery.

Supported employment services can be provided by a variety of agencies and individuals, such as rehabilitation facilities, workshops and day activity programs, state vocational rehabilitation agencies, state developmental disability and mental retardation agencies, mental health agencies, schools and education agencies, and private vendors. The flexibility of the model allows application across the various supported employment options as well as the wide range of potential programmatic and organizational configurations.

Process of Service Delivery

Six phases of service delivery are common to all supported employment options. They are: 1) initial assessment, 2) plan development, 3) job placement, 4) training, 5) ongoing support, and 6) periodic assessment. There is an overlap of activities among the phases due to the individual client focus and the inherent flexibility of supported employment. For example, a client receiving ongoing support in phase 5 may be provided with short-term intensive training due to a change in job duties or management at the job site. The relative positions of the phases within the service delivery process are indicated to the left of the vertical axis in Figure 1. Solid lines in the figure represent the normal service progression. Dotted lines represent responses to positive or negative changes in individual performance or in the employment situation. It is crucial to note that supported employment is planned to ensure independence and stability within the least restrictive environment.

The first four phases can be common to both supported employment and time-limited rehabilitation service delivery models. The services in each phase are applicable to a wide range of rehabilitation clients. For example, short-term training and support in phase 4 can be used to assist an individual with mild mental retardation in acquiring the skills necessary to obtain and maintain competitive employment. This same individual might not need the ongoing support services normally associated with supported employment. Or

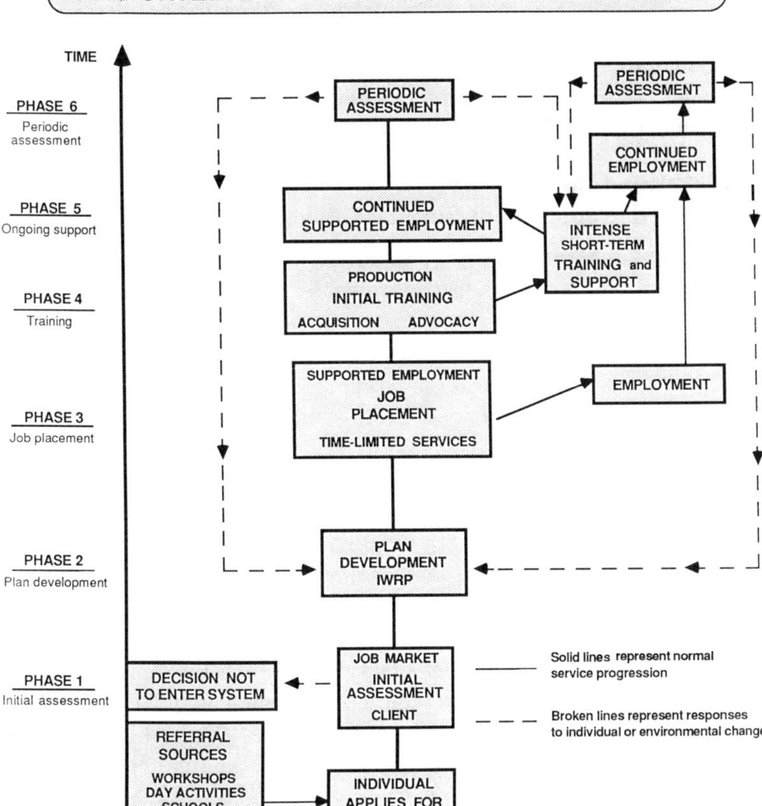

Figure 1. A model for the delivery of supported employment services.

phase 4 training and support could be used to assist another individual, already employed, to maintain a job jeopardized by poor performance on job tasks or inappropriate behavior in the work environment. A variety of possibilities exist for relating supported employment and traditional rehabilitation service delivery to better meet the individual needs of persons with disabilities.

An important difference between traditional or time-limited services and supported employment services is in the area of long-term individualized programmatic support. While many supported employment strategies might be used with individuals with mild disabilities, long-term support is reserved for those individuals with severe disabilities. This difference does not preclude agencies normally involved in time-limited services from delivering supported employment services for persons with severe disabilities. In such situations (e.g., state vocational rehabilitation [VR] agencies), long-term case management responsibility is transferred to another agency (e.g., mental health/mental retardation agencies). Case closure normally occurs during the ongoing support phase (5) with the potential for postemployment services or case reopening as a result of the periodic assessment phase (6).

Rehabilitation Counselor Activities in Supported Employment Service Delivery

Rehabilitation counseling is a profession requiring specific preparation and competence. Professionals trained as rehabilitation counselors can hold a variety of job titles related to supported employment; these titles may include vocational rehabilitation counselor, case manager, job placement specialist, and in some instances, employment training specialist. Since professional rehabilitation counselors holding diverse job titles share a common professional identification, they are referred to as rehabilitation counselors (RCs) throughout this chapter.

In the past, some rehabilitation counselors have performed some of the activities associated with supported employment. Often, however, those activities occurred within the framework of time-limited services and frequently from the more traditional perspective as described in Table 1. Potential rehabilitation counselor activities associated with each phase of supported employment are listed in Table 2. The activity list in Table 2 is not all inclusive. Due to the individually determined nature of supported employment, it would be difficult to anticipate all possible variations of RC activities. Also, activities vary substantially according to work setting, job title, and availability of community resources.

Rehabilitation counselor involvement in supported employment falls into one of two relatively distinct categories. The first, and more common, is the traditional case management, coordination, and counseling role. In this role, the RC works in close cooperation with an employment training specialist (or job coach) whose services have been purchased by the RC. The second, and less common, role of the RC is that of direct service as an employment training specialist. Either role contributes to supported employment service delivery and requires specific knowledge and competence. RCs in traditional roles may arrange for some of the activities listed in Table 2 to be accomplished by another service provider, such as an employment training specialist. The rehabilitation counselor remains, however, responsible for the quality and outcome of the service. As with other rehabilitation services, some of these activities are specific to supported employment while others are common to a wide range of rehabilitation services. The reader is referred to the previous chapter for a comprehensive discussion of the dynamic nature of the roles of rehabilitation counselors and other professionals involved in sup-

Table 2. Rehabilitation counselor activities by phase

I. Initial assessment phase
   A. Client: Identify or evaluate
      1. Past work experience
      2. General work-related interest areas
      3. Work hours available or preferred
      4. Social survival skills
      5. Mobility/transportation skills/availability
      6. Previous service history
      7. Relevant medical or psychological information
      8. Specific occupational skills or deficits
      9. Financial status, potential disincentives
      10. Work attitude/motivation
      11. General level of independence
      12. Parent or guardian level of support for employment
      13. Probable nature and level of ongoing support necessary for continued employment
      14. Potential reinforcers and relative strengths
   B. Job market: Identify, perform, and document
      1. Nature and scope of local work opportunities
      2. Specific jobs and work settings appropriate for supported employment
      3. Specific business/job requirements and flexibility
      4. Job analysis of potential supported employment jobs
      5. Specific job characteristics, such as wages, benefits, hours, level of social integration, potential transportation
      6. Potential for job accommodation
      7. Number of potential supported employment placements feasible or desired by employer
      8. Receptivity of employer to integration with co-workers and public
      9. Employer-specific hiring orientation and training process
      10. Job/employer-specific limitations on support/intervention
II. Plan development phase: Determine, document, and develop
      1. Available options
      2. Specific option to be developed if necessary
      3. Appropriate supported employment option for client
      4. Justification for choice
      5. Match of specific client to specific job
      6. Specific placement plan including schedule, wages, type and nature of support, specific vendors or individuals responsible
      7. Stabilization criteria, potential fading schedule
      8. Work-related, independent living, family, and social support
      9. Involvement and commitment of other agencies and funding sources for training and/or ongoing support

(*continued*)

Table 2. *(continued)*

III. Job placement phase
   1. Re-assess job requirements
   2. Place client on job
   3. Orient client and service providers to job
   4. Orient employer to program
   5. Implement identified accommodations
   6. Implement schedule and plan developed in phase II
   7. Ensure that all job components are task analyzed, taught, and evaluated
   8. Ensure that work-related behaviors are analyzed, taught, and evaluated
   9. Identify additional needs of client, service providers, and employer

IV. Training phase
   1. Ensure implementation of training schedule
   2. Monitor performance data
   3. Observe, advocate, and troubleshoot
   4. Monitor fading schedule and process
   5. Assess satisfaction of client, family, guardians, employers, and other providers
   6. Establish continuing feedback and communication schedule with all involved parties
   7. Reassess level of integration and suggest potential increases
   8. Identify potential problems which could warrant increased intervention

V. Ongoing support phase
   1. Reevaluate level of support needed to maintain employment
   2. Ensure orderly transfer of case management to long-term support agency if appropriate
   3. Evaluate and ensure stabilization
   4. Reassess satisfaction of all parties
   5. Reevaluate wages and integration
   6. Close VR case if appropriate

VI. Periodic assessment phase: Assess, analyze, and document
   1. Job performance
   2. Social integration
   3. Satisfaction of all parties
   4. Level of support
   5. Effectiveness of communication and feedback network
   6. Other appropriate placements
   7. If appropriate, develop plan to correct problems or move to another option

ported employment service delivery. A general description of each phase of service delivery listed in Figure 1 and potential rehabilitation counselor activities follows.

Initial Assessment (Phase 1) This phase involves the rehabilitation counselor in various developmental and analytical activities. There are two types of activities in this phase: 1) client assessment or the assessment of specific client characteristics, and 2) job market assessment or the assessment and development of supported employment opportunities within the community. The RC assembles needed client data and determines eligibility for vocational rehabilitation services. For some individuals with severe disabilities, this determination includes an evaluation of the appropriateness of supported employment. The rehabilitation counselor may perform the duties associated with job development or may refer specific clients to employment training specialists for assistance in placement. Supported employment generally utilizes a contemporary assessment approach that measures performance in the context in which the performance is expected, rather than relying on aptitudes and traits to forecast performance (Pancsofar, 1986). Often it includes an opportunity to observe an individual learning and/or performing one or more jobs in a real work environment.

Plan Development (Phase 2) The rehabilitation counselor bears the responsibility for coordination of the original individualized written rehabilitation plan (IWRP). The development of the plan involves the person with a severe disability, his or her family or guardians, and other individuals or agencies who are or will be involved in service delivery. The plan includes: 1) specific short-term and long-term objectives, 2) documentation of the assessment process and justification for choice of goal and services, 3) services to be rendered with specific designation of providers and schedule, 4) an indication as to how performance will be measured, and 5) criteria for stabilization. Plan development can recur at any time if changes in the individual or employment situation warrant a substantial revision in the original plan.

Job Placement (Phase 3) The rehabilitation counselor, in coordination with other service providers, is responsible for achieving the most appropriate match between client skills/needs and a supported employment job. The placement of an individual in such a job initiates the implementation of systematic training, ongoing support, and integration that should result in job retention. The placement phase tests the effectiveness of the multidisciplinary coordination that went into the IWRP.

Training (Phase 4) The rehabilitation counselor does not directly perform on-the-job training in the traditional model. This training can be performed by a qualified employment training specialist or job coach/trainer. The primary role of the traditional rehabilitation counselor in this phase is to determine the level of progress being made and to assist those working most closely with the individual in planning to further modify the environment or training techniques to improve progress. Some RCs, however, may be employed as employment training specialists and thus be involved in direct training of the client at the work site.

This phase includes: 1) training on the job for initial skill acquisition and development of production rate, 2) training in job-related tasks such as using public transportation and relating with co-workers, and 3) fading of support as the individual begins to master skills. It can also include a return to intense short-term support for remedial reasons or job advancement. The training phase is most commonly reentered as a result of changes in individual performance or employer expectations. This phase concludes the portion of the process traditionally referred to as time-limited services.

Ongoing Support (Phase 5) The goal of all supported employment activities is to enable an individual with a severe disability to maintain employment through the provision of necessary support. The role of the rehabilitation counselor in this phase involves the general monitoring of the "fading" process and determination of the degree to which initial goals have been met. For RCs in traditional roles, this phase may also involve: 1) assessment of satisfaction of all involved parties, 2) arrangement for a transfer of case management activities to a long-term support agency, and 3) case closure.

Periodic Assessment (Phase 6) In addition to ongoing support, a systematic follow-up program with periodic assessment is crucial for the identification of problems and the development of intervention strategies for job retention (Rusch, 1986b). Frequent reasons for retraining are a change in job duties, new supervision, or personal events. In addition, opportunities for movement into less restrictive employment options and increased independence will result from the continued assessment in Phase 6. The results of assessment dictate: 1) continuation of the current employment option, 2) additional short-term training, or 3) development of an amended plan to explore different options. The rehabilitation counselor is among those professionals uniquely qualified to determine the need to investigate other less restrictive forms of employment for the client, or to determine the ability of the supported employment employee to move into more advanced job roles usually associated with increases in pay.

SUPPORTED EMPLOYMENT OUTCOMES

Supported employment is in and of itself an outcome that results from the activities (as listed in this chapter) performed and/or monitored by rehabilitation counselors and other service providers. The success of an individual supported employment placement depends on the quality of these activities. The quality depends, of course, on the competence of the counselor and the other individuals involved in performing the activities.

The activities described in this chapter, indeed the six phases of service delivery, lead to specific supported employment outcomes. Each of the six phases is the beginning of a set of activities that are crucial steps in supported employment implementation. Even when the RC arranges for these activities to be performed by another service provider, she or he bears the ultimate responsibility for their quality. The outcomes listed below operationalize supported employment activities. They serve as criteria that prevent the professionals involved from becoming mired in *process*. These outcomes are as follows:

1. Permanent paid work is obtained for an individual who has a severe disability.
2. The individual receives long-term support of adequate intensity and frequency to continue employment.
3. The individual is integrated into the social network of the workplace.
4. Through coordination of appropriate agencies and professionals, client long-term service needs are assessed and met.

The activities described in this chapter are the tasks and tools of the competent rehabilitation counselor. The resultant outcomes enable the counselor, the client, and his or her parents and advocates, the other professionals involved, and employers to assess each supported employment placement.

An outcome orientation focuses on accomplishment rather than behavior. Competence is also assessed by evaluating outcomes and not the service process. The most important, yet perhaps most difficult, means of assessing professional competence is to focus on the professional's ability to foster the realization of supported employment outcomes, rather than on specific activities. By accepting the responsibility for training professionals, educators assume responsibility for the outcomes achieved as a result of their students' behavior. Thus an outcome orientation forms the basis of competency-based personnel preparation.

EDUCATION AND TRAINING OF REHABILITATION COUNSELORS IN SUPPORTED EMPLOYMENT

Preservice education in universities and in-service training in workshops and conferences represent two major modalities through which rehabilitation students and counselors can receive the information and practice the skills necessary to function in a supported employment program. The activities discussed earlier in this chapter suggest the potential content areas for preservice and in-service training programs. As with the special education approach to this topic (Renzaglia, 1986), both field- and knowledge-based content areas are addressed.

Preservice Training

Many of the suggested content areas are already present in many graduate rehabilitation counselor education program curricula. In order to identify areas not covered in graduate preservice programs, the graduate curriculum must first be considered.

Rehabilitation counselor education (RCE) curriculum has been intensively studied and developed since RCE was first funded by the federal government in 1954. During the 1960s, a number of professional organizations, including the American Rehabilitation Counseling Association (ARCA), collaborated on the development of curriculum standards. The outcome of these efforts was the formation of the Council on Rehabilitation Education (CORE), an incorporated body whose purpose includes evaluating and accrediting master's degree programs in rehabilitation counseling.

CORE (1983) identified 15 content areas necessary for program accreditation. For purposes of this chapter, the 15 content areas have been organized into five broad curriculum areas:

1. Foundation knowledge
   a. History and philosophy of rehabilitation and legislation affecting disabled persons
   b. The organizational structure of the vocational rehabilitation system, including public and private, for-profit and not-for-profit service delivery
   c. Rehabilitation research literature, research methods, and analysis
   d. Trends and issues in, and legal and ethical tenets for the practice of, rehabilitation counseling
   e. Rehabilitation counselor functions with disabled persons in a variety of settings
2. Core processes
   a. Counseling theories, issues and practices (individual and group), and theoretical basis of behavior and personality
   b. Case management process, including case finding, service coordination, referral to and utilization of other disciplines, and client advocacy
   c. Theories, methods and practices of career development, vocational assessment and evaluation, and work adjustment
   d. Medical aspects and functional limitations of disabilities
   e. Psychological aspects of disabilities; personal, social, and cultural impact on aspects of disabilities
3. Planning and delivering services
   a. Planning client vocational rehabilitation services
   b. Knowledge of community resources and services
4. Job engineering

   Understanding of requirements and characteristics of a variety of occupations, job analysis, job modification and restructuring
5. Job development, placement, and follow-along
   a. Utilizing occupational information and labor market trends
   b. Vocational placement, follow-up and/or follow-along services

Furthermore, these five broad curriculum areas can be assigned to each of the six phases in the supported employment service delivery model (Figure 1). Table 3 shows the most prevalent associations. In some supported employment settings it would be possible to establish the need for all five curriculum areas in all six phases of supported employment.

In addition to the curriculum areas typically covered by preservice RCE programs, students are required to take practica and a 600-hour internship. These courses offer an excellent opportunity for students to learn and practice the skills and competencies necessary to work in a supported employment setting.

The preceding material clearly demonstrates that CORE-accredited programs are required to have coursework covering all of the major areas necessary for graduates to function in supported employment programs. Nonetheless, there are several knowledge and competency areas that appear to require additional emphasis in many graduate RCE programs. For example, task analysis, job analysis, behavioral assessment, and behavioral training and self-management techniques are not given full attention in coursework, practica, and internships in many training programs. As is noted above, these competencies are required in most phases of supported employment. Because these areas are of utmost importance for rehabilitation counselors working in supported employment, new courses and/or new units in existing courses must be developed to prepare students for this role.

Modification of preservice programs obviously will not have an impact upon the skills of those individuals who have already graduated from RCE programs. For these persons, particularly those who will shortly be assigned to supported employment activities, in-service education is the solution to the problems they will most likely encounter.

Table 3. Curriculum areas required in each supported employment phase

	Curriculum content areas				
Service delivery phases	Foundation knowledge	Core processes	Planning and delivering services	Job engineering	Job development, placement, follow-along
Initial assessment	X	X		X	X
Plan development	X	X	X		
Job placement	X	X		X	X
Training	X	X	X	X	
Ongoing support	X	X		X	X
Periodic assessment	X	X			X

In-Service Training

In-service training will be necessary if persons with disabilities currently receiving rehabilitation services are to have access to this service option. Excellent materials or workshops for in-service training are available from such leading institutions as the Rehabilitation Research and Training Center at Virginia Commonwealth University; the Specialized Training Program at the University of Oregon, Eugene; the Secondary Transition Intervention Effectiveness Institute at the University of Illinois, Champaign; and the Rehabilitation Administration and Supported Employment Training Program at the University of San Fransisco.

Most supported employment in-service programs and materials to date have addressed audiences lacking employment orientation or familiarity. Rehabilitation counselors, however, will benefit from in-service programs that recognize their skills in job development and related areas and concentrate on less familiar topics like task analysis and behavioral training approaches. The activities listed in Table 2 of this chapter suggest additional in-service training topics.

The discussion of preservice preparation and in-service training indicates that the professional rehabilitation counselor has substantial preparation for the supported employment activities mentioned in this chapter. As with other professionals involved in supported employment, it is clear that additional preparation and role alterations will be necessary. To meet the new challenges, rehabilitation counselors will need to adopt more of an advocacy stance, and more of a focus on client needs rather than on the legislatively outmoded concept of feasibility of services. Additionally, some skill areas will need to be refined or adjusted. In-service training and modifications in RCE curricula will assist the profession in using supported employment to provide better services to persons with severe disabilities.

Continued upgrading of skills is a responsibility of all professionals. In addition to the two chapters on the topic in this book (Chapters 5 and 7), as well as in-service training, four general references are recommended to assist rehabilitation counselors in expanding their skills in supported employment. *The Supported Work Model of Competitive Employment for Citizens with Severe Handicaps: A Guide for Job Trainers* (Moon, Goodall, Barcus, & Brooke, 1986) offers a very practical guide to activities in all phases of service delivery. Specific training techniques are discussed and sample forms illustrate an organized approach to data collection at each phase. *Pathways to Employment for Adults with Developmental Disabilities* (Kiernan & Stark, 1986) offers a broad statement of supported employment service delivery, the current service system, and related issues. Included are chapters that offer valuable background information on legislative and economic characteristics. *Competitive Employment Issues and Strategies* (Rusch, 1986a) also offers a broad treatment of supported employment. It has chapters that focus on specific activities or phases such as assessment and service delivery coordination. Issues and methods for school-to-work transition are also discussed. *Supported Employment: A Community Implementation Guide* (Bellamy, Rhodes, Mank, & Albin, 1988) discusses the nature and purpose of supported employment and provides a practical guide for implementation. Relevant information is provided for professionals, agencies, parents, and others involved in preparation for supported employment.

COMMON QUESTIONS AND MISCONCEPTIONS

The recent development of supported employment and its difference from more traditional methods of service delivery has resulted in some confusion for rehabilitation counselors. This section addresses common misconceptions and areas of confusion through a question-and-answer format.

Are vocational transition, transitional employment, and supported employment interchangeable terms? Vocational transition, transitional employment, and supported employment are *not* interchangeable terms. While the goal of all three is to facilitate employment opportunities for individuals with disabilities, the type of service and method of delivery vary.

Vocational transition refers to services surrounding the transition from school to work. The employment outcomes of an individualized, systematically planned transition from school to work include employment with no special services, time-limited services, or ongoing services such as supported employment (Will, 1984a). For additional information on transition, consult the following resources: Brolin (1982); Brown et al. (1981); McCarthy, Everson, Moon, and Barcus, (1985); Szymanski and Danek (1985); and Wilcox and Bellamy (1982).

Transitional employment services, in one connotation, are time-limited services such as vocational evaluation, work adjustment, job placement, and training for individuals with a disability (Whitehead & Marrone, 1986). The work is part or full time, pays wages, offers opportunities for integration, and provides initial support. The phases of service delivery are initial assessment, plan development, job placement, and training. Services are terminated after phase 4 (see Figure 1) when the client becomes independent. Ongoing support and continuous assessment are not provided. Another connotation of transitional employment services refers to supported employment services specifically designed for persons with chronic mental illness (Rehabilitation Act Amendments, 1986).

Supported employment services are ongoing intensive services required for individuals with severe disabilities to gain and maintain paid employment in regular work settings. The features of supported employment include real work with all the benefits offered by work, ongoing support, emphasis on jobs instead of services for job preparation, full participation regardless of severity of disability, social integration, and flexibility in types of jobs and support (*Rehabilitation Research and Training Center Newsletter,* 1985). The phases of service delivery are initial assessment, plan development, job placement, training, ongoing support, and periodic assessment.

What is a job coach or employment training specialist? A job coach is a trained professional who provides supported employment services that can be purchased by a rehabilitation counselor. Recent literature has defined a job coach (also known as a job trainer) (Wehman & Melia, 1985) or employment training specialist (Cohen, Patton, & Melia, 1986) as a community-based person who provides individualized job placement, job-site training, and ongoing assessment and support for persons with severe disabilities. Operating out of nonprofit placement programs, special education programs, workshops, day activity centers, rehabilitation agencies, or on an individual vendor basis, the job coach or employment training specialist offers a service for rehabilitation counselors to purchase so that individuals with severe disabilities can be placed in employment. A job coach can provide the linkage between the client, employer, rehabilitation counselor, case manager, family or caregiver, school personnel, and rehabilitation agency staff. Competencies include a knowledge of client assessment, job analysis, job placement, behavioral training strategies, fading techniques, counseling, advocacy, interpersonal skills, employer needs, business procedures, parent/caregiver concerns, public and private agency regulations, staff roles, and evaluation techniques (Bellamy, O'Conner, & Karan, 1979; Kiernan & Stark, 1986; Moon et al., 1985; Rusch, 1986a; Wehman, 1981). Individual rehabilitation counselors may be employed as employment training specialists or job coaches in a variety of settings.

Are successful outcomes of supported employment programs determined by a client's ability to work independently without ongoing support? The definition of supported employment implies that most clients needing the service will *continue* to need some support in order to remain employed. Continued employment, wages, and levels of social integration, rather than complete independence, are the criteria for determining successful supported employment. The outcomes of employment for severely disabled individuals are the same as those for nondisabled individuals. These outcomes include wages and benefits, integration with nonhandicapped persons, normalization, job mobility, and improved perceptions by others (O'Neill & Associates, 1985; Wehman, 1981).

Is supported employment an acceptable goal on an individualized written rehabilitation plan and is it an allowed closure for rehabilitation counselors in state vocational rehabilitation agencies? Supported employment *is* an acceptable goal on an IWRP, and is an allowed 26 closure ("closed rehabilitated") for rehabilitation counselors working in state VR agencies (Rehabilitation Act Amendments, 1986). Supported employment services can be purchased by the rehabilitation counselor by redirecting the funds previously used for training at sheltered workshops or day activity centers. Purchase-of-service arrangements can be redirected to supported employment programs or individual job coaches as vendors who provide supported work services (Moon et al., 1985; Revell et al., 1984; Twelfth Institute on Rehabilitation Issues, 1985). These vocational rehabilitation dollars would be used to fund the *time-limited training services* in phase 4 (see Figure 1) (Hill et al., 1985). When the employee is completing the job to the company's standards and has reached the rehabilitation counselor's criteria for job stabilization, then vocational rehabilitation would receive case closure in status 26.

Although the state VR agency case may be closed, the supported employment client continues to receive services. Responsibility for case management and ongoing support is transferred from one agency to another. Interagency cooperation is essential to maintain the commitment for ongoing services that individuals with severe disabilities require for job retention. Funding for the ongoing support in phase 5 (see Figure 1) and periodic assessment in phase 6 (see Figure 1) would become the responsibility of state, local, public, or private agencies (Hill et al., 1987). Developmental disabilities or community mental health funding has been used in some areas. When appropriate, the state agency rehabilitation counselor can provide funds for more intense retraining by the job coach, using status 32 for the delivery of postemployment services. After job stabilization is resumed, the trainer responsible for ongoing support and periodic assessment would continue to monitor the worker's performance with funds from agencies financially responsible for ongoing support (e.g., mental retardation, developmental disabilities, or mental health agencies).

SUMMARY

Supported employment involves an adaptation of the traditional rehabilitation service delivery system to meet the needs of persons with severe disabilities. It is implemented in different options and agency configurations with the collaboration of various professions and funding sources. All supported employment service delivery includes six phases: 1) initial assessment, 2) plan development, 3) job placement, 4) training, 5) ongoing support, and 6) periodic assessment. Rehabilitation counselors can perform critical activities at each of these phases. The specific nature and extent of these activities varies according to the RC's employment setting.

Rehabilitation counseling preservice preparation offers a good foundation for the development of supported employment competencies. Modifications of preservice programs can help future graduates to use supported employment to increase employment possibilities for persons with severe disabilities. In-service training that builds on existing rehabilitation counselor knowledge and supported employment activities can meet the needs of current practitioners.

Leaders in the profession must continually seek new and improved service and employment possibilities for persons with disabilities. Supported employment is one such possibility. The profession of rehabilitation counseling, through its practice in a variety of agencies and service delivery systems, can play a major role in research and development in supported employment.

REFERENCES

Bellamy, G. T., O'Conner, G., & Karan, O. (1979). *Vocational rehabilitation of severely handicapped persons*. Baltimore: University Park Press.

Bellamy, G. T., Rhodes, L. E., & Albin, J. M. (1986). Supported employment. In W. E. Kiernan & J. A. Stark (Eds.), *Pathways to employment for adults with developmental disabilities* (pp. 129–138). Baltimore: Paul H. Brookes Publishing Co.

Bellamy, G. T., Rhodes, L. E., Bourbeau, P. E., & Mank, D. M. (1986). Mental retardation services in sheltered workshops and day activity programs: Consumer benefits and policy alternatives. In F. R. Rusch (Ed.), *Competitive employment issues and strategies* (pp. 257–271). Baltimore: Paul H. Brookes Publishing Co.

Bellamy, G. T., Rhodes, L. E., Mank, D. M., & Albin, J. M. (1988). *Supported employment: A community implementation guide*. Baltimore: Paul H. Brookes Publishing Co.

Bernstein, G., & Karan, O. (1979). Obstacles to vocational normalization for the developmentally disabled. *Rehabilitation Literature, 40*(3), 66–71.

Boles, S. M., Bellamy, G. T., Horner, R. H., & Mank, D. M. (1984). Specialized Training Program: The structured employment model. In S. Paine, G. T. Bellamy, & B. Wilcox (Eds.), *Human services that work: From innovation to standard practice* (pp. 185–205). Baltimore: Paul H. Brookes Publishing Co.

Brolin, D. E. (1982). *Vocational preparation of persons with handicaps*. Columbus, OH: Charles E. Merrill.

Brown, L., Pumpian, I., Baumgart, D., Van Deventer, P., Ford, A., Nisbit, J., Schroeder, J., & Gruenwald, L. (1981). Longitudinal transition plans in programs for severely handicapped students. *Exceptional Children, 47,* 624–630.

Buckley, J., & Bellamy, G. T. (1986). National survey of day vocational programs for adults with severe disabilities: A 1984 profile. In P. Ferguson (Ed.), *Issues in transition research: Economic and social outcomes* (pp. 1–11). Eugene, OR: Specialized Training Program.

Cohen, D., Patton S., & Melia R. (1986). Staffing supported and transitional employment programs: Issues and recommendations. *American Rehabilitation, 12*(2), 20–24.

Conley, R. W., Noble, J. H., & Elder, J. K. (1986). Problems with the service system. In W. E. Kiernan & J. A. Stark (Eds.), *Pathways to employment for adults with developmental disabilities* (pp. 67–83). Baltimore: Paul H. Brookes Publishing Co.

Council on Rehabilitation Education. (1983). *Accreditation manual for rehabilitation counselor education programs*. Chicago: Author.

Gold, M. (1975). Vocational training. In J. Wortis (Ed.), *Mental retardation and developmental disabilities: An annual review* (Vol. 7, pp. 254–264). New York: Brunner/Mazel.

Hill, M., Hill, J., Wehman, P., Revell, G., Dickerson, A., & Noble, J. (1987). Supported employment: An interagency funding model for persons with severe disabilities. *Journal of Rehabilitation, 53*(3), 13–21.

Hill, M., Revell, G., Chernish, W., Morell, J. E., White, J., & McCarthy, P. (1985). Social service agency options for modifying existing systems to include transitional and supported work services for persons with severe disabilities. In P. McCarthy, J. Everson, S. Moon, & M. Barcus (Eds.), *School to work transition for youth with severe disabilities* (pp. 195–218). Richmond: Virginia Commonwealth University, Project Transition into Employment.

Kiernan, W., & Stark, J. (Eds.). (1986). *Pathways to employment for adults with developmental disabilities*. Baltimore: Paul H. Brookes Publishing Co.

Lagomarcino, T. R. (1986). Community services: Using the supported work model within an adult service agency. In F. R. Rusch (Ed.), *Competitive employment issues and strategies* (pp. 51–63). Baltimore: Paul H. Brookes Publishing Co.

Mank, D. M., Rhodes, L. E., & Bellamy, G. T. (1986). Four supported employment alternatives. In W. E. Kiernan & J. A. Stark (Eds.), *Pathways to employment for adults with developmental disabilities* (pp. 139–153). Baltimore: Paul H. Brookes Publishing Co.

McCarthy, P., Everson, J., Moon, S., & Barcus, M. (Eds.). (1985). *School to work transition for youth with severe disabilities*. Richmond: Virginia Commonwealth University, Project Transition into Employment.

Moon, M. S., Goodall, P., Barcus, M., & Brooke, V. (Eds.). (1986). *The supported work model for competitive employment for citizens with severe handicaps: A guide for job trainers* (rev. ed.). Richmond: Virginia Commonwealth University, Rehabilitation Research and Training Center.

Moon, M. S., Orelove, F. P., & Beale, A. (1985). Self-test on competitive employment for mentally retarded persons. *Journal of Employment Counseling, 22*, 144–150.

O'Neill & Associates. (1985). *National leadership institute on supported employment*. Olympia, WA: Author.

Pancsofar, E. L. (1986). Assessing work behavior. In F. R. Rusch (Ed.), *Competitive employment issues and strategies* (pp. 93–102). Baltimore: Paul H. Brookes Publishing Co.

Pomerantz, D., & Margolin, D. (1980). Vocational rehabilitation, a time for change. In R. Flynn & K. Nitsch (Eds.), *Normalization, social integration, and community services* (pp. 215–258). Baltimore: University Park Press.

Rehabilitation Act Amendments of 1986, § 29 U.S.C. § 701 (1986).

Rehabilitation Research and Training Center Newsletter. (1985). *2*(2). Richmond: Virginia Commonwealth University, Rehabilitation Research and Training Center.

Rehabilitation Research and Training Center Newsletter. (1986). *3*(1). Richmond: Virginia Commonwealth University, Rehabilitation Research and Training Center.

Renzaglia, A. (1986). Preparing personnel to support and guide emerging contemporary service alternatives. In F. R. Rusch (Ed.), *Competitive employment issues and strategies* (pp. 303–316). Baltimore: Paul H. Brookes Publishing Co.

Revell, W. G., Wehman, P., & Arnold, S. (1984). Supported work model of competitive employment for persons with mental retardation: Implications for rehabilitative services. *Journal of Rehabilitation, 50*(4), 33–38.

Rhodes, L., & Valenta, L. (1985). Industry-based supported employment: An enclave approach. *Journal of the Association for the Severely Handicapped, 10*, 10–20.

Rusch, F. R. (Ed.). (1986a). *Competitive employment issues and strategies.* Baltimore: Paul H. Brookes Publishing Co.

Rusch, F. R. (1986b). Developing a long-term follow-up program. In F. R. Rusch (Ed.), *Competitive employment issues and strategies* (pp. 225–232). Baltimore: Paul H. Brookes Publishing Co.

Rusch, F. R., Mithaug, D. E., & Flexer, R. W. (1986). Obstacles to competitive employment and traditional program options for overcoming them. In F. R. Rusch (Ed.), *Competitive employment issues and strategies* (pp. 7–21). Baltimore: Paul H. Brookes Publishing Co.

Schalock, R., & Karan, O. (1979). Relevant assessment: The interaction between evaluation and training. In G. T. Bellamy, G. O'Conner, & O. Karan (Eds.), *Vocational rehabilitation of severely handicapped persons* (pp. 33–54). Baltimore: Paul H. Brookes Publishing Co.

Smith, M. (1986). *Supported employment for certain severely disabled persons.* Washington, DC: The Library of Congress, Congressional Research Service.

Snell, M. E. (Ed.). (1983). *Systematic instruction of the moderately and severely handicapped* (2nd ed). Columbus, OH: Charles E. Merrill.

Stainback, W., Stainback, S., Nietupski, J., & Hamre-Nietupski, S. (1986). Establishing effective community-based training stations. In F. R. Rusch (Ed.), *Competitive employment issues and strategies* (pp. 103–113). Baltimore: Paul H. Brookes Publishing Co.

Stokes, T., & Baer, D. (1977). An implicit technology of generalization. *Journal of Applied Behavior Analysis, 10,* 349–367.

Szymanski, E. M., & Danek, M. (1985). School to work transition for students with disabilities: Historical, current and conceptual issues. *Rehabilitation Counseling Bulletin, 29*(2), 81–89.

Twelfth Institute on Rehabilitation Issues. (1985). *Supported employment in rehabilitation.* Hot Springs: University of Arkansas, Arkansas Rehabilitation Research and Training Center.

Wehman, P. (1981). *Competitive employment: New horizons for severely disabled individuals.* Baltimore: Paul H. Brookes Publishing Co.

Wehman, P. (1986). Competitive employment in Virginia. In F. R. Rusch (Ed.), *Competitive employment issues and strategies* (pp. 23–33). Baltimore: Paul H. Brookes Publishing Co.

Wehman, P., & Kregel, J. (1985). A supported work approach to competitive employment of individuals with moderate and severe handicaps. *The Journal of the Association for Persons with Severe Handicaps, 10*(1), 3–11.

Wehman, P. H., Kregel, J., Barcus, J. M., & Schalock, R. L. (1986). Vocational transition for students with developmental disabilities. In W. E. Kiernan & J. A. Stark (Eds.), *Pathways to employment for adults with developmental disabilities* (pp. 113–127). Baltimore: Paul H. Brookes Publishing Co.

Wehman, P., & Melia, R. (1985). The job coach: Function in transitional and supported employment. *American Rehabilitation, 11*(2), 4–7.

Whitehead, C. (1979). Sheltered workshops in the decade ahead: Work and wages or welfare. In G. T. Bellamy, G. O'Conner, & O. Karan (Eds.), *Vocational rehabilitation of severely handicapped persons.* Baltimore: University Park Press.

Whitehead, C. W., & Marrone, J. (1986). Time-limited evaluation and training. In W. E. Kiernan & J. A. Stark (Eds.), *Pathways to employment for adults with developmental disabilities* (pp. 163–176). Baltimore: Paul H. Brookes Publishing Co.

Wilcox, B., & Bellamy, G. (1982). *Design of high school programs for severely handicapped students.* Baltimore: Paul H. Brookes Publishing Co.

Will, M. (1984a). *OSERS programming for the transition of youth with severe disabilities: Bridges from school to working life*. Washington, DC: U.S. Department of Education, Office of Special Education and Rehabilitation Services.

Will, M. (1984b). *Supported employment for adults with severe disabilities: An OSERS program initiative*. Washington, DC: U.S. Department of Education, Office of Special Education and Rehabilitation Services.

8

Rehabilitation Counseling and Client Transition from School to Work

Tennyson J. Wright, William G. Emener, and Joseph M. Ashley

RECENTLY, REHABILITATIONISTS, EDUCATORS, legislators and policy developers have confronted the dilemma of, "What will happen to [disabled youth] after they leave school?" (National Institute of Handicapped Research [NIHR], 1985, p. 1). Since 1970, more than 2.5 million youth with disabilities have left our nation's public school system; only 23% are either fully employed or enrolled in college; 40% are underemployed and earning wages at or near the poverty level; 26% are unemployed and on welfare; 8% are in their home community and idle much of the time; 3% are totally dependent and institutionalized (Project PERT Operations Manual, 1985). Additional empirical findings illustrate the post-school problem for developmentally disabled individuals: 1) only 5% of 1,450 developmentally disabled individuals in a Maryland study had jobs in business and industry (Crites, Smull, & Sachs, 1984); 2) of recent graduates of special education programs in the state of Colorado, 69% were reportedly employed; however, when the part-time job data were excluded from the analyses, the employment rate dropped to 32%, and the special education graduates' wages were much lower than those of nonhandicapped persons (Mithaug, Horiuchi, & Fanning, 1985); and 3) of 300 parents of mentally retarded young adults, 58% indicated that their child was unemployed; of those "children" who were employed, almost 75% earned less than $500 per month, most had never used professional job placement services, and their jobs had been obtained through family members and friends (Wehman, Kregel, & Seyforth, 1985).

Emener and Griswold (1986) have observed that the educational gains of disabled youth were not being utilized after graduation because rehabilitation agencies were poorly prepared to serve severely disabled students without pre-employment requisites. Unable to find remunerative employment, many developmentally disabled individuals turn to their local communities for vocational training and job placement assistance, but find their choices severely limited or nonexistent. Generally they find only three options: 1) regular workshop programs, 2) work activity centers, and 3) adult day programs. Research indicates that the majority of these options promote dependence, provide low wages, prompt slow or no movement into less restrictive employment options, and foster segregation from nondisabled peers and community resources (Bellamy, Rhodes, & Albin, 1986; *Project TIE,* undated).

It is important to note that the term *transition,* as used in special education, vocational education, and vocational rehabilitation today has come to denote the specific transition from school to work (Daniels, 1987; Will, 1984a, 1985). However, the usage of the term is not new, and since the turn of the century has been used to denote the concern with moving people from dependent to independent states (Cartwright, Cartwright, & Ward, 1984; Daniels, 1987; Rubin & Roessler, 1983). Schools were initially established as the mechanism for assisting persons to develop the literacy and socialization skills necessary for independence in society. Similarly, rehabilitation philosophy and practice are based on the notion of assisting each person to achieve independence in society.

Madeleine Will (1984a, 1985), Secretary of the Office of Special Education and Rehabilitation Services (OSERS), has championed the school-to-work transition initiative. Citing the large number of readiness programs and the paucity of productive collaborative planning and service delivery programs among special education, vocational education, and vocational rehabilitation programs, Will has advocated for change in the service delivery system (Emener & Griswold, 1986). In order to achieve change, Will (1985) has stated:

> The concept of transition should embody five separate features: [a] all individuals must be served; [b] employment is, in fact, the outcome of successful transition for disabled individuals, as well as their non-disabled peers; [c] the chronological time frame during which transition is provided is long, encompassing the high school years. Adolescence and young adulthood are also part of the transition process; [d] transition requires coordination among multiple and relatively complex services; and [e] the quality and appropriateness of each service provided under the transition umbrella is addressed. (p. 1)

Rehabilitation and education agencies have had a limited history of cooperation in transition programs since the 1940s, with a significant emphasis on work-study programs in the 1960s (Szymanski, 1984). Landmark legislation of the 1970s and subsequent amendments, along with the 1979 creation of the Office of Special Education and Rehabilitation Services, began a new and expanded era of transition services for youth with disabilities. The 1973 Rehabilitation Act, including Section 504; the Education for All Handicapped Children Act; and the Vocational Education Amendments form the current legislative base for most transition services (Fenton & Keller, 1985; Kallsen & Kidder, 1985; Szymanski & Danek, 1985).

With financial resources dwindling since 1980, special education, vocational education, and rehabilitation agencies have increased their attention to coordination of service delivery systems and use of dual program benefits (Szymanski, 1984). Szymanski pointed out that the coordination of services provided by a rehabilitation counselor can decrease costs while increasing positive outcomes. Service coordination is only one of many key roles that rehabilitation counselors can fill within transition from school to work programs. Thus, it is evident that professionals and legislators have recognized the need to provide appropriate services to a population of disabled individuals who need immediate and long-term comprehensive vocational services.

In light of this need, the purposes of this chapter are to: 1) discuss key experiences in the transition from school to work; 2) address the practice of rehabilitation counseling, focusing on the roles of the rehabilitation counselor in the transition from school to work; 3) discuss relevant professional preparation and continuing development issues in the field of rehabilitation counseling; and 4) conclude with the identification of several issues within the area of school-to-work transition that should be addressed in the future.

THE SCHOOL-TO-WORK EXPERIENCE

The passage of the Education for All Handicapped Children Act of 1975 (PL 94-142) marked the beginning of an era of concern with the transition from high school to adult life for a generation of special education students. Since that time, an almost overwhelming demand for services from vocational rehabilitation and other adult service providers has been created by the more than half a generation of special education students finishing school (Wehman, Wood-Pietruski, Everson, & Parent, 1985). The following two case examples from current literature illustrate the need for services.

> *Case 1:* Bill is 19 years old and has 14 years of education under his belt. Unfortunately, all he has to show for those years in school is a second-grade reading level; the ability to add, subtract, and sometimes multiply; and a quick temper. The most functional skill he has acquired is the ability to "hide" his learning disabilities. He accomplishes this mostly by staying away from other people. When he must interact with people he seems quite articulate, but be-

> comes annoyed if anyone imposes upon him to read, write, or calculate. His "cover-up" strategies have served him well; but now that he's out of school he must face the fact that his job opportunities are limited and that his learning disabilities will increasingly become obstacles to enjoying a productive and socially fulfilling life. (Drake & Witten, 1985, p. 34)
>
> *Case 2.* Michael is a 22 year old student in his last year of school who has attended special education school since he was 6 years old. Psychologists have assessed him as having moderate to severe mental retardation (IQ 26–51), according to standardized intelligence tests. Medical records report no significant sensory, perceptual, or motor problems, but a history of epilepsy, successfully controlled by medication for 3 years. School records indicate that his speech is clear, and he interacts minimally with others using short, incomplete sentences. He has acquired simple counting skills, basic word recognition skills, some coin discrimination, and can tell time to the hour. He has a history of aggressive behavior. His family is supportive and encourages him to interact with nonhandicapped peers and to use the public bus system. (Wehman, Wood-Pietruski, et al., 1985, p. 14)

Today, thousands of individuals like Bill and Michael with severe developmental disabilities are seeking adult services. These individuals and their parents want services that will lead to meaningful employment with decent wages. Too many young persons with disabilities leave public schools unemployed and remain unemployed (White & Smith, 1985). In 1983, the U.S. Commission on Civil Rights estimated the unemployment rate for these students to be as high as 50%–80% (Harold Russell Associates [HRA], 1984). Despite the cooperative agreements between schools and vocational rehabilitation agencies that provide work study, work adjustment and work sample evaluation programs in the public schools, there appears to be a continued lack of significant and measurable increases in the number and rate of disabled youth who enter meaningful and productive employment.

In a review of literature, White and Smith (1985) concluded:

> (a) . . . despite efforts to provide education in the least restrictive environment, less than 25% of disabled youth participate in vocational education; (b) . . . of those who do participate, an unacceptably small percentage find employment in their area of training; (c) . . . despite large investments of money and manpower, the employment picture for disabled youth and adults continues to be much worse than that of corresponding minority and special needs populations. (pp. 10–11)

An analysis of the long-term placements of work study students by White and Smith (1985) in the Great Falls School District in Montana indicated that:

1. Many learning disabled students found employment in occupations that reflected neither student interests nor abilities. Most positions were limited in type as well as in opportunities for training and advancement.
2. Students with employability deficits found the gap between the classroom and work experience too difficult to bridge. These students experienced frequent terminations and/or repeated sheltered employment, inhibiting the movement toward unsubsidized permanent employment. They "fell be-

> tween the cracks'' and subsequently graduated without any realistic prospects for employment. (p. 11)

White and Smith attributed these results to: 1) the low number of permanent private sector placements, 2) the high number of students involuntarily terminated annually, and 3) the low number of hard-to-place students placed in permanent private-sector employment annually. Despite the efforts of dedicated professionals in vocational rehabilitation, special education, vocational education, and community agencies, a number of factors may negatively affect the transition from school to work. Daniels (1987) has identified several:

> 1. The presence of a congenital disability may create a delay in all areas of development.
> 2. In some cases parents of youths with disabilities may be overly protective and, consequently, may not foster independence in their child.
> 3. Often persons with disabilities are restricted in the range of their experiences, which tends to restrict the development of independence.
> 4. Many people with disabilities require specialized ways of solving everyday life problems that necessitate specific training or equipment.
> 5. Negative attitudes toward persons with disabilities serve to limit their access to training programs, jobs, and interpersonal relationships.
> 6. Services for youth with disabilities tend to be fragmented and narrow in focus.
> 7. Certain disabilities are of a progressive or intermittent nature and require continual readjustment of plan and level of support. (pp. 285–286)

Coordination and cooperation among disciplines can expand knowledge, expertise, and resources. Vocational educators, special educators, and vocational rehabilitation staff have special experiences and skills specific to their discipline that, when shared cooperatively, can significantly facilitate education and rehabilitation programming. For example: 1) vocational educators can enhance the transition process by involving the rehabilitation counselor in formal and informal meetings of employer advisory groups and vocational training staff; 2) special educators can assist vocational educators by translating required goals and objectives into competency steps, and by adopting class activities so that students with disabilities can fully participate; and 3) vocational rehabilitation staff can identify the needs of the local labor market and assist in structuring sound career exploration and early work experience programs (Eleventh Institute on Rehabilitation Issues [EIRI], 1984). The major outcome desired of all disciplines involved in the transition process of disabled youth is employment—competitive or supported (consult Chapters 5 and 7 in this text on the role of rehabilitation counseling and supported employment). Vocational Occupational Rehabilitation in Special Education in Utica, New York has been very successful with transition from school to work programs due to the outstanding individual attention provided youth by vocational rehabilitation counselors who integrate special education, vocational education, and vocational rehabilitation services for special education students (Kallsen & Kidder, 1985).

The key to success is a coordinated team effort and an outcome-oriented focus on employment that utilizes the resources and services of each discipline. Key steps for students with disabilities as they move toward entering the labor market are:

> 1. Early educational preparation which provides students with the basic core skills required for them to develop their vocational potential.
> 2. Career exploration and awareness activities during pre and early adolescence which effectively frame a positive and realistic concept of the world of work for the student.
> 3. A series of formal and informal instructional plans such as the Individual Education Program (IEP) and the Individual Written Rehabilitation Program (IWRP). These plans are outcome oriented, built on evaluation of need and potential, and which consistently complement each other in planning for desired outcomes.
> 4. Work adjustment, vocational training, and work experiences which are integrated with nondisabled peers and which where possible, utilize community based work settings.
> 5. A systematic approach to building an understanding of the support required, whether it be minimal or extensive over time for the student with a disability to enter and remain in the labor market and to function at their [*sic*] potential level of independence in the community. (EIRI, 1984, p. 35)

THE ROLE OF THE REHABILITATION COUNSELOR IN TRANSITION FROM SCHOOL TO WORK

The transition of special education students from secondary school settings through post-secondary training options and employment has recently become a priority initiative throughout the education and rehabilitation community (Will, 1984a). The primary purpose of the school-to-work transition is to deliver the best possible services to develop a student's ability to become gainfully employed. The foundation of the transition process is a determination of each individual student's needs and of the best means of providing the necessary services, and the coordination and systematic planning of services deemed necessary for successful job placement (Project PERT Operations Manual, 1985; Szymanski & Danek, 1985; Wehman, Kregel, & Barcus, 1985).

A multidisciplinary team effort can ensure that all the necessary services are available to the disabled student. Members of the multidisciplinary team typically include a special educator, a vocational educator, a rehabilitation counselor, and selected other professionals from adult services, occupational therapy, and speech therapy, when needed (American Rehabilitation Counseling Association [ARCA], 1984; EIRI, 1984; HRA, 1984; Szymanski, 1984;

Wehman, Kregel, & Barcus, 1985). Through the multidisciplinary team approach, the special educator provides the leadership in the beginning stages of the transition process. Over time, the responsibility would shift to the vocational educator and then to the rehabilitation counselor. Although this model is not advocated by all professional disciplines, it has been accepted throughout the field of rehabilitation (ARCA, 1984; EIRI, 1984; Project PERT Operations Manual, 1985; Szymanski, 1984; Wehman, Kregel, & Barcus, 1985).

Daniels (1987) has noted that a priority of OSERS in its 1984 personnel preparation grant program was to increase cross-training between special education and vocational rehabilitation. Ten projects were funded to address the need for a sharing of skills among multidisciplinary teams at the preservice and inservice training levels; projects were intended to develop models that could be used to provide master's and doctoral level leadership personnel. The transitional leadership training program identified the following eight competencies that can facilitate successful transition from school to work:

1. Ability to plan effective independent living plans with youth with disabilities and their families
2. Mastery of content in the following areas on direct service, training and research levels:
   Career development
   Theories of personal social adjustment
   Job placement, job development, employment assistance
   Counseling strategies
   Functional skills and content
   Instructional design and delivery
   System change skills
   Vocational evaluation
   Family dynamics
3. Assessment of community resources in a given locale and identification of strengths and weaknesses of the service delivery system in the following areas:
   Employment
   Special education services
   Rehabilitation services
   Vocational education
   Leisure and recreation
   Housing
   Support services
4. Evaluation of the effectiveness of programs and services that serve youth with disabilities in transition from school to work
5. Awareness of the laws, rules and regulations concerning employment, education, and housing of youths with disabilities and ability to manage or influence those to the benefit of youth
6. Ability to conceptualize a change that will improve individuals' ability to function independently and to implement a change approach
7. Ability to design and deliver effective training to improve competencies of preservice and inservice personnel in providing service[s] to youth with disabilities in the transition period

8. Ability to plan and implement research projects that contribute to knowledge development about the problem encountered by disabled youth in moving from school to work (Daniels, 1987, pp. 305–306)

The above eight competencies will also be important for rehabilitation counselors in their role as primary members of transition planning teams, a role that will vary according to the policies of the vocational rehabilitation agency and secondary school personnel (HRA, 1984; Szymanski, 1984). Also, federal law and school system policy may determine the level of cooperation with a given rehabilitation agency in a specific locality (e.g., a school system) (ARCA, 1984). Examples of the roles of the rehabilitation counselor were identified by HRA (1984) in a study of exemplary transition programs in the United States. Of nine site visits to successful transition programs, the majority contained a rehabilitation counselor located in the school system or specifically assigned to a school case load. The rehabilitation counselors tended to be sophisticated and knowledgeable in the mechanisms of school systems as well as the rehabilitation process. As members of a multidisciplinary team, these rehabilitation counselors provided: 1) consultation with team members on determining vocational potential and vocational planning, 2) the analysis of the vocational and educational implications of the functional limitations and of the vocational and work adjustment needs, 3) input into the coordination of planning and service delivery, and 4) input into job placement and follow-up of each student. Thus, the rehabilitation counselor plays a major role in the transition process—providing consistency and a continuum of services from the secondary school experience through the adult service and job placement period. This continuum is extremely important in the transition process (ARCA, 1984; EIRI, 1984; HRA, 1984; Project PERT Operations Manual, 1985; Szymanski, 1984; Wehman, Kregel, & Barcus, 1985).

An additional function of the rehabilitation counselor is to provide input into the development of the individualized education program (IEP). The rehabilitation counselor can provide information on necessary curriculum modification and services that will help prepare a student for vocational success. This is extremely useful when the rehabilitation counselor begins to develop the student's individualized written rehabilitation program (IWRP), since it is important for the IEP and IWRP to complement one another. The multidisciplinary team will also be able to provide information to the rehabilitation counselor that will be useful in the development of the IWRP. The process of the multidisciplinary team approach allows all members to provide information and expertise to develop and maintain continuity between special education, vocational education, vocational rehabilitation, and the post-secondary school options.

The rehabilitation counselor should also manage the client through the transition program. According to Szymanski and Danek (1985), the rehabilitation counselor's knowledge and experience in the world of adult services can help "navigate" a student through the maze of service delivery systems in the postsecondary realm. Daniels (1987) has suggested that clinical interventions (e.g., counseling strategies) and social interventions (e.g., removing architectural barriers) need to be applied on the individual, service delivery, and leadership levels. He delineates seven general processes that are important: 1) task analysis, 2) behavioral analysis, 3) decision making, 4) discrepancy analysis, 5) networking, 6) advocacy, and 7) sales. As more agencies are involved in the transition process, case management increases in importance. Effective case management requires the identification and utilization of appropriate personnel and services to achieve maximum vocational success. In short, it means achieving the greatest results with the least amount of effort and resources. As an advocate, the rehabilitation counselor is uniquely qualified to assist the multidisciplinary team. For example, as a client advocate during job placement, the rehabilitation counselor can give technical assistance to prospective employers, and counseling to the newly placed employee (student). This can be especially important to the adolescent placed in a summer job or in a vocational education course. Proper placement of the special education student in the vocational education setting can be facilitated by the rehabilitation counselor through technical assistance to vocational instructors in the modification of course materials and in counseling the student.

Vocational training and the community provide work experiences that allow a student an opportunity to participate in meaningful employment situations with real demands (Wehman, Kregel, & Barcus, 1985). The rehabilitation counselor's knowledge in matching a disabled individual's abilities to job requirements is instrumental in helping a student gain access to these opportunities. The rehabilitation counselor also provides assistance to school personnel, and may authorize supportive services such as attendants, job-site training, transportation, and additional supervision. The rehabilitation counselor is able to provide vocational educators with information on employment options in a particular vocational area, including the job modifications, work behaviors, and mobility demands of a particular work environment. The rehabilitation counselor's knowledge, training, and experience dictate that vocational options extend beyond the traditional placement of special education students into custodial and food service occupations. Rehabilitation counselors can use their knowledge of vocational alternatives to expand the career opportunities of special education students through community training, and by coordinating the effects of community and state employment agencies. Training provided in the environment where the behavior is ultimately expected to be performed is the most effective (Wehman, 1981). Therefore, for students with transfer of training problems, training in the real work environment would seem to be the preferred option. While the ideal vocational development continuum is not clearly evident, progress toward the ideal will probably result from earlier career preparation and more training in real work environments (Wehman, 1981; Will, 1984b).

The rehabilitation counselor provides vocational planning expertise to the school system and the parents of the special education student (Project PERT Operations Manual, 1985; Wehman, Kregel, & Barcus, 1985). Communication between the rehabilitation counselor, parents, and student is the preferred method of developing a working relationship. The rehabilitation counselor interacts with the parents and the special education student to increase awareness of vocational options and the potential of the student for employment. This orientation is consistent with the presuppositions and purposes of the education system—to provide the most appropriate education to the special education student (Wehman, Kregel, & Barcus, 1985). Working with parents and students, the rehabilitation counselor can promote development of a "work attitude"—a positive feeling toward work (Project PERT Operations Manual, 1985). The rehabilitation counselor's relationship with parents is best conceived as part of the advocate function. The rehabilitation counselor must be proactive in helping the multidisciplinary team develop parental and student attitudes that are challenging yet realistic for the student's vocational development. Work ability and independent functioning should be developed concurrently as the desired outcome.

The rehabilitation counselor can ensure that all possible services are delivered to the student. Through interagency coordination, more students can be served as programs become more cost effective when duplicate agency services are eliminated. The rehabilitation counselor can facilitate program cost effectiveness by monitoring various agencies' services, ensuring that no service gaps exist, and that duplication of services is eliminated or minimized.

The rehabilitation counselor must understand and utilize the concept of least restrictive environment (EIRI, 1984). Specifically, the education regulations of PL 94-142 mandate the least restrictive environment. The regulations state:

> 1. To the maximum extent appropriate, handicapped children including children in public or private institutions or other care facilities, are educated with children who are not handicapped.
> 2. That special classes, separate schooling or other removal of handicapped children from the regular educational environment occurs only when the nature or severity of the handicap is such that education in regular classes with the use of supplementary aids and services cannot be achieved satisfactorily. (*Federal Register*, 1977, p. 42497)

The least restrictive environment allows the student a greater opportunity for positive social interaction and vocational outcomes, emphasizing increased independence and community integration. The rehabilitation counselor facilitates vocational development in the least restrictive environment by assisting the student's integration into the world of work. Such integration can provide the following benefits: 1) opportunities for integration and socialization with co-workers and supervisors without disabilities, 2) normal role modeling opportunities, and 3) opportunity for employers and the community as a whole to realize the work potential and ability of developmentally disabled individuals (EIRI, 1984).

PROFESSIONAL PREPARATION AND CONTINUING DEVELOPMENT OF THE REHABILITATION COUNSELOR

The vocational rehabilitation counselor has traditionally received preservice education and continuing education through the auspices of university based programs accredited by the Council on Rehabilitation Education (CORE). CORE-accredited rehabilitation counseling programs are appropriate for the preservice education and continuing education of transition-oriented rehabilitation counselors. Given the relatively recent development of this specialty in rehabilitation counselor education, emphasis should be placed on developing and offering elective courses in cooperation with the disciplines of special education, vocational education, and psychology at the preservice and continuing education levels. These courses should emphasize special education services, vocational education, adolescent development, applied behavior analysis, and service delivery methodologies, including transitional and supported employment, that emphasize cooperation and programming to meet the special needs of disabled individuals (consult Chapters 5, 6, and 7 in this text for additional details on transitional and supported employment). Education should also include the purpose and eligibility criteria for each of the service delivery systems, the points of overlap of each of these services, and the vocational planning process of the IEP and the IWRP.

Rehabilitation counselors and other professionals in the educational system need to increase their familiarity with and knowledge of each discipline's organizational structures and systems. The mission of the school system is not limited merely to the education of handicapped students, but the education of all students. Rehabilitation counselors must understand school system dynamics in order to work more effectively within these systems. As a consultant in the educational system, it is important that the rehabilitation counselor learn the methodologies for providing technical assistance and consultation (HRA, 1984; NIHR, 1985; Szymanski, 1984).

In order for the rehabilitation counselor to remain a knowledgeable, competent, and contributing member of the multidisciplinary team, continued preservice and continuing education must be designed to develop the requisite skills to function effectively in educational, vocational, employment, and training settings. Continuing identification and modification of the rehabilitation counselor's job roles must remain an ongoing priority of rehabilitation educators and practitioners.

CONTINUING ISSUES

Fenton and Keller (1981) summarize the short-sightedness of special education and vocational rehabilitation as having a "tunnel vision" approach to their own areas of responsibility and to how they look at each other. The narrow and independent approach of each discipline has frequently focused on the limited needs of persons with disabilities at specific ages, with little or no recognition that the common concern and mission of rehabilitation is for the same person—the disabled student. Both professions assist people with handicapping conditions to develop their physical, emotional, educational, social, and vocational potential to the fullest. Thus, professionals from both disciplines possess the skills to assist people with handicapping conditions to achieve a maximum level of productivity and function.

Fenton and Keller (1981) identified nine areas that remain as critical issues that need to be addressed. They are: 1) the role and functions of vocational rehabilitation personnel and school personnel; 2) mutual understanding and appreciation of/between rehabilitation personnel and school personnel; 3) organization, policies, and procedures of school systems; 4) goals for which school personnel are accountable; 5) communication and support between rehabilitation counselors and special educators; 6) assurance of support and backing of the vocational rehabilitation agency for the rehabilitation counselors; 7) special training for rehabilitation counselors working in schools; 8) knowledge of special educators and guidance counselors in the school district by rehabilitation counselors; and, 9) sensitivity, group processes, and facilitation skill development for rehabilitation counselors implementing cooperative agreements.

To increase the success of transition services, current issues professionals should address include: 1) the relationships between transition and supported employment; 2) independent living programs and transition; 3) considerations by state and local agencies to assist vocational rehabilitation counselors with increased client loads; 4) appropriate education of rehabilitation and education personnel to prepare them for collaborative programming; 5) evaluation of the effects of collaborative programming agreements; 6) the relationships between vocational rehabilitation, special education, and vocational education at the federal, state, and local level; 7) the system changes needed to accommodate new agencies and individuals in the process of transition, such as the concept of *parents as partners;* 8) transition services from the adult support system; and 9) increased funding for new and innovative transition services. These current issues are not inclusive of all issues concerning professionals in transition from school to work programs. However, they do represent a sampling of the many concerns expressed by professionals (Daniels, 1987; Drake & Witten, 1985; Emener & Griswold, 1986; Fenton & Keller, 1981; Hasazi, 1985; Szymanski, 1984).

It is the opinion of the authors that there are eight issues in need of immediate attention:

1. Phenomena such as "transition," "meaningful work," and "employment" currently exist with diverse conceptualizations. How these phenomena are conceptualized, operationally defined, and measured represents a set of issues in need of functional resolution (see Szymanski & Danek, 1985).
2. Unfortunately, very little is known about special career-related needs (see Chubon, 1985) and developmental concerns and tasks relevant to employment (see Davis, Anderson, Linkowski, Berger, & Feinstein, 1985), and the attitudes and motives of adolescents with disabilities toward work (McCarthy, 1983). There would appear to be a plethora of possible research topics in these areas, the results of which could be critical to school-to-work programs.
3. Given the variety of professional disciplines and service delivery program units involved in school-to-work programming, the need is evident for synergistic and interrelated policy (see Emener & Griswold, 1986), ultimate systems changes to support transition (Kallsen & Kidder, 1985; Will, 1985), and establishment of unity among special education and rehabilitation programs (Daniels, 1987; Nadolsky, 1985). For example, vocational rehabilitation counselors have not always been welcome in the schools. Ambiguity, confusion, and misinformation regarding the role of the rehabilitation counselor have to be replaced with mutual understanding and appreciation by multidisciplinary team members. Moreover, rehabilitation personnel must become familiar with the organizational components of the schools and ways in which they can be accessed.
4. At the local level, interagency cooperation and participation, including the public schools and other human service agencies, are clearly needed (see Cavanagh, 1983; Hasazi, 1985). Vocational rehabilitation counselors must not only know the vocational educators, special educators and guidance counselors in their geographic service area but also remain "close" to the leaders in the industrial and business sectors of the community.
5. The identification and refinement of theoretical bases of alternative service delivery programming, coupled with improved measures of program efficiency and effectiveness, present numerous research and demonstration issues (NIHR, 1983, 1985). For example, meeting the educational and vocational needs of students with disabilities is only one of several significant goals for which school personnel are held accountable. Lack

of funds, untrained personnel, and increasing public criticism for the failure to respond properly have caused educators to be particularly sensitive to being asked to do more and more with fewer facilities, funds, and personnel.

6. Effective rehabilitation counselors and other professionals (e.g., special educators and vocational educators) need similar knowledge, attitudes, skills, and competencies. Thus, there are numerous issues relevant to the preparation and training of such professionals (see Daniels, 1987; Emener, 1986; Fenton & Keller, 1985; Riggar & Riggar, 1978; Szymanski, 1984).
7. While professionals agree that the family plays a significant role in the development of a disabled child, much still needs to be discerned about that role(s) (see Seligman, 1985).
8. The United States Senate report language on rehabilitation counseling accompanying the 1986 Handicapped Act Amendments clearly indicated that rehabilitation counseling was to be considered as a related service and that such a service must be provided where necessary to assist students in benefitting from special education services consistent with their individualized education programs (Kirk, 1986). Despite the encouraging report language, barriers still remain in many states for school districts wishing to hire rehabilitation counselors. Professionals in rehabilitation counseling and special education will need to work together to enable students with disabilities to benefit from the expertise of school-employed rehabilitation counselors.

These eight issues, at the very least, are crucial to the efficiency and effectiveness of school-to-work programs and the work of the rehabilitation counselors with disabled youth.

CONCLUDING COMMENT

The need for and benefits of efficient and effective services for disabled youth have been clearly documented. Moreover, the need for the continuing cooperative development of programs, such as the school-to-work program, has also been documented—specifically in the areas of policy, legislation, and cooperative service delivery programming. The roles and functions of the rehabilitation counselor are certainly pivotal in school-to-work initiatives and efforts. The rehabilitation counselor should feel compelled not only to provide effective professional services but also to advocate for cooperative initiatives and efforts with all professional disciplines and groups engaged in the process. Essentially, rehabilitation counselors can *lead by example* and provide the energy, synergy, and drive that will marshal the collective efforts of many toward working with individuals with disabilities as they strive to better their lives.

REFERENCES

American Rehabilitation Counseling Association (ARCA). (1984). *Transition from school to work for students with disabilities (ARCA position on PL 98-199).* Alexandria, VA: Author.

Bellamy, G. T., Rhodes, L. E., & Albin, J. M. (1986). Supported employment. In W. E. Kiernan & J. A. Stark (Eds.), *Pathways to employment for adults with developmental disabilities* (pp. 129–138). Baltimore: Paul H. Brookes Publishing Co.

Cartwright, G., Cartwright, C., & Ward, M. (1984). *Educating special learners.* Belmont, CA: Wadsworth.

Cavanagh, R. M., Jr. (1983). Cooperative programming with the schools: A proposal. *Journal of Rehabilitation, 49*(1), 33–36.

Chubon, R. A. (1985). Career-related needs of school children with severe physical disabilities. *Journal of Counseling and Development, 64,* 47–51.

Crites, L., Smull, M., & Sachs, M. (1984). *Demographic and functional characteristics of respondents to the mentally retarded community needs survey: Persons living at home with family.* Unpublished manuscript, University of Maryland, School of Medicine, Baltimore.

Daniels, J. L. (1987). Transition from school to work. In R. M. Parker (Ed.), *Rehabilitation counseling: Basics and beyond* (pp. 283–317). Austin, TX: PRO-ED.

Davis, S. E., Anderson, C., Linkowski, D. C., Berger, K., & Feinstein, C. F. (1985). Developmental tasks and transitions of adolescents with chronic illnesses and disabilities. *Rehabilitation Counseling Bulletin, 29,* 69–80.

Drake, G. A., & Witten, B. J. (1985). Facilitating learning disabled adolescents' successful transition from school to work. *Journal of Applied Rehabilitation Counseling, 17*(1), 34–37.

Eleventh Institute on Rehabilitation Issues. (1984). *Continuum of services: School to work.* Menomonie: University of Wisconsin–Stout, School of Education and Human Services, Stout Vocational Rehabilitation Institute, Research and Training Center.

Emener, W. G. (1986). *Rehabilitation counselor preparation and development: Selected critical issues.* Springfield, IL: Charles C Thomas.

Emener, W. G., & Griswold, P. P. (1986). Rehabilitation programs and the need for synergy and interrelated policy development: The OSERS school-to-work initiative. *Journal of Rehabilitation Administration, 10*(2), 40–47.

Federal Register. (August 23, 1977). Education of Handicapped Children, 121a 550. Washington, DC: U.S. Department of Health, Education and Welfare, Office of Education.

Fenton, J., & Keller, Jr., R. A. (1981). Special education—vocational rehabilitation: Let's get the act together. *American Rehabilitation, 11*(3), 26–30.

Gold, M. W. (1975). Vocational training. In J. Wortis (Ed.), *Mental retardation and developmental disabilities: An annual review.* (Vol. 7, pp. 254–264). New York: Brunner/Mazel.

Harold Russell Associates. (1984). *Report on cooperative programs from school to work* (Contract No. 300-83-0158). Washington, DC: U.S. Department of Education, National Institute of Handicapped Research.

Hasazi, S. B. (1985). Facilitating transition from high school: Policies and practices. *American Rehabilitation, 11*(3), 9–11, 16.

Hasazi, S., Gordon, L., & Roe, C. (1985). Factors associated with the employment status of handicapped youth exiting high school from 1979–1983. *Exceptional Children, 5,* 455–469.

Kallsen, P. G., & Kidder, S. B. (1985). Vocational rehabilitation: Perspective on transition. *American Rehabilitation, 11*(3), 25–31.

Kirk, F. S. (1986). Notes from Washington. In J. F. Scorzelli & R. Wolfe, (Eds.), *ARCA-NRCA Newsletter, 14*(2). Boston: Northeastern University.

Kokaska, C., & Brolin, D. (1985). *Career education for handicapped individuals.* Columbus, OH: Charles E. Merrill.

McCarthy, H. (1983). Understanding motives of youth in transition to work: A taxonomy for rehabilitation counselors and educators. *Journal of Applied Rehabilitation Counseling, 14*(1), 52–61.

Mithaug, D., Horiuchi, C., & Fanning, P. (1985). A report on the Colorado statewide follow-up survey of special education students. *Exceptional Education, 51,* 397–404.

Nadolsky, J. M. (1985). Achieving unity in special education and rehabilitation. *Journal of Rehabilitation, 51*(1), 22–23.

National Institute of Handicapped Research. (1983). Cooperative work preparation for students with disabilities. *Rehab Brief, 6*(4).

National Institute of Handicapped Research. (1985). School to work: A model for vocational preparation. *Rehab Brief, 8*(7).

Project PERT Operations Manual. (1985). *Postsecondary education/rehabilitation transition for the mildly mentally retarded and the learning disabled.* Unpublished manuscript, Woodrow Wilson Rehabilitation Center, Fishersville, VA.

Project TIE (Transition Into Employment). (undated). *1*(1). Richmond: Virginia Commonwealth University, Rehabilitation Research and Training Center.

Riggar, T. F., & Riggar, S. W. (1978). The rehabilitation counselor in an educational setting. *Personnel and Guidance Journal, 57*(1), 58–60.

Rubin, S. E., & Roessler, R. (1983). *Foundations of the vocational rehabilitation process.* Austin, TX: PRO-ED.

Seligman, M. (1985). Handicapped children and their families. *Journal of Counseling and Development, 64,* 274–277.

Szymanski, E. M. (1984). Rehabilitation counselors in school settings. *Journal of Applied Rehabilitation Counseling, 15*(4), 10–13, 56.

Szymanski, E. M., & Danek, M. M. (1985). School-to-work transition for students with disabilities: Historical, current, and conceptual issues. *Rehabilitation Counseling Bulletin, 29,* 81–89.

Wehman, P. (1981). *Competitive employment: New horizons for severely disabled individuals.* Baltimore: Paul H. Brookes Publishing Co.

Wehman, P., Kregel, J., & Barcus, J. M. (1985). From school to work: A vocational transition model for handicapped students [Monograph]. *Competitive Employment for Persons with Mental Retardation: From Research to Practice, 1,* 171–196.

Wehman, P., Kregel, J., & Seyforth, J. (1985). Employment outlook for young adults with mental retardation. *Rehabilitation Counseling Bulletin, 29,* 90–99.

Wehman, P., Wood-Pietruski, W., Everson, J., & Parent, W. (1985). A supported employment approach to transition. *American Rehabilitation, 11*(3), 12–16.

White, S. H., & Smith, H. L. (1985). Vocational skills training: Increasing employment for disabled youth. *Journal of Job Placement, 1*(1), 10–14.

Will, M. (1984a). *OSERS programming for the transition of youth with disabilities:*

Bridges from school to working life. Washington, DC: U.S. Department of Education, Office of Special Education and Rehabilitation Services.

Will, M. (1984b). *Supported employment for adults with severe disabilities: An OSERS program initiative*. Washington, DC: U.S. Department of Education.

Will, M. C. (1985). Statement on transition. *American Rehabilitation, 11*(3), 1.

9

Rehabilitation Counseling Considerations with Sensory-Impaired Persons

Sue E. Ouellette and James A. Leja

WHILE COMPARATIVELY SMALL in numbers, individuals with sensory impairments present a major challenge in the delivery of quality rehabilitation services. Although this population has great potential for rehabilitation success, few rehabilitation personnel receive any specialized training to serve them. As a result, these professionals may feel uncomfortable or inadequately prepared to serve sensory-impaired clients, resulting in a historical lack of appropriate services for this population and frustration for the professionals who seek to provide quality services.

When first developing appropriate client services, counselors are hindered by a lack of informative research and publication on successful strategies with these clients. Later, effective service delivery is limited when specialized resources are not consistently available, or when counselors who identify sensory-impaired clients cannot gain access to the in-service professional training they need.

To improve services to this group, therefore, rehabilitation professionals will need to examine how the special characteristics of this population determine critical issues in the provision of quality rehabilitation services. Sensory-impaired persons as a group are similarly affected by particular problems and limitations in gaining access to and benefiting from rehabilitation services. Therefore, service issues are examined in view of the generic needs of sensory-impaired persons. Too often, literature has addressed sensory-impaired subpopulations—hearing-impaired, vision-impaired, and deaf-blind persons—as separate entities needing separate rehabilitation approaches, oblivious of the common factors of communication loss.

DEFINING THE POPULATION

The sensory disabilities are similar in that each spans a range of impairment from partial to more profound loss. In addition, there is also a shared difficulty in the measurement and definition of the various types of losses.

Hearing impairment, for example, is defined by Schein and Delk (1974) to include all significant deviations from normal hearing, including deafness. A functional definition of deafness is more difficult to arrive at and has been debated at length in the professional literature (Schein, 1964). *Dorland's Illustrated Medical Dictionary* (1984), for example, defines deafness as "lacking the sense of hearing or not having the full power of hearing; moderate lack of hearing is often called hearing loss" (p. 409). Audiological definitions of deafness, which focus on a measurement of hearing loss in decibels across specific frequencies of sound, also vary, and there may be difficulty in accounting for the effect of a specific loss (in decibels) at a specific frequency or frequencies.

Most professionals in the field of deafness rehabilitation counseling have adopted Schein and Delk's (1974) definition of deafness as "the inability to hear and understand speech" (p. 133), thus providing a more function-oriented definition. Similarly, Levine (1960), citing a definition of deafness developed by the Convention of Executives of American Schools for the Deaf, defines deaf persons as "those in whom the sense of hearing is nonfunctional for the ordinary purposes of life" (p. 311). A recent effort by Austin (1983) has moved further in the direction of a functional model by classifying deafness by specific levels of independent and dependent functioning.

While little agreement exists regarding the definition of deafness, even less agreement exists regarding the condition commonly referred to as "hard-of-hearing." In general, this term is defined by exclusion; that is, all hearing-impaired persons who are not deaf are considered to be hard-of-hearing. A simplistic, but useful, distinction is drawn by the deaf community, which considers hard-of-hearing persons to be those who have sufficient hearing to use the telephone, while deaf persons are those who cannot use the telephone even with amplification.

Just as the definitions used to describe deafness and hearing impairment are elusive, so are those used to describe blindness. A nationwide survey of rehabilitation agencies found no common definition of visual impairment (Robinson, 1983). The term *blindness* typically evokes an image of total sight loss. But those with no vision are estimated to account for only 25% of the legally blind population (Vander Kolk, 1981). The remaining 75% have some useable vision. It is this latter group that appears to defy accurate labeling.

The National Society for the Prevention of Blindness (NSPB) (1966) defines blindness as "visual acuity for distant vision of 20/200 or less in the better eye with best correction, or visual acuity of more than 20/200 if the widest diameter of field of vision subtends an angle no greater than 20 degrees." This definition has been adopted as the current legal definition of blindness in the U.S. The World Health Organization (WHO) uses two vision categories: low vision (20/80 to 20/500) and blindness (20/500 or less) (Colenbrander, 1976). However, Genensky (1978), while adopting the definition of legal blindness used by the NSPB, adds yet another numerical and clinically descriptive category: partial sightedness. He states that a person is partially sighted if the acuity in the better eye, even with ordinary corrective lenses, does not exceed 20/70, or if the maximum diameter of the visual field does not exceed 20 degrees, and further describes persons who are functionally blind as those who are either totally blind or have light perception or light projection.

The term *visual impairment* is also used as a functional measure of sight loss. In an educational context, visual impairment can be divided into categories of mild, moderate, or severe vision loss (Scholl, 1983). Mild impairment refers to visual problems that can be ameliorated by ordinary corrective lenses. Persons who are considered moderately vision impaired learn primarily through sight, but benefit from modifications to instructional materials. Finally, those with severe visual impairments must use senses other than vision in the educational process (Bradley-Johnson, 1986).

The National Center for Health Statistics (NCHS) (1975) uses yet another definition in its gathering of prevalence data to describe visual functioning. They use the term *severe functional vision,* and define it as "inability to read ordinary newsprint even with the aid of corrective lenses or, if under 16 years of age, blind in both eyes or having no useful vision in either eye" (pp. 4–5).

The final constituent of the population of sensory-impaired persons, those who are deaf-blind, have a disability that is also subject to variations and controversy in definition. Taff-Watson (1984) cites both functional and ophthalmological/audiological methods for defining deaf-blindness. A functional definition, for example, is provided by the Regional Centers for Deaf-Blind Children:

> . . . children who have auditory and visual handicaps, the combination of which cause severe communication and other developmental and educational problems that cannot be properly accommodated in special education programs solely for the hearing handicapped child or the visually handicapped. (*Federal Register,* Vol. 38, #196, October 11, 1973)

In contrast, the Helen Keller National Center employs a more clinical, ophthalmological/audiological definition:

> Central visual acuity of 20/200 or less in the better eye with corrective lenses or central acuity greater than 20/200 if a peripheral diameter of the visual field subtends at angular distance of no greater than 20 degrees, and a chronic hearing impairment so severe that most speech cannot be understood with optimum amplification and/or speech discrimination score of 40% or less in the better ear. (Taff-Watson, 1984, p. 3)

EPIDEMIOLOGY

In considering the characteristics of the sensory-impaired population as a whole, it is useful to understand the prevalence of each impairment. Using the legal definition of blindness in gathering statistics on blindness in 16 states for the Model Reporting Area (MRA), the National Institute of Neurological Diseases and Blindness in 1970 identified 96,252 legally blind persons. Of these, 27% were under the age of 45, 26.8% were between 45 and 64 years of age and 46.2% were 65 and over (Kahn & Moorhead, 1973).

The National Center for Health Statistics offers an even greater prevalence rate of blindness and visual impairment. Using the term *severe functional vision* as defined earlier, the NCHS estimated 1,306,000 severely visually impaired persons in 1971. Of this number, 9.2% were under 45 years of age, 21.1% were between the age of 45 and 64, and 67.7% were 65 years of age or older. However, as this is both self- and proxy-reported data, its reliability is suspect (Vander Kolk, 1981, p. 4).

Schein and Delk (1974), reporting the results of the most recent census of hearing-impaired persons in the United States, report that 13,362,842 individuals have some form of hearing loss, yielding a prevalence rate of 16,603 per 100,000. Of these persons, 6,548,842 have significant bilateral hearing loss. Deaf persons, those who cannot hear and understand speech, number 1,767,046. A total of 410,522 individuals are prevocationally deaf (onset prior to the age of 19) and 201,625 are prelingually deaf (onset prior to the age of 3 years). It is this prelingually deaf population that, to a large degree, constitutes the majority of hearing-impaired persons seen for specialized rehabilitation services.

Schein and Delk (1974) further report that the largest prevalence rate for prevocational deafness is found in the north central region of the United States (Illinois, Indiana, Iowa, Kansas, Michigan, Minnesota, Missouri, Nebraska, North Dakota, Ohio, South Dakota, and Wisconsin). The lowest incidence of prevocational deafness occurs in the northeast section, including Connecticut, Maine, Massachusetts, New Hampshire, New Jersey, New York, Pennsylvania, Rhode Island, and Vermont. The south and west sections of the country have nearly identical prevalence rates, 194.6 persons per 100,000.

Efforts to provide a demographic profile of deaf-blind persons in the United States have been hampered by the previously described difficulties in defining deaf-blindness and by the lack of a comprehensive national data base containing information on deaf-blind persons of all ages (Ouellette, 1984). The Helen Keller National Center, using its own definition of deaf-blindness, has as of 1987 identified 9,300 deaf-blind persons living in the United States. It estimates, however, that the total number of deaf-blind persons in this country is between 30,000 and 40,000.

A recent study by Wolf, Delk, and Schein (1982) estimated a prevalence of 747,457 persons in the U.S. with some combination of hearing and sight impairments. Of these individuals, 45,310 were classified as deaf-blind, 25,923 as deaf and severely impaired visually, 359,366 as blind and severely impaired auditorially, and 316,858 as severely impaired both auditorially and visually.

Finally, it must be noted that the size of the sensory-impaired population in this country is expected to increase dramatically in the near future as the percentage of older citizens increases. The United States Bureau of the Census (1977) has projected that by the year 2000, 31 million persons will be 65 years of age or older, compared with 23 million in 1977. Lowman and Kirchner (1979) estimate that nearly 900,000 Americans over the age of 65 are unable to read newsprint and, by the year 2000, this number should rise to 1,767,000. This also suggests that a larger proportion of persons requesting rehabilitation services in the future will be sensory impaired as the aging process takes its toll on sight and hearing. As a result, rehabilitation professionals will be serving clients who have acquired sensory losses late in life as a result of aging. While these individuals may not experience the educational and developmental consequences of growing up with a sensory deficit, they may be presented with a variety of concerns that will vary depending upon the severity of the impairment.

CRITICAL ISSUES IN PROVIDING SERVICES TO SENSORY-IMPAIRED PERSONS

Prevocational and Transitional Issues

Prevocational and transitional concerns are of major importance in the rehabilitation of sensory-impaired persons because of the developmental nature of the disabilities involved. Since the major portion of individuals who need rehabilitation services lose their sight and/or hearing at an early age, vocational rehabilitation personnel must deal not only with the physical limitations of the disability, but also with the linguistic, educational, psychological, and social effects of growing up without the crucial assistance of one or more senses. In this population, early intervention is essential if later rehabilitation efforts and the transition from school to work are to be successful.

The need for early identification of children with significant hearing impairments continues to be emphasized in the professional literature. Mindel and Vernon (1971), Schlesinger and Meadow (1972), Furth (1973), and Levine (1981) have effectively documented the need for early intervention to avoid delay in the child's development of language and communication skills. Rehabilitation professionals working with persons who are hearing-impaired have found that the most effective rehabilitation strategy includes prevention of many of the sequelae of hearing loss, including poor academic skills, limited communication ability, inadequate social skills, and lack of awareness of the world of work. These developmental deficits have the potential to severely limit the ability of hearing-impaired individuals to seek and maintain employment and to live independently.

Another potential developmental barrier that can be addressed through early identification and intervention has been identified by Schein and Delk (1974). They state that 90% of all hearing-impaired children are born to parents with normal hearing. Further, 88% of hearing parents of deaf children do not know sign language (Rainer, Altshuler, & Kallman, 1969; Rawlings, 1973), and therefore are often unable to communicate effectively with their children. The resulting lack of communication between parents and child results in a delay in the development of critical language and communication skills, and a lack of important parent-child bonding during the early years of the deaf child's life.

In addition to early identification and intervention programs, there is a need for programs to assist hearing-impaired young adults in transition from public and private schools to the world of work. In general, the Office of Special Education and Rehabilitation Services (OSERS) and the rehabilitation profession as a whole have strongly supported the need for transitional services for disabled youth. The need for a cooperative relationship between special education, vocational education, and vocational rehabilitation is evident for the hearing-impaired population, as for all disabled youth. Studies by Bolton (1975), McHugh (1975), and Brolin (1976) have suggested that hearing-impaired youths, in particular, experience a lack of early vocational experience that creates barriers to eventual employment and habilitation.

A specific need in the area of transitional services is the early involvement of a vocational rehabilitation agency with hearing-impaired children prior to their exit from mainstreamed or residential school programs. However, state rehabilitation agencies may actually discourage early involvement with school-age children, since successful closure of a case opened when a child is 14 or 15 years old might not occur for several years. Thus, many hearing-impaired youths may not be seen by a state agency counselor until after their graduation from high school.

Additionally, hearing-impaired youth, particularly those with severely limited language, education, and vocational skills, are often not able to find entry-level positions for summer work and other prevocational activities that would assist in formulating future career options. These experiences are particularly important to hearing-impaired youth who may lack sufficient linguistic and communication skills to acquire even the most basic information about the world of work. This issue has been delineated by Veatch (1984), who suggested a number of specific interventions to ease the school-to-work transition.

Persons who are visually impaired or blind face problems similar to children and young adults who are deaf or hearing impaired with regard to prevocational and transitional services. As with the hearing-impaired population, early identification of and early intervention with children with visual impairments can significantly reduce delays in cognitive, social, and personality development (Warren, 1984).

It is widely accepted that infants, within the first 2 years of life, pass through significant developmental stages. Though there are numerous theories of the human development process, such as the personality developmental theories of Freud and the social learning theories of Bandura and Walters, perhaps the most widely accepted theory of intellectual development is the cognitive developmental theory of Piaget (Piaget, 1952). Piaget described four stages of cognitive development, of which the first stage, sensorimotor development, is particularly applicable to the understanding of subsequent intellectual and motor deficits in blind and visually impaired persons. In this stage, the infant develops an understanding of the world through sensory information, gained through an interaction with the environment. The visually impaired child, having greatly reduced or no visual stimulation, must rely on the other senses to acquire this understanding. If the child is prevented from other sensory input by either an overprotective parent or the lack of stimulation ordinarily provided by visual cues, one or more of the sensorimotor stages may be skipped. To skip any one of the critical segments of this stage may mean the loss of specific skills and abilities (Langley, 1980; Moore, 1984). For example, the visually handicapped child who passes over the crawling stage and has not, as a consequence, practiced weight shifting or hip and trunk rotation, will later exhibit wide and rigid leg movements during walking (Ferrel, 1985). Eventually, such inappropriate posture, gait, and other nonverbal maneuvers can impede employment (Lombana, 1980).

Other deficits may also become apparent if early intervention (and remediation) does not occur. As one theory suggests (Knight, 1972; Scott, 1969), stereotypic behavior may develop in blind children as a result of reduced physical and sensory stimulation in early childhood. Also, insufficiencies in language stimulation for visually impaired infants may impede expressive language (Ferrel, 1985). In addition, without early intervention, inhibitory parents and teachers who expect the child's development to be somewhat retarded may unconsciously create a self-fulfilling prophecy, restricting the child's opportunity to learn because the time was not right (Warren, 1984).

Developmental deficits acquired in childhood not only affect further developmental stages, but also, because of incomplete cognitive development, affect the blind and the visually impaired person's ability to pursue and sustain employment and live independently. The problem-solving abilities used continually in adult life begin to be mastered in childhood challenges.

Another concern in the area of prevocational and transitional services for blind and visually impaired persons is the existence of a gap between education and rehabilitation services. Though educators and rehabilitation counselors have sought to close this gap through uniting in the Association of Education and Rehabilitation of Blind and Visually Impaired Persons (AER), and in publishing jointly in professional journals, both disciplines continue to be uneasy with each other. Erickson and Wyrick (1984) suggest that, in part, this dichotomy exists because education and rehabilitation professionals each persist in their own kind of "tunnel vision," limiting the ability of the specialists to see beyond their special objectives (p. 20). Where special education primarily concerns itself with the academic needs of students, vocational and self-care training needs may go unmet. In contrast, vocational rehabilitation services, designed to prepare clients for employment and independent living, have given little attention to correcting deficits in social adjustment to the work place (Erickson & Wyrick, 1984).

This gap between rehabilitation and education also manifests itself in the philosophical differences between public schools and residential schools for the visually impaired student. The primary goal of the residential school has been the preparation of students to achieve a full introduction into adult life (Spungin, 1982, p. 231). While some students are prepared to enter job training programs or college, others are prepared to work in noncompetitive employment.

Undoubtedly, the public school system has similar goals, but they are not applied quite as comprehensively. For example, according to Scholl (1981), vocational and social skills are usually given the lowest priority in a student's high school program. Because not enough time is available daily to include all of these activities, academic skills become the major focus of the education program (Scholl, 1981). Spungin (1982), however, believes that the residential school of the future will assist the public school in this dilemma by providing part-time instruction in prevocational and vocational activities.

The need for early identification and intervention with deaf-blind children would seem evident from the preceding discussion of long-term deficits resulting from visual or hearing impairments alone. Difficulties in identifying deaf-blind children complicate the provision of prevocational services to deaf-blind individuals who were born with both impairments. Although some states have sought to develop a registry of deaf-blind children, the only national registry is maintained by Helen Keller National Center. Transitional programs have been successfully developed, such as a subsidized work program for rubella-caused deaf-blind teenagers reported by Busse, Romer, Fewell, and Vadasy (1985). Their subjects, who were also mentally retarded, demonstrate the use of existing work programs adapted through individualized programming to meet the needs of deaf-blind adolescents.

Vocational Issues

Also of considerable importance to the delivery of quality services to sensory-impaired persons are identified gaps in the provision of vocational services. Three segments of the vocational rehabilitation process are particularly relevant for this population: vocational evaluation, vocational training, and job placement. Other issues relating to the employment of sensory-impaired persons are also discussed in this section.

Vocational Evaluation While various issues regarding the vocational evaluation of hearing-impaired persons have been discussed in detail in the professional literature (see, for example, Watson, 1977; Watson, Anderson, Marut, Ouellette, & Ford, 1983), this area warrants additional attention. Although a directory of services for hearing-impaired clients listed over 90 programs providing work evaluation services to this population (Marut, Watson, & Buford, 1984), there remains a need to develop guidelines to ensure that hearing-impaired clients receive important evaluation services which will be accurate and appropriate to their needs. Such guidelines should stress the need for repetition of instruction, simplification of written language, and the difficulty of maintaining test standardization when using sign language. These factors affect not only how well the client understands what is expected of him or her during the evaluation, but also how the evaluator interprets the results. Furthermore, as a result of the 1963–1967 rubella epidemic, a large number of severely hearing-impaired and often multiply disabled persons are currently entering the rehabilitation process in need of comprehensive diagnostic services, including vocational evaluation.

The literature on visual impairment discusses the obstacles to consistent and efficacious testing methods in vocational evaluation. As with other sensory impairments, the very tools with which vocational evaluators work sometimes can fall short of providing standard, transferable data, and must be used with understanding and precision. The means of conducting testing (Braille, sign language), matched to the communication abilities of the client, may, by differences in interpretation, itself create differences in results. The evaluator's inability to find appropriate normative data for the test results of a visually impaired client may also impede a useful analysis of the client's functional skills.

Literature in the field is often critical of the validity of vocational evaluation for visually impaired persons, and of the ability of current evaluation tools to give accurate information about a client's potential. M. Peterson (1985) points to the limitations of standard commercial vocational evaluation systems in usefully measuring the vocational aptitude of any visually impaired worker. Such tests, he notes, are designed to be administered via pencil and paper, rather than through performance of hands-on tests of job-related tasks. As vocational evaluation testing becomes less and less concerned with experiential trials, Peterson predicts a concomitant loss of "face validity and vocational exploration" (p. 478).

The use of work samples as a tool in the vocational evaluation process has also come under criticism. Work samples administered in a fabricated situation do not reflect a client's performance in an actual situation, but like other tests create anxiety for the client (Lorenz, 1975). Furthermore, the client may have very little input into the planning or preparation of the assessment tool (Lorenz, 1975). If this is the case and the evaluator has insufficient training in conducting valid evaluations of visually impaired persons, the results may be invalid and the recommendations may perpetuate occupational stereotyping (M. Peterson, 1985). Work samples have also been developed for only a limited range of jobs. There is a need to develop work samples for skilled, technical careers and professional jobs, employment that visually impaired persons may undertake if they receive specialized training.

To examine how work evaluations can be more relevant to visually impaired persons, the American Foundation for the Blind is sponsoring a task force to develop recommendations. The Rehabilitation Research and Training Center on Blindness and Low Vision is also involved in research and development related to vocational evaluation. It will be interesting to see how these organizations address some of the problems that have been cited.

Providing vocational evaluation services to deaf-blind clients is even more complex and difficult. Few assessment instruments have been specifically designed for this population. Often, instruments and procedures standardized for use with blind, deaf, or general client groups must be adapted for use with deaf-blind clients, and yield results of questionable validity (Eleventh Institute on Rehabilitation Issues [EIRI], 1984). While the development of appropriate assessment tools and techniques must remain a priority for future research, current assessment practices focus on observation and experience with the client, and rely on the experience of the evaluator with this population (EIRI, 1984). Unfortunately, not enough experienced and competent evaluators exist, and misdiagnosis, particularly of mental retardation and mental illness, is common (Nelipovich & Naegele, 1984).

Training In the past 15 years, there has been a tremendous increase in the number of training programs available to hearing-impaired persons, particularly at the postsecondary level (Rawlings, Karchmer, & DeCaro, 1983). From 1864 to 1968, hearing-impaired persons wishing to pursue higher education had only two choices: attend Gallaudet College or select an institution of higher learning that does not offer supportive services such as interpreters or notetakers. In 1964 the National Technical Institute for the Deaf was established, followed by additional programs throughout the country spurred by Title V of the 1973 Rehabilitation Act. By 1983 the number of postsecondary educational programs offering a full range of services for hearing-impaired students had increased from one to 61, with additional schools offering partial services to this population (Rawlings et al., 1983). As a result, more hearing-impaired students are attending postsecondary educational programs. Additionally, institutions of higher learning are playing a more active role in providing vocational training services that were previously provided to hearing-impaired clients by rehabilitation facilities and trade schools.

Postsecondary education services for this population are extremely expensive, resulting in a current federal expenditure of over $60 million per year, with additional tens of millions of state dollars also contributed to community college programs (Ouellette, El-Khiami, & Schroedel, 1984). Despite this massive expenditure of funds, little research has been conducted to investigate the effectiveness and efficiency of various training options. Continued federal funding should be encouraged to support research efforts, such as a current project undertaken by the University of Arkansas Rehabilitation Research and Training Center on Deafness and Hearing Impairment (Ouellette et al., 1984). This project is investigating the types of postsecondary educational services available to hearing-impaired persons and assessing their effectiveness by examining the opinions of current students, graduates, parents, vocational rehabilitation counselors, and other professional groups. Such research is critical to enabling rehabilitation counselors to make cost-effective decisions regarding appropriate training options for hearing-impaired clients.

Job Placement Placement in competitive employment, as the ultimate goal of the vocational rehabilitation process, requires special consideration with the hearing-impaired and deaf-blind population. These individuals often lack the communication skills, linguistics competencies, and experiential knowledge base essential for successful job seeking and placement.

Traditional selective placement practices, in which the counselor assumes major responsibility for securing employment for the client, have had limited long-term effects (Torretti, 1983). In this system, sensory-impaired clients lacking appropriate job-seeking knowledge and skills often must return to the vocational rehabilitation system each time a job change is necessary or desired.

Current literature has recognized the soundness of approaching placement efforts with this population by teaching the client appropriate job-seeking skills, including use of the popular "job club" model (Azrin & Beasel, 1980). However, Amrine and Bullis (1985) suggest that the standard job club approach is heavily dependent upon communication skills and must, therefore, be modified for hearing-impaired and deaf-blind clients. Torretti (1983), West-Evans and Shiels (1983), and Dwyer (1983) all report substantial benefits from such a client-directed approach. However, further research is needed to determine necessary modifications that will optimize the effectiveness of a client-centered approach with sensory-impaired persons (Amrine & Bullis, 1985).

Watson (1985) also indicates a need for broadening the range of placement services traditionally available to hearing-impaired persons. He suggests that job retraining services be made available ''to assist mature deaf workers in obtaining timely new skills required by the changing labor market'' (p. 288). Watson also emphasizes the need for career education and guidance in addition to standard placement services. The full range of preplacement, placement, and postplacement services must be made available, including a full spectrum of services ranging from selective placement to job clubs, job-seeking skills training, job analysis and modification, on-the-job coaches, job development, cooperative programs between rehabilitation and industry, and statewide placement services.

Employment Issues

In addition to issues related to specific phases of the rehabilitation process, several issues regarding employment warrant discussion. One concern is disincentives to employment, including easily available Social Security payments. As a result of the underemployment that often results from the compounding effects of sensory impairments, many individuals may find it more advantageous to remain nonworkers and collect various available benefits than to accept low-paying, entry-level employment. Further, to maintain their social service benefits, students enrolled in post-secondary educational programs may attempt to lengthen their academic programs and postpone graduation.

A second issue, specific to hearing-impaired persons, is the need for job retraining services. Because communication deficits often create barriers to the hearing-impaired worker's advancement in employment, many individuals remain in entry-level positions and may be particularly vulnerable to being laid-off or losing their positions to new technology. In-service training programs provided to employees to learn new skills and upgrade existing knowledge may be less accessible to hearing-impaired workers whose reading skills may be minimal or who depend on interpreters for training meetings. Thus, it is recommended that job retraining and upgrading programs be developed to meet the unique needs of these individuals.

A discussion of issues related to the employment of blind and visually impaired persons is compounded by a difficulty in determining the number of individuals who are employed. Employment estimates tend to vary depending on the definition of disability used in each study. There is little debate, however, that unemployment and underemployment among persons who are blind is a significant issue (Lombana, 1980; Vieceli, 1972). Moreover, there exists some variability in estimates of the number of visually impaired and blind persons who are available for work and would be eligible for assistance in securing and maintaining employment. For example, through estimates of the legally blind population in 1978, and the 1970 statistics on legally blind persons from the state registers of the six states that participated in the Model Reporting Area, Kirchner (1981) estimated that there were 210,000 legally blind working adults across the United States in 1978. The National Center for Health Statistics, using the criterion of "inability to see to read ordinary newsprint even with glasses on," estimated that in 1977 there were 364,000 severely visually impaired working-age adults in the United States (Kirchner & Lowman, 1978; Kirchner & Peterson, 1979). A survey conducted by the Bureau of the Census in 1976 estimated that there were 776,000 visually handicapped working-age adults in the U.S. This estimate, though appearing inflated, took into account persons age 18–64 for whom visual problems are secondary or tertiary factors, in addition to persons for whom it is the primary disability. The census figures also revealed that in 1976, 17% of the visually handicapped persons in the labor force were unemployed, compared to only 7% of the rest of the labor force.

In addition to experiencing high unemployment as a group, legally blind persons also have traditionally been significantly underemployed or employed in low-paying jobs. The Rehabilitation Services Administration, which compiles and summarizes descriptive data on persons who have been rehabilitated, found that in 1981 the cases of 9,506 men and women who were blind in both eyes were closed as rehabilitated. Of these, 5,364 cases were closed as clients moved on to homemaking, 386 to sheltered employment, 110 as unpaid family workers, and 3,646 to competitive employment. However, salaries for those who had entered employment were reported to be much lower than the national average for all households.

What are the reasons for this? Bauman (1975) suggests that many visually impaired and blind persons are vocationally unsuccessful because they are minimally involved in career planning and decision-making activities. Spain (1981) believes that job training programs do little to encourage the disabled population in general to develop the necessary skills needed to secure and maintain employment.

Kirchner and Peterson (1980) state that in general, visually impaired persons continue to be disadvantaged in work even after they have obtained employment. They obtain jobs that are less permanent and any skills or academic achievements do not necessarily translate into a rise in occupational status.

A review of current program efforts reveals limited use of any comprehensive approach to job development and job placement for working-age blind persons. This may be, in large part, due to the limited knowledge that placement specialists and counselors have of visual impairment and blindness.

The employment outlook for deaf-blind persons is limited by misconceptions of the combined disabilities that often result in the belief, even by rehabilitation personnel, that deaf-blind persons are incapable of obtaining and sustaining employment. Data provided by the Helen Keller National Center (HKNC) for July, 1982 to June, 1983 indicate that 42.4% of 139 individuals who received training from HKNC entered employment, while 57.6% remained unemployed. Further, only 23.0% of those working were competitively employed, while 61.2% worked in sheltered workshops, 13.7% in work activity centers, and 2.1% in family enterprises or homebound employment (Helen Keller National Center for Deaf-Blind Youth and Adults, 1983). A document prepared by the EIRI (1984) stresses the need to consider the employability of each deaf-blind person as a distinct individual, and to expand professional consciousness regarding jobs that deaf-blind persons are capable of doing.

Independent Living Issues

Ouellette and Lloyd (1980), reporting the findings of a national conference on independent living services for hearing-impaired persons, document the need for comprehensive programming to meet the needs of deaf adults who have often grown up in sheltered family environments or within the protective atmosphere of residential school programs. These dependency-inducing environments, coupled with the communication, language, and experiential limitations that often accompany early severe hearing impairment, can result in a lack of knowledge and skills essential to independent living. While great legislative change has occurred in recent years, many hearing-impaired persons, particularly prelingually deaf young adults, still lack access to appropriate independent living skills schools training programs.

Although the 1978 Rehabilitation Act Amendments provided for the establishment of independent living services for all disabled persons, most programs developed as a result of this landmark legislation have been targeted to the needs of mobility-impaired and other physically disabled persons (Crewe & Zola, 1983). Few independent living centers offer skill training designed to meet the more subtle developmental deficits encountered by deaf young adults, or have staff members who are specially trained to communicate with hearing-impaired persons.

Information about one comprehensive independent living program specifically designed for hearing-impaired persons has recently been reported in the literature; this program may serve as a model for other such programming. Holt (1985) describes a statewide program involving 10 independent living counselors specifically trained in deafness rehabilitation, and able to communicate with hearing-impaired clients. These counselors, dispersed strategically throughout the state, provide a "cradle to grave" continuum of services that includes casefinding, intake, evaluation, advocacy, referral to vocational rehabilitation, services to deaf children and their families, services to deaf adults, and services to older deaf adults.

In addition to comprehensive independent living programs for hearing-impaired persons, there is a need to develop independent living skill training programs specifically for low-achieving deaf clients. Such programs are needed to teach the basic skills needed for daily living, including personal grooming and care, managing a budget and banking, using public transportation, food shopping and preparation, clothing care, household management, child care, driver's education, and knowledge of the legal system (Ouellette & Lloyd, 1980).

Many clients could also benefit from group home arrangements to ease the transition from high school to employment. Many deaf clients do not have families to turn to, and therefore supervised housing is needed. Such group home experience can enable clients to use and absorb independent living skills for their own individualized needs. Concern exists that many hearing-impaired clients currently served in rehabilitation facilities will be unable to carry over independent living skills into actual independent living situations. Often, instruction is given in a classroom setting with the assumption that clients will transfer skills learned in the classroom to "real life" situations. Such transfer of learning often does not occur, and skills are forgotten in an actual independent living situation. Facilities should be encouraged to investigate methods of optimizing the carryover of independent living skills training, perhaps through programs based in the group home. There is also a need to provide sufficient staff to work individually with hearing-impaired clients rather than solely in classroom environments.

The provision of independent living training for deaf-blind individuals remains a high priority for state-federal vocational rehabilitation programs. The EIRI (1984) defined 25 needs for independent living training for deaf-blind clients, including teletypewriter and Braille teletypewriter services, interpreting services, reader and/or mobility services, attendant care, housing, communication, and recreation services.

Similarly, Doyle, Burch, Paoletti-Schelp, and Richards (1984) list a broad range of independent living services needed by deaf-blind persons, including community education/awareness, family services, transportation, housing information and referral, accessibility compliance review and modification, legal services information and referral, telephone relay, health service referral, recreation, group homes, vocational rehabilitation, job banks, peer counseling and peer resource personnel, interpreters, personal care attendants and companions, volunteer services, counseling, orientation and mobility training, respite care, advocacy, and information and referral services.

Congenitally blinded or early-blinded and visually impaired individuals frequently reach adulthood with severe social and emotional difficulties, as well as deficits of self-concept and of concepts of the world and others in it (Luxton, 1981). Social skills deficits and emotional immaturity make it difficult for blind persons to become integrated into society and to achieve success in school or work environments.

Parents and teachers of visually impaired children may become overprotective and, unknowingly, isolate the child from necessary services. Furthermore, segregation of the visually impaired child in the educational setting may be unintentionally prolonged. Subsequently, when these children are placed in classes to negotiate the academic environment and become "successfully mainstreamed," they often fail at social skills (Scholl, 1981).

The literature and opinions of professionals are occasionally contradictory on these issues. Resnick (1983), in a study of the responses of 74 congenitally and totally blind respondents to an integration questionnaire, found that, on the average, these persons felt accepted in early childhood and had a combination of segregated and integrated school experiences. These individuals belonged to both sighted and blind groups, graduated from college, and mainly had sighted friends with no visual impairment. Despite the limitations of the study, such as self-reporting and a rather homogeneous sample, Resnick suggests the results showed that respondents had a predominantly positive self-image. It becomes apparent that the issue of severe social and emotional difficulties among congenitally blinded or early-blinded individuals is problematic, due to the lack of a clear focus on the parameters of the problem, and to the varying experiences of rehabilitation counselors in handling such problems.

Service Delivery Issues

In addition to the need for specific services for sensory-impaired persons, there is also a need for improvements in the coordination and quality of the entire service delivery system. In the area of hearing impairment, it appears that the service delivery system has moved away somewhat from the suggestions of the model state plan (MSP) for rehabilitation of deaf clients (Schein, 1980). The MSP, developed to address the unique needs of hearing-impaired rehabilitation clients, and readily endorsed by the Council of State Administrators in Vocational Rehabilitation (CSAVR) and major professional organizations, calls for state coordinators of services for the deaf (SCDs) and rehabilitation counselors for the deaf (RCDs) in each state. These specialized personnel are considered essential in meeting the need for highly specialized and coordinated services for this population. With the current limitations in available funding, however, some states have eliminated the SCD position or have combined it with other duties, potentially weakening the effectiveness of the position. Similar actions have been taken with RCD positions, often replacing the specialized counselor with a generalist who may lack appropriate communication skills and specialized knowledge needed to appropriately serve this population.

A second issue involves the lack of standards regarding hiring criteria for RCDs that can have a negative impact on the provision of services to hearing-impaired clients, particularly the lower functioning deaf client. In order to provide quality services, RCDs must have a broad range of skills and knowledge, including communicative competence and a thorough understanding of the educational, vocational, social, and psychological implications of the disability. These skills and knowledge are required above and beyond the competencies necessary for all rehabilitation counselors. However, less than half of all state agencies have developed competency-referenced job descriptions for RCDs (Danek, 1984). Among states with such job descriptions, there is no universal standard against which to measure actual performance.

Similarly, blindness and visual impairment are severe disabilities that inherently require specialized services (Maxson, 1984). Since 1879, a network of services for blind and visually impaired individuals has provided services to persons in the United States (Koestler, 1976). Agencies and individuals, through education and experience, develop the skills unique to counseling, instruction, and program management in blindness.

Professionally qualified workers are often not available to provide quality services to blind individuals who seek rehabilitation services from state and private agencies in the United States. A study by Uslan, Asenjo, and Peck (1982) examined the demands for rehabilitation teachers (RTs) in 1981. Two measures were used in this study to document the demands for RTs: economic demand (budgeted vacancies) and perceived need (desired new positions above and beyond budgeted vacancies).

State and private agencies, veterans' administrations, and residential schools were surveyed. Of the 259 agencies surveyed, 219 responded. The results revealed over twice as many budgeted vacancies for rehabilitation teachers as there were graduates of university training programs. With projections to 1990 indicating a growth in the numbers of blind and visually impaired persons needing rehabilitation services, the shortage could become greater.

In a similar study of orientation and mobility (O&M) personnel needs in 1980, Uslan, Peck, and Kirchner (1981) found a "tight balance" (p. 8) between the supply and demand of O&M specialists. Despite projections of increased numbers of visually impaired and blind persons, monies set aside to increase the numbers of qualified professionals has decreased. For example, a

1981 poll of university training programs revealed a 55% drop in federal funding (Gruman, 1982). The negative impact of these cuts on the enrollment in training programs should further reduce the supply of qualified persons.

The reductions in federal-state funding for rehabilitation services are also having an adverse affect on the quality of personnel in rehabilitation agencies, and on the quality and comprehensiveness of services. For example, many vocational rehabilitation (VR) agencies are asking their counselors to work with blind and visually impaired persons without providing additional training. Few agencies require their counselors, rehabilitation teachers, or orientation and mobility specialists to be certified (Nelipovich, Godley, & Vieceli, 1982). Currently, because of budgetary constraints (among other reasons), one state is considering having its state O&M employees provide outdoor instruction to more than one client at a time, a directive that may expose clients, instructors, agencies, and states to increased liability. It is evident that those who employ counselors to work with blind clients do not yet adequately recognize the need for special skills and education to provide high quality, comprehensive services.

The EIRI (1984) identified a number of similar services provision issues affecting the delivery of services to deaf-blind persons. Of major concern is the question of which agency (i.e., that serving blind, deaf, or general clients) should serve deaf-blind persons. The EIRI document urges that a clear policy be developed on this issue to meet the service needs of deaf-blind persons, and that resources needed by the deaf-blind persons be made accessible. Where possible, the primary service provider should be the agency serving the deaf-blind person's disability identity group: as a deaf person with a visual loss, or a blind person with a hearing loss.

Other issues involved in providing rehabilitation services to deaf-blind persons center around the low incidence of the combined disabilities. Factors to be considered include geographic accessibility, staff-to-client ratio, time allotment, family service needs, and communication issues (EIRI, 1984). Also of concern is the need for interagency cooperation to meet the range of needs of deaf-blind persons. Since these needs are often too broad and too extensive for any single agency to meet, Gottula (1984) suggests the need for development of a state plan for this population with a major change in orientation, one in which agency personnel look beyond their own particular sphere to consider the whole spectrum of a deaf-blind person's life. Only through such an approach can a deaf-blind person's needs be discovered and the best agencies for addressing those needs identified. One such model for interagency cooperation is available in the Kansas P.L.A.N. (Participating Life-Long Plan for Affecting Needs), which employs a state coordinator of deaf-blind services and a number of resource service coordinators. The state coordinator's salary is shared by five cooperating agencies, and clear responsibilities for each agency are defined (EIRI, 1984).

Special Need Subpopulations

Historically, sensory-impaired persons have been treated in the literature as a homogeneous group, with few distinctions regarding unique subgroup needs. More recently, however, a growing recognition that sensory-impaired persons have a full range of traits, abilities, and limitations has been emerging in the profession. There is also a growing recognition that certain subsections of this population have special needs. It is the belief of the authors that four special-need subpopulations require specialized attention and services from the rehabilitation community. These subgroups and the special problems they present include persons with sensory impairment: 1) who are elderly, 2) who live in rural areas, 3) who have disabilities mild enough to be considered ''hidden,'' and/or 4) who have multiple disabilities.

Elderly Persons With Sensory Impairments The U.S. Bureau of the Census (1977) has projected that by the year 2000, 31 million people will be 65 years of age or older, compared to 23 million in 1977. Many of these individuals will develop sensory impairments and, thus add to the population of elderly persons with hearing and/or visual loss. Few existing programs are available to meet the needs of elderly sensory-impaired persons. While many individuals can turn to volunteer community organizations such as deaf senior citizens groups, significant needs remain that require social service interventions. Criswell (1979) listed isolation, financial concerns, stereotypes about both deafness and growing old, and substandard housing as some of the major problems faced by older hearing-impaired individuals. Becker (1980) noted that old age is itself like a disability, in that it affects one's role and social status—older hearing-impaired persons may be multiply handicapped by both age and hearing impairment.

The increase in the availability of independent living services has lagged behind the increased numbers of elderly sensory-impaired persons. Reasons given for this lack of concern center around the philosophy that rehabilitation services are oriented toward employability and vocational skill development (Dickman, 1977). Gross (1979) and others (Asch, 1980; Beattie, 1976) note that rehabilitation services are primarily ''geared towards young and working blind persons because the return on investment will be higher than if the same sum of money is invested in services for the elderly, where little or no monetary profit is feasible'' (p. 50). However, Gross (1979) argued that, given the findings that home or community care represents definite cost savings over nursing home care, policy makers should be inclined to apportion monies to the former.

In addition, older persons who might choose to continue to contribute actively to society find the choice taken out of their hands. As more Americans enjoy good health longer than their parents, many find age 65 to be an arbitrary cut-off date and, instead of retiring, begin new careers, as either paid workers or highly experienced volunteers. As a greater percentage of the population becomes elderly in the next century, not only will society depend on older citizens to continue functioning, but the retirement age may well rise; expectations for activity over 65 will change; and it may be "in" to be over 65 and active.

Older people also may not receive needed services because of their concern about being identified as deaf or blind (Kaarlela, 1978; Kass, 1980). Because elderly blind persons cease discussing their vision problems, many who would benefit from a variety of services are unknown to the service providers (Kass, 1980). Further, Asch (1980) suggests that services are unavailable because there is a high cost associated with the services needed by this population. A study of residents of buildings for elderly and handicapped persons in New York City suggests that the health-related social and psychological service needs of the elderly blind population may exceed those of their sighted counterparts (Gillman, Simmel, & Simon, 1986).

Despite these negatives, a number of agencies, both private and public, have begun to respond to the needs of this growing population. Programs have included in-service training programs to nursing home and church personnel, peer counseling discussion groups, aids such as writing guides and white canes, and home teaching programs where clients may learn adaptive living techniques (Asch, 1980; Beyers-Lang, 1984).

In addition to discussing the independent living needs of older sensory-impaired persons, consideration should also be given to those confined to institutional settings due to illness or accident. Mobility training and other adaptive techniques can increase independence, thereby decreasing dependence on institutional staff, and lowering the risk to health that so often follows surrendering one's self-reliance (Hill & Harley, 1984).

Rural Populations While the needs of potential rehabilitation clients residing in rural communities have begun to be recognized in the literature, virtually no research or writing exists on the needs of sensory-impaired individuals in rural settings. Already isolated by the nature of their disability, these individuals may not receive vocational rehabilitation and other crucial services. Transportation is often a major problem in rural areas, a fact that has implications not only for rehabilitation services related to independent living, but also for access to work, shopping, and health care. Another problem experienced by rural disabled persons is simply the lack of information about resources.

Partial Sensory Impairment The lack of literature available on the special needs of partially sensory-impaired clients is striking in comparison to the rapidly growing body of knowledge about more severely hearing-impaired and deaf individuals. Jackson (1979) noted that the hard-of-hearing individual is, ironically, often faced with additional difficulties because his or her handicap is not obvious. As a result, the individual may have diverse needs that are often overlooked. Persons who are hard-of-hearing may be particularly disadvantaged in receiving vocational rehabilitation services, in that they do not fit into the traditional case loads consisting of either mildly hearing-impaired persons who need only a hearing aid to function optimally, or profoundly deaf clients who need highly specialized services to address their developmental deficits and sign language communication needs. Often, hard-of-hearing individuals are in need of comprehensive vocational services, including development of appropriate work skills, habits, and attitudes. While the language skills of these individuals may be superior to those of clients who are deaf, they may have severe gaps in their knowledge of work and independent living. These gaps are often more apparent when the severely hard-of-hearing individual has been mainstreamed into special education classes and is making the transition from school to work.

Multiply Disabled/Low-Functioning Persons with Sensory Impairments Sensory-impaired persons with multiple disabilities often require specialized facilities for appropriate services. Traditionally, however, emphasis has focused on the more numerous clients who have only one impairment. For example, since 1938, legislation such as the Wagner-O'Day Act has created and expanded employment opportunities for blind and visually impaired persons. Consequently, the workshops serving blind persons have become a valuable resource for the evaluation, training, and employment of rehabilitation counselors serving blind individuals.

The referral and cooperative agreements between counselors and facilities have encouraged rehabilitation for many blind persons through short-term and long-term employment opportunities. But many rehabilitation agencies have attempted to serve multiply disabled persons much as they do the traditionally targeted population (Cotton & Wade, 1984). As a consequence, numerous inappropriate institutional placements have occurred with persons who might have otherwise successfully participated in a sheltered workshop or community work/living environment (Cotton & Wade, 1984).

Also underserved are individuals with singular sensory impairments who function at the lower end of the spectrum of vocational, independent living, and social skills. For example, most available vocational services for hearing-impaired persons, including post-secondary training programs, are geared to serve the higher-functioning client. In FY 1980, $38,977,000 in federal funds was appropriated for post-secondary education of deaf persons (Peterson, 1981). In sharp contrast, appropriations for programs serving severely handicapped multiply disabled deaf clients totalled only $357,158.

Most vocational rehabilitation counselors find it easier to serve the college-bound hearing-impaired person than the lower-functioning client, despite the federal emphasis on serving severely disabled persons. Hanson (1980) notes that it is easier to support a 5-year college program for a capable deaf client than it is to support a 6-month work adjustment program for a multiply handicapped deaf client. The deaf college student need only demonstrate a "C" average to warrant the continuation of rehabilitation funds, whereas there is an expectation that lower-functioning deaf clients should demonstrate substantial improvement on detailed progress reports every 4 weeks. As Hanson (1980) notes, "Panic sets in if that client isn't showing dramatic progress at the end of 12 weeks" (p. 1).

In addition to the critical lack of funding for these individuals and the limiting effects of state agency policies, there is a paucity of facilities available to meet the needs of low-functioning and/or multiply handicapped, sensory-impaired persons. Quality rehabilitation centers, independent living programs, group homes and halfway houses, and sheltered workshops geared to their needs are desperately needed.

Conclusion

While the needs of sensory-impaired persons are varied and complex, the attention of the rehabilitation profession should immediately focus on four primary areas. First, there is a need to adjust the service delivery system to address the unique concerns of this population. The rehabilitation profession must consider the complexity of providing services to sensory-impaired persons, as well as the fact that rehabilitation of these individuals may often require a greater than average expenditure of time, energy, and money. Case load sizes need to be reduced and appropriate support services provided to enable counselors and other rehabilitation professionals to be maximally effective in serving this population. Further, there is a need for a strong and coordinated service delivery system that will meet their unique needs. This system should take into account the developmental nature of these disabilities and coordinate services with clients and their families, the educational system, and the adult service delivery network, including vocational rehabilitation.

Second, the existence of subgroups of sensory-impaired persons must be recognized and their needs addressed. There is a mandate to respond to special-need subgroups within the sensory-impaired population, including elderly persons, multiply disabled individuals, and sensory-impaired persons who reside in rural areas. Independent living training is of concern to these and other segments of the sensory-disabled population, as are issues related to gainful employment. Toward this goal, a series of studies is recommended to determine functional levels of clients with different types, degrees, and combinations of sensory impairments. The results of these studies could be used to develop a standardized case difficulty index that would correlate the functional level of a sensory-impaired client with the time and financial expenditure needed to provide appropriate services. Such a tool would enable administrators to accurately assess the adequacy of an agency's staff and budget to meet the unique and complex needs of sensory-impaired persons.

Third, both long- and short-term training opportunities are needed to increase the skills and knowledge of professionals serving this population. Both rehabilitation counseling and program administration training programs should include specific instruction and, if possible, practical experience in providing services in addition to other specialization or general rehabilitation training. This comprehensive training would also cover the provision of appropriate services to persons with partial sensory impairments, including hard-of-hearing persons and those with partial sight. More emphasis in training should also be placed on the need of multiply disabled persons and individuals with sensory impairments who are low functioning. To adopt these more comprehensive and more demanding training objectives, university and specialty rehabilitation training programs will require increased federal funding as well as aggressive planning and implementation.

Among practicing rehabilitation professionals, continuing training opportunities will increase their ability to give clients with varying impairments a broad continuum of rehabilitation services. Continuing education programs that will foster understanding and cooperation between education and rehabilitation professionals are of particular importance to the provision of quality services to this population. Additional training in the areas of transition from school to work and supported employment is needed. In-service training programs for blindness specialists are needed to better acquaint these specialists with the specific problems and communication issues related to serving deaf-blind persons. Similarly, specialists who work with deaf clients need professional training in issues related to visual impairment.

In-service training is also valuable for professionals from allied human service disciplines whose expertise is needed by sensory-impaired persons. Independent living instructors could benefit from programs that address the adaptation of existing services to sensory-impaired persons. Mental health professionals, including counselors, social workers, and psychologists, could gain communication skills and awareness of the special issues facing their sensory-impaired clients. By sensitizing these individuals to the special considerations involved in serving sensory-impaired persons, serious gaps in service delivery can be closed. Finally, short-term training programs could train sensory-impaired and other interested persons who could provide many services as peer counselors or fill other paraprofessional roles, such as job coaches.

Finally, research and demonstration projects are needed to develop a strong knowledge base and appropriate tools to assist rehabilitation professionals in serving this population. Research is needed to identify discrete and specific competencies needed by specialists who serve hearing-impaired, visually impaired, and deaf-blind persons. The results of such an effort would be useful in the professional certification process and to accreditation bodies evaluating professional preparation programs.

Research and demonstration projects in the area of prevocational and transitional services are also needed. Early involvement of state rehabilitation agencies with sensory-impaired youth (prior to age 15) in both mainstreamed and residential settings is mandatory for effective transitioning. Such involvement is facilitated when state rehabilitation agencies and school programs work together to develop summer evaluation, career awareness, and work adjustment programs targeted toward early vocational experiences for school-aged youth. Mason and West (1979) suggest that such cooperation could result in the creation of a joint individualized education program/individualized written rehabilitation program (IEP/IWRP) or a "written individualized education and rehabilitation program" (WIERP).

Independent living research could include a survey of existing centers and programs to determine their accessibility to sensory-impaired persons. Additional funding is also needed for independent living services authorized by Title VII, Part C of the Rehabilitation Act to include assistance to visually impaired persons through the provision of eye glasses, visual aids, medical treatment, orientation and mobility training, rehabilitation teaching, counseling, reader services, Braille instruction, and transportation (PL 93-112 as amended).

Research is also needed to identify the most effective methods and techniques for serving special subpopulations, including the partially sensory-impaired, multiply disabled and low-functioning individuals, elderly persons, and those who reside in rural areas. It is particularly important that the service delivery system now begins cooperatively to prepare to identify and serve the growing number of elderly persons with sensory impairments. Finally, research is needed regarding the possibility of developing rural rehabilitation and independent living specialists to serve outlying areas, perhaps using an itinerant model.

There is also a need for research and demonstration projects related to specialized services for sensory-impaired persons. Additional vocational and psychological assessment instruments appropriate to the needs of sensory-impaired persons need to be developed, standardized, and validated. Suggested criteria might also be developed to assist counselors in determining a particular facility's capability for serving sensory-impaired persons. Exemplary facilities that might be able to provide technical assistance in this area could be identified. Guidelines for service could potentially be included in such standards as those of the Commission of Accreditation of Rehabilitation Facilities (CARF). Finally, a national directory of qualified resource persons who provide mental health services to this population could be assembled and disseminated.

With regards to employment, research is needed on job placement methodologies and techniques. Additional curricula and teaching materials for job-related vocabulary, concepts, and job-seeking procedures are needed, as are studies of the effectiveness of job clubs and other client-centered placement efforts. There is also a need to firmly establish the numbers of working-age blind and visually impaired persons—whether visual impairment is a primary or secondary disability—and to identify the occupations and jobs currently being performed by those who are working.

Another objective in promoting employment among sensory-impaired persons would be the establishment of a priority system to protect the interests of multiply disabled workers and support the three-tiered system of priorities under the Javits-Wagner-O'Day Act. Separate appropriations for Randolph-Shepard Act programs should be secured to create additional employment opportunities (Randolf-Sheppard Vending Stand Act, 1936; Erickson & Wyrick, 1984). Medicaid and Medicare reimbursement for low-vision services is also recommended.

REFERENCES

Amrine, C., & Bullis, M. (1985). The job club approach to placement: A viable tool? *Journal of Rehabilitation of the Deaf, 19,* 18–22.

Asch, C. (1980). Training senior citizens center staff in blind rehabilitation techniques. *Journal of Visual Impairment and Blindness, 74*(5), 183–185.

Austin, G. F. (1983). Independent and dependent characteristics and service needs of deaf people: A levels model. In D. Watson, G. Anderson, P. Marut, S. Ouellette, & N. Ford (Eds.), *Vocational evaluation of hearing-impaired persons: Research and practice* (pp. 7–24). Little Rock: University of Arkansas, Rehabilitation Research and Training Center on Deafness and Hearing Impairment.

Azrin, N., & Besalel, V. A. (1980). *Job club counselor's manual: A behavioral approach to vocational counseling.* Baltimore: University Park Press.

Bauman, M. K. (1975). Guided vocational choice. *New Outlook for the Blind, 69,* 354–360.

Beattie, W. M. (1976). Aging and the social services. In R. H. Binstock & E. Shanas (Eds.), *Handbook of aging and the social sciences* (pp. 619–642). New York: Van Nostrand Reinhold.

Becker, G. (1980). *Growing old in silence.* Berkeley: University of California.

Beyers-Lang, R. (1984). Peer counselors: Network builders for elderly persons. *Journal of Visual Impairment and Blindness, 78*(5), 193–197.

Bolton, B. (1975). Preparing deaf youths for employment. *Journal of Rehabilitation of the Deaf, 9,* 11–16.

Bradley-Johnson, S. (1986). *Psychoeducational assessment of visually impaired and blind students.* Austin, TX: PRO-ED.

Brolin, D. E. (1976). *Vocational preparation of retarded citizens.* Columbus, OH: Charles E. Merrill.

Busse, D. G., Romer, L. T., Fewell, R. R., & Vadasy, P. F. (1985). Employment of deaf blind rubella students in a subsidized work program. *Journal of Visual Impairment and Blindness, 79*(2), 59–64.

Colenbrander, A. (1976). VH, visually impaired: What's the difference? *The California Transcriber, 18*(3), 106.

Cotton, R. D., & Wade, J. P. (1984). A demonstration work activities center for multiply handicapped, visually impaired persons. *Journal of Visual Impairment and Blindness, 78*(7), 303–306.

Crewe, N. M., & Zola, I. K. (1983). *Independent living for physically disabled people.* San Francisco: Jossey-Bass.

Criswell, E. C. (1979). Deaf Action Center's senior citizens program. *Journal of Rehabilitation of the Deaf, 12,* 36–40.

Danek, M. (1987, May). *Deafness rehabilitation needs and competencies.* Paper presented at the meeting of the American Deafness and Rehabilitation Association, Minneapolis, MN.

Dickman, I. R. (1977). *Outreach to the aging blind: Some strategies for community action.* New York: American Foundation for the Blind.

Dorland's illustrated medical dictionary. (1984). Philadelphia: W. B. Saunders.

Doyle, S., Burch, D., Paoletti-Schelp, M., & Richards, L. (1984). Independent living services. In D. Watson, S. Barret, & R. Brown (Eds.), *A model service delivery system for deaf-blind persons* (pp. 15–24). Little Rock: University of Arkansas Rehabilitation Research and Training Center on Deafness and Hearing Impairment.

Dwyer, C. (1983). Job seeking and job retention skill training with hearing impaired persons. In D. Watson, G. Anderson, N. Ford, P. Marut, & S. Ouellette (Eds.), *Job placement of hearing-impaired persons: Research and practice* (pp. 17–26). Little Rock: University of Arkansas Rehabilitation Research and Training Center on Deafness and Hearing Impairment.

Eleventh Institute on Rehabilitation Issues. (1984). *Strategies for serving deaf-blind clients.* Hot Springs: Arkansas Rehabilitation Research and Training Center.

Erickson, G. D., & Wyrick, D. (1984). The national trend of cooperation in services to deaf-blind multi-handicapped persons. In G. L. Goodrich (Ed.), *Yearbook of the Association for Education and Rehabilitation of the Blind and Visually Impaired* (pp. 20–37). Alexandria, VA: Association for Education and Rehabilitation of the Blind and Visually Impaired.

Federal Register, Volume 38, Number 196, Part 121.C.37, October 11, 1973.

Ferrel, K. (1985). Infancy and early childhood. In G. T. Scholl (Ed.), *Foundations of education for blind and visually handicapped children and youth.* New York: American Federation for the Blind.

Furth, H. G. (1973). *Deafness and learning: A psychosocial approach.* Belmont, CA: Wadsworth.

Genensky, S. (1978). Data concerning the partially sighted and functionally blind. *Journal of Visual Impairment and Blindness, 72,* 177–180.

Gillman, A. E., Simmel, A., & Simon, E. P. (1986). Visual handicap in the aged: Self-reported visual disability and the quality of life of residents of public housing for the elderly. *Journal of Visual Impairment and Blindness, 50*(2), 588–590.

Gottula, P. (1984). Interagency cooperation. In D. Watson, S. Barrett, & R. Brown (Eds.), *A model service delivery system for deaf-blind persons* (pp. 39–43). Little Rock: University of Arkansas Rehabilitation Research and Training Center on Deafness and Hearing Impairment.

Gross, A. M. (1979). Preventing institutionalization of elderly blind persons. *Journal of Visual Impairment and Blindness, 72,* 49–53.

Gruman, D. (1982). A survey of teacher training programs. *Journal of Visual Impairment and Blindness, 76,* 377.

Hanson, J. (1980, March). *SCD News* [Des Moines, IA], p. 1.

Helen Keller National Center for Deaf-Blind Youths and Adults. (1983). *Annual report.* Sands Point, NY: Author.

Hill, M., & Harley, R. K. (1984). Orientation and mobility for aged visually impaired persons. *Journal of Visual Impairment and Blindness, 78*(2), 49–54.

Holt, E. W. (1985). *A statewide model of delivering independent living services to deaf persons.* In B. Heller & D. Watson (Eds.), *Mental health and deafness: Strategic perspectives* (pp. 24–32). Silver Spring, MD: American Deafness and Rehabilitation Association.

Jackson, P. J. (1979). Special problems of the hard-of-hearing. *Journal of Rehabilitation of the Deaf, 12,* 13–26.

Kaarlela, R. (1978). A survey of the characteristics and needs of two selected groups of older blind persons (Doctoral dissertation, University of Michigan). *Dissertation Abstracts International, 39,* 813A–814A.

Kahn, H. A., & Moorhead, H. B. (1973). *Statistics on blindness in the model reporting area, 1969-70.* Washington, DC: U.S. Government Printing Office.

Kass, G. M. (1980, October). The elderly blind and the plain brown wrapper. *Braille Monitor,* pp. 402–406.

Kirchner, C. (1981). National statistics on employment of blind and visually handicapped persons: Developing some baselines to measure the effects of mainstreaming. *AAWB Annual,* 119–134.

Kirchner, C., & Lowman, C. (1978). Sources of variation in the estimated prevalence of visual loss. *Journal of Visual Impairment and Blindness, 72*(8), 329–333.

Kirchner, C., & Peterson, R. (1979). Employment: Selected characteristics. *Journal of Visual Impairment and Blindness, 73*(6), 239–242.

Kirchner, C., & Peterson, R. (1980). Worktime, occupational status, and annual earnings: An assessment of underemployment. *Journal of Visual Impairment and Blindness, 74*(5), 203–205.

Koestler, F. (1976). *The unseen minority.* New York: David McKay.

Knight, J. (1972). Mannerisms in the congenitally blind child. *New Outlook for the Blind, 66,* 297–302.

Langley, M. B. (1980). *The teachable moment and the handicapped infant.* Reston, VA: Council for Exceptional Children, CROC Clearing House on Handicapped & Gifted Children.

Levine, E. (1960). *Psychology of deafness: Techniques of appraisal for rehabilitation.* New York: Columbia University.

Levine, E. S. (1981). *The ecology of early deafness: Guides to fashioning environments and psychological assessments.* New York: Columbia University.

Lombana, J. H. (1980). Career planning with visually handicapped students. *Vocational Guidance Quarterly, 28,* 219–224.

Lorenz, J. R. (1975). Work samples and the growing challanges of evaluation. In M. K. Bauman (Ed.), *Use of work samples with blind clients.* Philadelphia: Nevil Interagency Referral Service.

Lowman, C., & Kirchner, C. (1979). Elderly blind and visually impaired persons: Projected numbers in the year 2000. *Journal of Visual Impairment and Blindness, 73,* 69–73.

Luxton, K. (1981). A jigsaw puzzle: Constructing a sound bridge to adulthood for visually handicapped adolescents. *AAWB Annual,* 97–105.

Marut, P., Watson, D., & Buford, D. (1984). *The national directory of rehabilitation facilities offering vocational evaluation and adjustment training to hearing-impaired persons.* Little Rock: University of Arkansas Rehabilitation Research and Training Center on Deafness and Hearing Impairment.

Mason, A., & West, J. H. (1979). *The written individualized rehabilitation and education program.* Unpublished manuscript. (Available from South Central Regional Center for Services to Deaf-Blind Children, 2930 Turtle Creek Plaza, Suite 107, Dallas, TX 75219.

Maxson, J. (1984, June). *Winning isn't everything—It's the only thing.* Paper presented at AAWB-AEVH Alliance, Nashville, TN.

McHugh, D. (1975). A view of deaf people in terms of Super's theory of vocational development. *Journal of Rehabilitation of the Deaf, 9,* 1–11.

Mindel, E., & Vernon, M. (1971). *They grow in silence: The deaf child and his family.* Silver Spring, MD: National Association of the Deaf.

Moore, S. (1984). The need for programs and services for visually impaired handicapped infants. *Education of the Visually Impaired, 16,* 48–57.

National Center for Health Statistics. (1975). *Prevalence of selected impairments: United States, 1971* (DHEW Publication No. 75-1526). Washington, DC: U.S. Government Printing Office.

National Society for the Prevention of Blindness. (1966). *Estimated statistics on blindness and visual problems.* New York: Author.

Nelipovich, M., Godley, S. H., & Vieceli, L. (1982). Job descriptions of rehabilitation teachers and O & M specialists in state agencies. *Journal of Visual Impairment and Blindness, 76*(5), 191–194.

Nelipovich, M., & Naegele, L. (1984). Communication. In D. Watson, S. Barrett, & R. Brown (Eds.), *A model service delivery system for deaf-blind persons* (pp. 25–32). Little Rock: University of Arkansas Rehabilitation Research and Training Center on Deafness and Hearing Impairment.

Ouellette, S. (1984). Deaf-blind population estimates. In D. Watson, S. Barrett, & R. Brown (Eds.), *A model service delivery system for deaf-blind persons* (pp. 7–10). Little Rock: University of Arkansas Rehabilitation Research and Training Center on Deafness and Hearing Impairment.

Ouellette, S., El-Khiami, A., & Schroedel, J. (1984, November). *A study of postsecondary education for deaf people in the United States.* Paper presented at the regional Conference on Postsecondary Education for Hearing-Impaired Persons, Knoxville, TN.

Ouellette, S., & Lloyd, G. T. (Eds.). (1980). *Independent living skills for the severely handicapped deaf person preparing to enter gainful employment.* Silver Spring, MD: American Deafness and Rehabilitation Association.

Peterson, E. (1981). The two sides of habilitation/rehabilitation services for the deaf. *Journal of Rehabilitation of the Deaf, 14,* 14–25.

Peterson, M. (1985). Work evaluation of blind and visually impaired persons for technical, professional, and managerial positions. *Journal of Visual Impairment and Blindness, 79*(10), 478–480.

Piaget, J. (1952). *The origins of intelligence in children* (2nd ed.). New York: International Universities.

Rainer, J., Altshuler, K., & Kallman, F. (1969). *Family and mental health problems in a deaf population* (2nd ed.). Springfield, IL: Charles C Thomas.

Randolf-Sheppard Vending Stand Act of 1936 (PL 74-732), as amended by PL 83-565 and PL 93-516, § 20 U.S.C., Ch. 6A, § 107.

Rawlings, B. (1973). *Characteristics of hearing-impaired students by hearing status, United States: 1970–71* (Series D., Number 10). Washington, DC: Gallaudet College, Office of Demographic Studies.

Rawlings, B., Karchmer, M. A., & DeCaro, J. J. (1983). *College and career programs for deaf students.* Washington, DC: Gallaudet College.

Resnick, R. (1983). An exploratory study of the lifestyles of congenitally blind adults. *Journal of Visual Impairment and Blindness, 77*(10), 476–481.

Robinson, L. W. (1983). A survey study to develop and demonstrate feasibility of a national data base for visual impairment (Doctoral dissertation, Brigham Young University). *Dissertation Abstracts International, 44,* 1392A–1393A.

Schein, J. D. (1964). Factors in the definition of deafness as they relate to incidence and prevalence. In *Proceedings of the conference on the collection of statistics of severe hearing impairments and deafness in the United States* (Public Health Service Publication No. 1227). Washington, DC: U.S. Government Printing office.

Schein, J. D. (Ed.). (1980). *Model state plan for vocational rehabilitation of deaf clients* (2nd rev.). New York: Deafness Research and Training Center.

Schein, J. D., & Delk, M. T. (1974). *The deaf population of the United States.* Silver Spring, MD: National Association of the Deaf.

Schlesinger, H. S., & Meadow, K. P. (1972). *Sound and sign: Childhood deafness and mental health.* Berkeley: University of California Press.

Scholl, G. T. (1981). Impacts of mainstreaming during career building: Ages 13–21. *AAWB Annual,* 72–80.

Scholl, G. (1983). Assessing the visually impaired child. In S. Ray, M. J. O'Neil, & N. T. Morris (Eds.), *Low incidence children: A guide to psychoeducational assessment* (pp. 67–90). Natchitdoches, LA: Steven Ray.

Scott, R. (1969). The socialization of blind children. In D. A. Goslin (Ed.), *Handbook of socialization theory and research* (pp. 1025–1046). Chicago: Rand McNally.

Spain, J. B. (1981). Employment of handicapped people: An enigmatic future. *Journal of Visual Impairment and Blindness, 75,* 122–125.

Spungin, S. J. (1982). The future role of residential schools for visually handicapped children. *Journal of Visual Impairment and Blindness, 76*(6), 229–233.

Taff-Watson, M. (1984) Population definition. In D. Watson, S. Barrett, & R. Brown (Eds.), *A model service delivery system for deaf-blind persons* (pp. 3–5). Little Rock: University of Arkansas Rehabilitation Research and Training Center on Deafness and Hearing Impairment.

Torretti, W. T. (1983). The placement process with severely disabled deaf persons. In D. Watson, G. Anderson, N. Ford, P. Marut, & S. Ouellette (Eds.), *Job placement of hearing-impaired persons: Research and practice* (pp. 51–69). Little Rock: University of Arkansas Rehabilitation Research and Training Center in Deafness and Hearing Impairment.

U.S. Bureau of the Census. (1977). *Projections of the population of the United States: 1977–2050.* Current population reports, Series P-25, No. 204. Washington, DC: U.S. Government Printing Office.

Uslan, M. M., Asenjo, J. A., & Peck, A. F. (1982). Demand for rehabilitation teachers in 1981. *Journal of Visual Impairment and Blindness, 76*(10), 412–416.

Uslan, M. M., Peck, A. F., & Kirchner, C. (1981). Demand for orientation and mobility specialists in 1980. *Journal of Visual Impairment and Blindness, 75*(1), 8–12.

Vander Kolk, C. (1981). *Assessment and planning with the visually impaired.* Baltimore: University Park Press.

Veatch, D. (1984). Intervention strategies to ease the transition from school to work for deaf adolescents. In G. B. Anderson & D. Watson (Eds.), *The habilitation and rehabilitation of deaf adolescents* (pp. 317–325). Washington, DC: The National Academy of Gallaudet College.

Vieceli, L. (1972). Placement in competitive employment. In R. Hardy (Ed.), *Social and rehabilitation services for the blind* (pp. 58–69). Springfield, IL: Charles C Thomas.

Warren, D. (1984). *Blindness and early childhood development* (2nd ed.). New York: American Federation for the Blind.

Watson, D. (Ed.). (1977). *Deaf evaluation and adjustment feasibility*. New York: Deafness Research and Training Center.

Watson, D. (1985). Strategic interventions for the job placement of deaf persons. In B. Heller & D. Watson (Eds.), *Mental health and deafness: Strategic perspectives* (pp. 286–296). Silver Spring, MD: American Deafness and Rehabilitation Association.

Watson, D., Anderson, G., Marut, P., Ouellette, S., & Ford, N. (Eds.). (1983). *Vocational evaluation of hearing-impaired persons: Research and practice*. Little Rock: University of Arkansas Rehabilitation Research and Training Center on Deafness and Hearing Impairment.

West-Evans, K., & Shiels, J. W. (1983). Projects with industry: A model for placement of deaf clients. In D. Watson, G. Anderson, N. Ford, P. Marut, & S. Ouellette (Eds.), *Job placement of hearing-impaired persons: Research and practice* (pp. 71–82). Little Rock: University of Arkansas Research and Training Center on Deafness and Hearing Impairment.

Wolf, E., Delk, M., & Schein, J. (1982). *Needs assessment of services to deaf-blind individuals* [Final report to the U.S. Department of Education]. Silver Spring, MD: Rehabilitation and Education Experts.

10

Neoplastic Disease

Considerations for the Rehabilitation Profession

John D. Dolan, Harry A. Allen, and Terry Tregle Bell

The Commission on Chronic Illness has defined chronic illness as

> any impairment or deviation from normal that has one or more of the following characteristics: (1) is permanent; (2) leaves residual disability; (3) is caused by non-reversible pathological alteration; and (4) may be expected to require a long period of observation, supervision or care. (Mayo, 1956, p. 9)

Neoplastic disease, commonly known as cancer, falls within this definition, as its victims often manifest not just one but all four of these characteristics (Dolan, 1983).

Cancer is a general term for more than 100 diseases that are characterized by an abnormal and uncontrolled growth of cells. The resulting mass or tumor possesses the capacity to invade and destroy surrounding normal tissue, thus interfering with the body's normal functioning. To further complicate matters, these cancer cells have the ability to metastasize or travel through the body (National Cancer Institute, 1981).

While cancer strikes any age and kills more children between the ages of 3 and 14 than any other disease, it strikes more frequently with advancing age. About 71 million Americans alive today will eventually be confronted with the disease, which strikes three out of every four families.

Of all diseases, cancer evokes the greatest fear. Even though twice as many Americans die from heart disease each year, more people fear death by cancer than by heart disease (National Cancer Institute, 1981). Cancer has a devastating impact on the individual as well as on the family. The intense fear this disease evokes, coupled with its ever-increasing incidence and the enormous expense to the individual and society, dictate that efforts be directed toward understanding the psychological, social, and physical implications of cancer. The American Cancer Society reports that over 5,000,000 Americans have had a history of cancer. Three million of these Americans are considered cured, and their life expectancies are equal to the life expectancies of individuals who have not had cancer (American Cancer Society, 1985). As a result of improved treatment methods the survival trend is expected to improve and the probability of 5-year survival will likewise improve. As survival rates increase, more individuals and families will face adjustment issues related to the disease and its treatment. Rehabilitation professionals must address the rising needs of this population.

This chapter addresses the economic considerations of cancer and its treatment; current modes of treatment, including psychobehavioral treatment modalities; the psychological impact of cancer on the individual and the family; the vocational considerations of cancer; and, finally, implications for rehabilitation counselors.

ECONOMIC COSTS OF CANCER

Direct and Indirect Costs

The precise costs of cancer are difficult to estimate. Nevertheless, direct costs (hospital, doctors, drugs) in the United States have been estimated at greater than $10 billion for the year 1980. Indirect economic costs (lost wages and assets) have been estimated at between $15 and $25 billion per year (American Cancer Society, 1985). A 1978 SEER report estimated the average cost for individual direct medical services for cancer to be $20,000 (National Cancer Institute, 1980b).

Costs to the Individual

Costs to the individual with cancer, and to his or her family, include direct monetary loss of income, medical and nonmedical expenses, and psychosocial costs. In families incurring greater than $10,000 in expenses, less than 50% receive medical insurance payments for their expenses (McNaull, 1985). Nonmedical expenses associated with treatment include transportation, food, lodging, clothing, and family care. In addition to the direct medical and nonmedical costs, psychosocial costs are incurred, resulting from loss of bowel and/or bladder control, loss of sexual and motor function, disfigurement, suicide, loss of savings, relocation, divorce, and family disintegration. Individuals undergoing treatment often exhaust all available sick leave, annual leave, and income, thus increasing the indirect costs of cancer. In extreme cases, loss of the family home and of life savings may result.

MODES OF TREATMENT

Surgery

The purpose of surgery, the oldest and most tested therapeutic modality for the treatment of cancer, is complete removal of the tumor. The patient's general health and age are considered, in addition to the histologic type, anatomic location, size, and stage of the tumor, in determining whether surgery will be the chosen mode of treatment. The patient's medical and social history must also be considered.

Radiation

Radiation therapy uses ionizing radiation in the treatment of cancer patients, and is directed at the tumor with a minimal effect on surrounding tissue. However, other types of treatment may be employed if substantial damage will be done to surrounding tissue (Shimkin, 1973). Hospitalization and anesthesia are rarely required in treatment. Side effects from treatment, depending on the body site treated and the amount of radiation delivered, include anorexia, nausea, vomiting, diarrhea, and skin reactions. Severe secondary results of radiation therapy may become evident months or years after treatment.

Chemotherapy

Advances in medical science have resulted in a new method of cancer treatment chemotherapy. Approximately 50,000–60,000 cases of cancer annually are now curable with chemotherapy as the primary means of treatment. This trend, while encouraging, is nevertheless mitigated by numerous factors. For example, almost all chemicals used in treating the conditions are toxic, not only to cancer cells but to normal cells as well. Consequently, many patients suffer agonizing side effects such as fear, anxiety, pain, nausea, insomnia, hair loss, diarrhea, loss of appetite, loss of weight, and muscular tension (Barckley, 1968; Golden, 1975; Redd, 1980; Rusk, 1971). The ordeal can be so devastating to some patients that they literally choose to die rather than continue with treatment. In fact, some actually die from treatment before its beneficial effects can be realized.

Psychological Implications of Treatment

The recognition of these facts, and inception of the Rehabilitation Act of 1973, has meant that comprehensive rehabilitation and continuing care services for persons experiencing cancer have received increased attention (Lebow, Maisiak, Sanders, Soong, & Cain, 1982). Consequently, increased attention has been focused on those psychological implications of cancer that emphasize quality of survival (Diller et al., 1979; Lehmann et al., 1978). The American Cancer Society (1979), Diller et al., and Lehmann et al. proposed that intervention by a single individual or program may be of assistance in the rehabilitation process. In addition, McAleer and Kluge (1978) suggested that the rehabilitation counselor, serving as a liaison between the patient and the medical team, may help reduce some of the patient's anxiety and, therefore, facilitate the rehabilitation process.

Psychobehavioral Treatment Modalities

Behavioral interventions to reduce the devastating effects of cancer and its treatment involve techniques such as deep muscle relaxation, cue-controlled relaxation, systematic desensitization, guided imagery, and hypnosis (Burish & Lyles, 1981; Dolan, Allen, & Sawyer, 1982; Lyles, Burish, Krozely, & Oldham, 1982; Morrow & Morrell, 1982; Redd, Andresen, & Minagawa, 1982). Relaxation techniques such as deep muscle relaxation, cue-controlled relaxation, and systematic desensitization help patients to reduce muscle tension associated with anxiety and physiological arousal (Lyles et al., 1982). The anxiety experienced by cancer patients may increase the negative experiences (e.g., pain, nausea, and vomiting) of the individual (Dolan, 1983). By reducing muscle tension, anxiety and the negative experiences associated with it are reduced. Guided imagery and hypnosis allow patients to focus their attention on pleasant thoughts and scenes, rather than on the anxiety and fear associated with the chemotherapy and its aftermath. Patients are, in fact, distracted from their present situation and worries.

In addition to feelings of anxiety and fear, a sense of helplessness and loss of control is prevalent among cancer patients. Many feel there is little they can do to help themselves, and they become despondent (Meyerowitz, 1980). Learning behavioral techniques provides patients with the requisite skills to bring about a relaxed state and reduce the experience of nausea, emesis, anxiety, and fear. Subjects in a number of studies reported gaining some sense of control over their predicament (Burish & Lyles, 1981; Dolan et al., 1982; Lyles et al., 1982; Morrow & Morrell, 1982; Redd et al., 1982). Some patients who used relaxation tapes also gave the tapes to family members to help relieve their stress (Fleming, 1985). This feeling of control, which begins with learning how to manage one's own responses to pain and treatment, can generalize to other realms of life as patients continue their new life with cancer.

Dolan (1983) conducted a study designed to alleviate the stress often associated with the cancer experience and frequently responsible for exacerbating such symptomatology as sleep interruptions, pain, and nausea. The program was designed to reduce the frequency of sleep interruptions and the frequency, duration, and intensity of pain and nausea experienced by adult oncology outpatients due either to their condition or to invasive chemotherapy treatment. Components of the program included a number of well-tested psychobehavioral procedures such as assessment and education, deep muscle relaxation, cue-controlled relaxation, thought stopping, focused attention, and positive coping statements. The subjects represented five different types of cancer, different forms of treatment, different symptoms, and different prognoses. Results revealed that overall the program had utility in reducing negative side effects associated with cancer and its treatment.

Morrow and Morrell (1982) examined the use of systematic desensitization and deep muscle relaxation to eliminate anticipatory nausea and emesis with a group of 60 patients at the University of Rochester Cancer Center. Subjects were assigned to one of three groups. One group received systematic desensitization and progressive muscle relaxation; another group received a Rogerian type of counseling. Group three served as a control group, and received no treatment. Patients instructed in progressive muscle relaxation and systematic desensitization reported a significantly greater decrease in anticipatory nausea and emesis than did the other two groups.

Burish and Lyles (1981) worked with 16 clients receiving chemotherapy and anti-emetics for nausea and vomiting. Pulse rates and blood pressure were monitored during three stages: pretraining, training, and posttraining. Patients were taught deep muscle relaxation and guided imagery techniques during the training stage. Then chemotherapy treatments were administered during the guided imagery. During the posttreatment phase, the patients relaxed on their own, independent of the therapist. Patients' self-reports, nurses' reports, and physiological measures all showed a decrease in the adverse side effects of treatment.

Redd et al. (1982) investigated the effect of hypnosis on six women experiencing anticipatory nausea. The women were taught a relaxation and distraction procedure. The patients focused on an object and on the therapist's voice and suggestions. The therapist taught deep muscle relaxation and guided imagery suggesting feelings of comfort and absence of nausea. These sessions were taped, and the patients were instructed to listen to the tapes daily. One week later the patients returned, and the above procedures were repeated to induce hypnosis. Results clearly showed hypnosis to be effective in controlling anticipatory nausea and emesis.

Supportive group treatment and hypnotic pain control exercises proved effective in reducing mood disturbances in metastatic breast cancer patients (Spiegel & Bloom, 1983). Members of the treatment group who learned a self-hypnosis exercise expressed no increase in pain for 1 year following treatment. Patients who were not instructed in the self-hypnosis exercise, but who were provided supportive group treatment, experienced a slight increase in pain during the year, and a control group experienced a substantial increase in pain. The frequency and duration of pain, however, was not significantly different in any of the groups. The manner in which the individuals responded to the sensation of pain and the associated suffering caused by the pain was positively altered when group support was available to them.

In advanced cancer, an increase of tension may precipitate or exacerbate pain, and increase the anxiety and mental stress of the patient. In a study conducted by Fleming (1985) in a hospice environment, patients learned relaxation therapy that consisted of: 1) developing an awareness of the interaction of tension throughout the body, and how the tension may be controlled by relaxing one's breathing; 2) postural re-education; 3) emotional control, showing the patient there is a choice in how one responds to a situation; 4) concentrating attention on immediate sensations to exclude anxious and distressing thoughts; 5) learning to control pain by altering the pattern of shallow and irregular breathing when pain is present, to create a more relaxed state; and 6) using relaxation tapes, that were available to the patients when needed. Patients eventually functioned independently of the therapist and the tapes. This relaxation program helped reduce anxiety that was previously unresponsive to drugs. Patients also reported the ability to control their own pain and prevent its recurrence.

Similar interventions have been implemented with children and adolescents experiencing negative reactions to chemotherapy treatment (Ellenberg, Kellerman, Dash, Higgins, & Zeltzer, 1980; Olness, 1981; Zeltzer, Kellerman, Ellenberg, & Dash, 1983). In another study, video games were used with three adolescent boys undergoing chemotherapy treatment who were experiencing anticipatory, as well as posttreatment, nausea (Kolko & Rickard-Figueroa, 1985). Symptom distress reduction occurred in all three boys. This method also employed thc distraction of attention from the anxiety-eliciting stimulus present in the environment at the time of treatment.

Common components found in the above studies included some form of relaxation and imagery. The application of these techniques is far-reaching for a number of reasons: 1) they can be learned easily in a short period of time; 2) they are cost efficient, in that no special equipment is required; 3) they can be practiced with minimal effort; and 4) they are minimally intrusive and need not interfere with the patient's daily routine or the physician's therapeutic regimen. Once the rehabilitation counselor has become proficient in the use of these techniques, he or she may use them in almost all situations where the patient is experiencing difficulties caused or exacerbated by anxiety (Dolan et al., 1982).

PSYCHOLOGICAL IMPACT OF CANCER

The Individual with Cancer

To understand an individual's reaction to cancer, one must understand what cancer means to that individual. Each person responds in a unique fashion. Although survival rates are increasing and attitudes are gradually changing, many still view cancer as "totally incurable, horribly painful and always fatal" (McNaull, 1985). However, a diagnosis of cancer no longer automatically places one in the category of "dying persons." People with cancer continue to function in a social network of family, friends, and work, and/or within the medical system.

Moos and Tsu (1977) identified two specific categories of problems faced by individuals with chronic illnesses. The first category is associated with biomedical and environmental factors; that is, with life alterations resulting from pain and incapacitation, from dealing with the hospital environment and developing relationships with medical personnel, and from treatment. The second category is associated with a broader scope of problems, such as maintaining emotional balance and a positive self-image; continuing relationships within the family, as well as with friends; and, finally, preparing for an uncertain future. Others have identified similar stresses. Barton (1977) found fear of loss of future to be a common experience of individuals with life-threatening illness. Carey (1976) identified four major concerns of terminally ill patients, including fear of pain, separation from loved ones, fear of burdening loved ones, and concern about care of loved ones. Meyerowitz (1980) found that cancer patients experience emotional distress, including anger, depression and/or anxiety; physical disturbances, including psychosomatic effects as well as those resulting from the disease itself or from treatment; disruption of marital and sexual relationships and activity levels; and fears regarding the progression of the disease and death.

Patient adjustment to cancer is considered to be directly related to coping mechanisms. Moos and Tsu (1977) identified the following four measures patients employ to overcome the complexities of the illness: 1) denying or minimizing the gravity of the illness; 2) suppressing, projecting, or displacing emotions; 3) finding a purpose or meaning in the illness; and 4) rehearsing all of the possible outcomes of the illness to prepare for any conceivable result. Some individuals turn to faith in a divine person for consolation (National Cancer Institute, 1980a).

As advances in medicine prolong the potential life expectancy of cancer patients, psychosocial problems and rehabilitation issues increasingly become more important long-term concerns (Novotony, Hyland, Coyne, Travis, & Pruyser, 1984). Rehabilitation counselors can provide services necessary to enhance the coping abilities of individuals confronted with cancer. Rehabilitation counselors can provide emotional support to allow the venting of feelings in a safe and empathetic environment. For some clients, the setting of goals, whether as short-term as a weekend trip, or as long-term as returning to a job, even on a part-time basis, may provide opportunities to achieve a sense of meaning or accomplishment that might otherwise be lacking in their current life situations. Finally, techniques described in the "Psychobehavioral Treatment Modalities'' section of this chapter are often effective in reducing anxiety and creating a relaxed state that can enhance the patient's overall coping ability.

Cancer in the Family

A diagnosis of cancer affects the entire family, as well as the individual. The structure of most family units is generally stable, with specific roles, relationships, and expectations. A diagnosis of cancer usually disrupts this balance within the family.

Northouse (1984) identifies the difficulties experienced by the family during the cancer patient's illness. During the initial phase, when the patient is hospitalized for treatment and the attention of the hospital staff is focused on the patient, the family is no longer responsible for the care of their ill family member and may begin to feel excluded. This feeling of exclusion may not always stem from the actions of the staff, but may be the result of the patient's embarrassment about the illness or need to protect the family from emotional strain. Family members, in fact, may be responsible for excluding themselves from the patient because of their inability to handle their anxieties or accept the illness.

Communication among family members, as well as with hospital staff, is essential during the initial hospitalization. New information about the disease and its effects must be digested and understood by the family. Obtaining information from hospital staff, however, may be difficult. Studies by Bond (1982) and Speedling (1980) found that physicians and nurses generally did not initiate discussions with family members. Family members reported feeling that physicians and nurses were too busy to bother with them. Koenig (1968) reported that families may be reluctant to initiate conversations with physicians and staff due to fear of the possible information they could receive. Often the language used by the health care professional, and particularly the physician, is foreign to the patient and family. Plain and simple explanations are crucial to help all understand the diagnosis and its implications.

Patients report difficulties in communicating within the family as well. Gordon et al. (1977) found the absence of open communication within the family as the second most frequently reported problem by 136 respondents in their study. Patients also reported concealing their true emotions to avoid upsetting family and friends; family members found it difficult to discuss openly with the patient their emotions concerning the disease and diagnosis, because of a need to protect the patient and others from the realities of cancer.

Lack of communication with children in families with one ill parent affects the child's coping abilities. The child who is not told about the disease will become aware of the disruptions in household routine, the prolonged absence of the ill parent, and the well parent's lack of emotional availability to the child. Coping and good familial relationships were better in families where the children were informed and the family routine was maintained with minimal disruption. In families where parents were unable to deal effectively with their own anxieties, and where they withheld the truth about the disease and its progression, children experienced higher levels of stress than children within families where communication was open and caring (Cancer Care, Inc. & The National Cancer Foundation, Inc., 1977).

For patients experiencing the terminal phase of cancer, communication centers on the issue of death. Hinton (1981) found dying patients and spouses engaged in three communication patterns. The first pattern consisted of maintaining hope by not speaking the truth about the approaching death. The second pattern involved the avoidance of any communication in an effort to limit the amount of distress experienced; and the third pattern consisted of nondiscussion of emotional-laden issues. Individuals who fell into this third pattern had consistently avoided communication about emotional issues throughout their lives together. Others have reported similar findings of guarded communication about death between patient and spouse (Vachon et al., 1977; Krant & Johnson, 1977–1978). The value of open communication concerning death has also been reported. Cohen, Dezenhuz, and Winget (1977) found that when family members were able to communicate openly, there was better adjustment after the loss of the spouse. The question of open communication in the family facing death is one that must be tailored to meet each family's needs. Preexisting patterns will frequently determine the post-illness communication style. Families who wish to communicate about death but are unable to may require assistance. When one member of the family feels the need to communicate while others do not, special attention should be directed to that member to allow the venting of feelings.

Oberst and James (1985) found the major difficulty for the spouse of cancer patients during the initial hospitalization to be the disruption of the family's life-style. Subjects reported that traveling back and forth to the hospital interrupted their employment, household schedules, child care patterns, and social activities. These demands on spouses, coupled with the shock and disbelief associated with the diagnosis, drained their emotional reserves. When the patients were discharged, spouses initially felt in control in their own homes, but as time passed they experienced high emotional distress, feelings of vulnerability, and ineffective coping styles. Concern for the patient's health turned to concern for their own health because of lack of sleep and the inability to eat. Increased physical problems were also reported by family members (Welch, 1981).

Reorganization of family roles also may be necessary as the ill member may be unable to resume his or her previously held role while recuperating from surgery or undergoing treatment. In the Oberst and James study (1985), spouses reported a change from a mutually supportive relationship to one in which they were supportive but received nothing in return.

Adolescent children of cancer patients experience particular difficulties, as they may be required to assume the role of caregiver. At this time of life, the adolescent begins to develop an identity separate from the family. The alteration in patterns of relating in the family, as well as the emotional turmoil of cancer, increases the incidence of behavior problems (Cancer Care, Inc. & The National Cancer Institute, 1977). New household and child care responsibilities may be imposed. Some adolescents respond by accepting the added burden. Others may act out their resentment by refusing to visit the hospital, drinking, or using drugs (Wellisch, 1979). Other disturbances such as poor school performance, eating or sleeping disturbances, aggressive behavior, refusal to obey, and sexual acting out may appear.

Family members must sacrifice their own time in order to take care of the patient in the hospital and at home. Unable to spend much time with each other and engage in outside social activities, they may begin to feel isolated. Emotional support previously available to them is no longer available (Giacquinta, 1977).

When the patient has progressed enough to return home, hope and expectations rise. The patient is expected to resume some prior responsibilities, and the special attention provided in the hospital is often withdrawn. Visitors may come frequently at first, but less often as time passes. Spouses of cancer patients experience anger, frustration, and distress about their perceived lack of support, not only from friends and relatives but also from professionals such as doctors and nurses (Oberst & James, 1985).

The family experiences some of the same feelings of loss of control, uncertainty, and helplessness that are experienced by the patient. Often, the family's needs are overshadowed by the needs of the patient through the ordeal of cancer.

VOCATIONAL CONSIDERATIONS

In Western society, an individual's sense of identity and self-worth are often derived from work. The ability to work and hold a job entitles the individual to independence, a means of controlling one's own affairs, and a sense of worth (Feldman, 1984). What happens, then, to the person with cancer who has been raised in this work-related value system and who must relinquish this role?

Many people survive after treatment for cancer and return to their previous life-styles. These individuals face a new challenge on the job. King (1984) found blatant job discrimination to be rare, but job problems were not uncommon. Patients were told they were being relieved of certain duties to ease their job strain, and then were urged to quit their job for the sake of their health. In addition, some patients were required to surrender health insurance benefits in order to keep a job. Other difficulties included patients being excluded from any type of promotion and, in some cases, demoted.

Individuals attempting to find new jobs experienced similar difficulties. Employers were reluctant to hire them because their insurance rates would increase, patients would miss too much work because of the disease, or the treatment or the job would be too stressful. Patients were advised to return after being symptom free for 5 years. Employers did not discriminate between different types of cancer, and viewed all types of cancer as deadly. In addition, employers expected all cancer patients to relapse. Patients who returned to their previous job felt trapped in the job, and were afraid to change because they would lose medical insurance or sick leave (Feldman, 1984).

Studies by Wheatley and Cunnick (1972) and Stone (1975) examined absenteeism rates and work performance of employees with cancer histories employed by Metropolitan Life Insurance Company and Bell Telephone Company. No significant differences were found in absenteeism rates between employees who had undergone treatment for cancer and those who had no history of a diagnosis or treatment of cancer. Further, cancer patients were more likely to come to work even when they were sick, and had fewer excuses for absences than non–chronically ill employees. Absences of cancer patients were related to surgery or subsequent therapy, and were generally less than 6 weeks. Respondents who were the main source of support for a family endured pain and fatigue and pushed themselves beyond physical capacity.

Feldman (1984) found that cancer patients frequently used work as a method to relieve their anxieties by occupying their minds. They viewed work as a way of demonstrating that they were still capable of being productive members of society. Returning to work served as an anchor that provided stability and a sense of control. Nevertheless, the possibility of dismissal due to illness was a constant threat. Job uncertainty coupled with the unpredictable aspects of the disease posed continuing coping problems for the patient.

IMPLICATIONS FOR REHABILITATION COUNSELORS

Cancer is a disease that affects the individual psychologically, socially, and vocationally. In addition, its impact on the family disrupts family structure and functions. Because survival rates are increasing, many more people will require services to help them adjust to the disease and to the effects of treatment. Rehabilitation counselors can implement a variety of behavioral interventions to help patients and families cope with the anxieties and fear brought about by a diagnosis of cancer. They can also provide the emotional support needed by both the patient and family during hospitalization; and when the patient returns home, can act as a liaison between the patient and family and the hospital staff. Explanation of the implications of the disease and treatment can be offered in a manner that facilitates understanding. Today, more and more cancer patients are returning to prior employment or attempting to find new employment, and are meeting difficulties on the job. Rehabilitation counselors can serve as liaison between the client and the employer to help overcome any attitudinal barriers concerning cancer and its prognosis. In addition, counselors can help the individual overcome job discrimination and isolation from co-workers because of the disease.

REFERENCES

American Cancer Society. (1979). Report on social, economic and psychological needs of cancer patients. In *Cancer: Major findings and implications.* San Francisco: Author.

American Cancer Society. (1985). *1985 cancer facts & figures.* New York: Author.

Barckley, V. (1968). Grief, a part of living. *Ohio's Health, 20,* 34–38.

Barton, D. (1977). *Dying and death: A clinical guide for caregivers.* Baltimore: Williams & Wilkins.

Bond, S. (1982). Communicating with families of cancer patients. *Nursing Times, 78,* 1027–1029.

Burish, T. G., & Lyles, J. N. (1981). Effectiveness of relaxation training in reducing adverse reactions to cancer chemotherapy. *Journal of Behavioral Medicine, 4*(1), 65–78.

Cancer Care, Inc., & The National Cancer Foundation. (1977). *Listen to the children! A study of the impact on the mental health of children of a parent's catastrophic illness.* New York: Author.

Carey, R. G. (1976). Counseling the terminally ill. *Personnel & Guidance Journal, 55,* 124–126.

Cohen, P., Dezenhuz, I. M., & Winget, C. (1977). Family adaptation to terminal illness and death of a parent. *Social Casework, 58,* 223–228.

Diller, L., Gordon, W. A., Freidenbergs, I., Ruckdeschel-Hibbard, M., Levine, L. R., Wolf, C., Ezrachi, O., Lipkins, R., Lucido, D., & Francis, A. (1979, March). Demonstration of benefits of early intervention of psychosocial problems and early intervention toward rehabilitation of cancer patients. *Final Report, New York University Medical Rehabilitation Research & Training Center,* No. 1.

Dolan, J. (1983). Cancer and chemotherapy: A psychological approach to coping. *Journal of Applied Rehabilitation Counseling, 14*(3), 36–39.

Dolan, J., Allen, H. A., & Sawyer, H. W. (1982). Relaxation techniques in the reduction of pain, nausea and sleep disturbances for oncology patients: A primer for rehabilitation counselors. *Journal of Applied Rehabilitation Counseling, 13*(4), 35–39.

Ellenberg, L., Kellerman, J., Dash, J., Higgins, G., & Zeltzer, L. (1980). Use of hypnosis for multiple symptoms in an adolescent girl with leukemia. *Journal of Adolescent Health Care, 1,* 132–136.

Feldman, F. L. (1984). Wellness and work. In C. L. Cooper (Ed.), *Psychosocial stress and cancer* (pp. 173–200). New York: John Wiley & Sons.

Fleming, U. (1985). Relaxation therapy for far-advanced cancer. *The Practitioner, 229,* 471–475.

Giacquinta, B. (1977). Helping families face the crisis of cancer. *American Journal of Nursing, 77,* 1585–1588.

Golden, S. (1975). Cancer chemotherapy and management of patient problems. *Nursing Forum, 14,* 216–221.

Gordon, W., Feidenberg, I., Diller, L., Rothman, L., Wolf, C., Ruckdeschel-Hibbard, M., Ezrachi, O., & Gerstman, L. (1977, September). *The psychosocial problems of cancer patients: A retrospective study.* Paper presented at the American Psychological Association Meeting, San Francisco.

Hinton, J. (1981). Sharing or withholding awareness of dying between husband and wife. *Journal of Psychosomatic Research, 25,* 337–343.

King, M. (1984, Autumn). After cancer: Trouble on the job? *Cancer News,* pp. 6–8, 22.

Koenig, R. (1968). A survey of social service needs. *Social Work, 13,* 85–90.

Kolko, D., & Rickard-Figueroa, J. L. (1985). Effects of video games on the adverse corollaries of chemotherapy in pediatric oncology patients: A single case analysis. *Journal of Consulting and Clinical Psychology, 53*(2), 223–228.

Krant, M. J., & Johnson, L. (1977–1978). Family members' perceptions of communication in late stage cancer. *International Journal of Psychiatry in Medicine, 8,* 203–216.

Lebow, J., Maisiak, R., Sanders, E., Soong, S-J., & Cain, M. (1982). Rehabilitation counseling needs of cancer patients. *Rehabilitation Counseling Bulletin, 25*(4), 231–234.

Lehmann, J. F., DeLisa, J. A., Warren, C. G., DeLateur, B. J., Bryant, P. J., & Nicholson, C. G. (1978). Cancer rehabilitation assessment of need, development and evaluation of a model of care. *Archives of Physical Medicine and Rehabilitation, 59,* 410–419.

Lyles, J. N., Burish, T. G., Krozely, M. G., & Oldham, R. K. (1982). Efficacy of relaxation training and guided imagery in reducing the aversiveness of cancer chemotherapy. *Journal of Consulting and Clinical Psychology, 50,* 509–524.

Mayo, L. (1956). *Problems and challenges in guidelines to action in chronic illness.* New York: National Health Council.

McAleer, C. A., & Kluge, C. A. (1978). Counseling needs and approaches for working with a cancer patient. *Rehabilitation Counseling Bulletin, 21,* 238–245.

McNaull, F. (1985). The social and economic costs of cancer. In S. & S. Garb (Eds.), *Cancer treatment and research in humanistic perspectives* (pp. 94–103). New York: Springer-Verlag.

Meyerowitz, B. E. (1980). Psychosocial correlates of breast cancer and its treatment. *Psychological Bulletin, 87,* 108–131.

Moos, R., & Tsu, V. (1977). The crisis of physical illness: An overview. In R. H. Moos (Ed.). *Coping with physical illness* (pp. 246–268). New York: Plenum.

Morrow, G., & Morrell, C. (1982). Behavioral treatment for the anticipatory nausea and vomiting induced by cancer chemotherapy. *New England Journal of Medicine, 307*(24), 1476–1480.

National Cancer Institute. (1980a). *Coping with cancer* (DHHS Publication No. [NIH] 80-2080). Bethesda, MD: Author.

National Cancer Institute. (1980b). *Surveillance, epidemiology, and end results report (SEER), incidence and mortality data: 1973–1977.* Bethesda, MD: Author.

National Cancer Institute. (1981). *Chemotherapy and you: A guide to self-help during treatment* (DHHS Publication No. [NIH] 81-1136). Bethesda, MD: Author.

Northouse, L. (1984). The impact of cancer on the family: An overview. *International Journal of Psychiatry in Medicine, 14*(3), 215–242.

Novotny, E. S., Hyland, J. M., Coyne, L., Travis, J. W., & Pruyser, H. (1984). Factors affecting adjustment to cancer. *Bulletin of the Menninger Clinic, 48*(4), 318–328.

Oberst, M. T., & James, R. H. (1985, April). Going home: Patient and spouse adjustment following cancer surgery. *Topics in Clinical Nursing,* pp. 46–57.

Olness, K. (1981). Imagery (self-hypnosis) as adjunct therapy in childhood cancer: Clinical experience with 25 patients. *American Journal of Pediatric Hematology/Oncology, 3,* 313–321.

Redd, W. H. (1980). *In vivo* desensitization in the treatment of chronic emesis following gastrointestinal surgery. *Behavior Therapy, 11*(3), 421–427.

Redd, W. H., Andresen, G. V., & Minagawa, R. Y. (1982). Hypnotic control of anticipatory emesis in patients receiving cancer chemotherapy. *Journal of Consulting and Clinical Psychology, 50*(1), 14–19.

Rusk, H. A. (1971). Rehabilitation of patients with cancer related disability. *Rehabilitation Medicine* (3rd ed.). St. Louis: C.V. Mosby.

Shimkin, M. B. (1973). *Science and cancer* (DHEW Publication No. [NIH] 75-568). Bethesda, MD: National Cancer Institute.

Speedling, E. J. (1980). Social structure and social behavior in an intensive care unit: Patient-family perspectives. *Social Work in Health Care, 6,* 1–15.

Spiegel, D., & Bloom, J. R. (1983). Group therapy and hypnosis reduce metastic breast carcinoma pain. *Psychosomatic Medicine, 45,* 333–339.

Stone, R. W. (1975). Employing the recovered cancer patient. *Cancer,* (July Supplement), 36.

Vachon, M. L., Freedman, K., Formo, A., Rogers, J., Lyall, W., & Freeman, S. (1977). The final illness in cancer: The widow's perspective. *Canadian Medical Assocation Journal, 117,* 1151–1153.

Welch, D. (1981). Planning nursing interventions for family members of adult cancer patients. *Cancer Nursing, 4,* 365–370.

Wellisch, D. K. (1979). Adolescent acting out when a parent has cancer. *International Journal of Family Therapy, 1,* 230–241.

Wheatley, G. M., & Cunnick, W. R. (1972). *The employment of persons with a history of treatment for cancer.* New York: Metropolitan Life Insurance Co.

Zeltzer, L., Kellerman, J., Ellenberg, L., & Dash, J. (1983). Hypnosis reduction of vomiting associated with chemotherapy and disease in adolescents with cancer. *Journal of Adolescent Health Care, 4,* 77–84.

11

Basic Issues and Trends in Head Injury Rehabilitation

Brian T. McMahon and Robert T. Fraser

In 1985, the National Head Injury Foundation (NHIF) signed a cooperative agreement with the U.S. Office of Special Education and Rehabilitation Services, the Council of State Administrators of Vocational Rehabilitation, and the National Association of State Directors of Special Education (NHIF, 1985a). The goals of this arrangement are:

1. Recognize traumatic brain injury (TBI) as a specific disability
2. Develop and provide increased knowledge and information regarding TBI to agency administrators, case managers, counselors, educators, rehabilitation specialists, service providers, and the general public
3. Increase accessibility and awareness of existing services for clients and improve methods to gain such services
4. Enhance coordination and transition among existing services so that individuals may reach maximum potential
5. Expand and stimulate the array of innovative services and strategies in rehabilitation and education, including independent living services and job opportunities, to respond to the needs of individuals with TBI
6. Expand upon scientific knowledge through research and development procedures to collect data that will assist in developing treatment strategies, programs, services, and models for rehabilitation, education, and services
7. Encourage the expansion of public and private policies that stimulate and foster the above goals
8. Encourage the development of meaningful activities and vocational opportunities for this population

9. Encourage the development and implementation of state and local agreements between NHIF state associations that will foster all of the above goals
10. Encourage a fixed point of responsibility for planning, coordination, and delivery of appropriate services as needed

With this as a backdrop, the Twelfth Institute on Rehabilitation Issues (TIRI) selected "Rehabilitation of TBI (traumatic brain injury)" as a prime study topic in 1985. The resulting monograph of the same name, published by the University of Wisconsin–Stout Vocational Rehabilitation Institute, became the fastest selling monograph in the history of the IRI process. It is the definitive publication to date for rehabilitation counselors interested in head injury (TIRI, 1985).

Also in 1985, American Rehabilitation Counseling Assocation President Edna Szymanski appointed a special task force on head injury rehabilitation, with this chapter's authors as co-chairs, to study issues pertinent to rehabilitation counseling in the rapidly expanding field of head injury rehabilitation. This chapter and Chapter 12 represent the final report of this group.

By 1985, the number of categorical head injury programs nationally had grown from a handful in 1980 to approximately 500 (NHIF, 1985b). Three federally funded research and training centers on head injury and stroke continued their efforts at New York University, the University of Washington, and Baylor University. The NHIF, founded only in 1980, has expanded its mailing list to 25,000 persons, its support groups to over 275, and its state chapters to over 37. Through the promptings of these state chapters, a number of state-federal vocational rehabilitation agencies have begun to improve service delivery to head-injured persons.

As the survival rate for head-injured persons continued its dramatic climb, the head injury rehabilitation industry came of age. In recent years, the inevitable occurred; that is, the representatives of vocational rehabilitation service delivery systems (public and private sector) and this new health care/human services field met head to head over a variety of mutual concerns. Clearly established today as one of the major trends in rehabilitation for the 1980s, the practice of the rehabilitation of clients with head injury requires a reemphasis of some age-old rehabilitation themes, and a thorough understanding of some new issues as well. The development of these themes and issues is the goal of this chapter.

LEVELS AND TYPES OF REHABILITATION PROGRAMS FOR PERSONS WITH HEAD INJURY

Rehabilitation programs for head-injured persons may be conceptually divided into various levels of care that correspond generally to the level of functioning and service needs of the clients they are designed to assist. The following represents one version of these programs and its typical components. Note that not every program in head injury rehabilitation has all of the components listed. Pervading all quality programs, however, regardless of level, are assessment and reassessment, as well as family, behavioral, and cognitive restoration services.

Acute Rehabilitation Programs

Acute rehabilitation is frequently confused with acute hospitalization; that is, the community hospital or trauma unit into which the head-injured client was initially received and medically stabilized, often after neurosurgical or other lifesaving measures. In head injury rehabilitation, this term is more often used to refer to any medical environment that addresses the medical rehabilitation needs of the head-injured person, and in which additional measures for cognitive and behavioral restoration are also available. The overwhelming majority of the categorical head injury programs nationally (i.e., with beds designated for the treatment of head-injured individuals) are involved in the acute rehabilitation phase. Typical settings include rehabilitation hospitals, rehabilitation units of general hospitals, and specially equipped skilled nursing facilities (Jennett, 1975). Subprogram offerings within the acute rehabilitation facility might include one or more of the following.

Coma Intervention and Sustained Coma Care Designed for recently injured clients still in coma, the clinical objectives in these programs are to heighten and strengthen the recovery process through intensive health, nutritional, and physical interventions, as well as controlled sensory stimulation (Lasden, 1982). Coma management is a sophisticated endeavor that, if properly handled, can accelerate the rehabilitation process after consciousness is regained. Often the need for supportive family services in the forms of education and therapy are greatest at this time.

Active Rehabilitation As the client's medical condition stabilizes, early and active intervention by a complete interdisciplinary team is begun. This includes physical, occupational, behavioral, psychosocial, cognitive, recreational, and speech and language therapies appropriate to the client's cognitive status and physical tolerance. Prevocational programming is not unusual in these programs (Smith, 1983). The rate of progress toward independent functioning in a number of areas, such as mobility and independent living skills, appears to be positively related to the timing and appropriateness of these interventions.

Sustained Development These programs are available for individuals who appear to have attained maximum benefit from intensive therapy, but who still need continued, less intensive services to maintain their status or to continue progress at a slower rate. The focus is on social, emotional, and recreational programming as well as services to families.

Extended Care These programs provide long-term supportive care for medically involved individuals not likely to return to the community, or individuals who might otherwise be placed in skilled nursing facilities designed exclusively for geriatric populations.

Residential Community Reentry or Transitional Living Programs

Residential community reentry or transitional living programs are designed for medically stable clients with good potential for independent living but whose behavioral or ongoing cognitive problems are not well managed in the home community on an outpatient basis (Hackler & Tobis, 1983). Generally higher functioning than acute rehabilitation clients, these clients typically require behavior management, independent living, and/or vocational rehabilitation services, which are the primary themes of these programs. Additional services such as allied health, psychosocial, recreational, cognitive, and family therapies are provided according to individual need, but only as they support the three major themes. Subprograms may include one or more of the following:

Intensive Retraining Programs These provide a goal-oriented program of therapies designed to improve the physical, cognitive, vocational, communicative, behavioral, and interpersonal functioning of residents. The goal of such programs is singular—community re-entry; that is, a return to the home community or the least restrictive alternative. Based upon their readiness, residents progress through a series of progressively more homelike living situations en route to community placement (Pancsofar & Blackwell, 1986).

Behavioral Rehabilitation Programs These are systematic, goal-oriented programs of behaviorally anchored training designed to develop prosocial behaviors among the residents (Wood, 1984). Progressive applied behavior analysis principles and techniques (relying heavily on intensive teaching, contingency contracts, and the use of social praise) are the primary methods by which residents are taught to monitor and control their conduct.

Supervised Living Programs These programs provide for the care and supervision of residents who require some assistance in meeting their basic needs. The supervised living arrangement may be long term, or even indefinite for those who might well be managed at home with minimal monitoring or supervision, but who have no home available. Sometimes these arrangements are respite oriented (temporary placement for less than 60 days) to provide relief for family members and/or to focus on limited treatment objectives. In either situation, supervised living programs are designed to provide a comfortable, homelike atmosphere in which a full, healthy life can be continued with a reasonable degree of community participation and a high quality life-style.

Vocational Rehabilitation (VR) Programs These appear to be headed toward supported employment models. They provide actual employment opportunities, ongoing assessment, job coaching, work hardening, and social integration for residents (Wehman, 1981). "Place and train" approaches, with prescriptive training aimed at specific placement targets, are likely to dominate the VR picture for the reasons provided in the following chapter.

Comprehensive Outpatient Rehabilitation Facilities (CORFs)

For clients whose behavioral and cognitive problems are not so severe as to prohibit community living, CORFs provide the full range of retraining services required to maintain and enhance independent living capabilities. The focus is typically upon reimbursable allied health and case management services, although psychosocial or vocational issues are sometimes addressed (Prigatano & Fordyce, in press).

Intensive Services Programs These offer full-day rehabilitation programs as intense as one would find in a community reentry program, except that the clients reside within their usual family environments.

Concentrated Services Programs These provide 1–4 hours of daily skill-building services in specific areas needed to attain long-term independence. Such programs are designed for head-injured individuals deficient in one or two areas, for whom training could make a significant difference in their daily lives.

Academic/Educational Services Programs These programs offer study skills training, academic support, and counseling for clients seeking to complete educational requirements. Setting realistic educational goals and developing strategies for their attainment are the primary professional activities. The linkages between training directions and national job trends are reviewed by vocational program staff.

Group and Vocational Programs These are two interrelated, full-day programs concerned with such areas as money management, social skills development, vocational evaluation, training, and job placement, in classes of roughly five clients each.

CONSIDERATIONS FOR CASE FINDING

The wide range of services for head-injured individuals described above has only recently become available, and very few areas of the country have the full spectrum of services in place. Head-injured individuals have had an unfortunate history in terms of options for recovery. When the survival rate was relatively low for severely head-injured persons (less than 15% only 10 years ago), very few treatment programs existed that were specific to their needs. The NHIF estimates that there still remain between 1 and 1.8 million head-injured persons who have never received rehabilitation services (NHIF, 1982).

Additionally, misdiagnoses and inappropriate placements were commonplace. Physical restoration programs were often ill equipped to manage the cognitive and behavioral problems that head-injured clients presented. Placement in inpatient psychiatric environments would ensue, where primary diagnoses of organic brain syndrome, schizophrenia, major depression, or "other neurological disorder" would be followed by chemotherapeutic interventions with neuroleptic and/or antidepressant medications, often without consideration for the client's neurological status. Additionally, most psychiatric programs were ill equipped to address the needs for physical and cognitive restoration. Family members became progressively confused by the plethora of diagnoses, prognoses, and treatment approaches, and were particularly disturbed by the lack of effectiveness of traditional psychiatric approaches. Frequently, after multiple placements in both rehabilitation and psychiatric environments, many head-injured persons whose needs could not be met at home were placed in long-term nursing facilities, where chronic depression, sensory deprivation, learned helplessness, and physical deterioration became typical experiences.

To the extent that aggressive, comprehensive outreach and case finding are priority activities for the rehabilitation counselor, one need look no further than the nearest nursing home, state or private psychiatric facility, developmental disability center, or sheltered care home to discover unserved and underserved head-injured persons. Local chapters of the NHIF and National Easter Seal Society, neurology and intensive care units of local hospitals, neurologists, neurosurgeons, physiatrists, rehabilitation and neurology nurses, and allied health professionals will all appreciate one's interest and participation in services to head-injured persons. Most will describe clients who are "just not the same" or "just not fitting in" since their hospital discharge.

IMPORTANT COMPONENTS OF REHABILITATION PROGRAMS FOR PERSONS WITH HEAD INJURY

The following critical components in effective head injury rehabilitation programs, although not unheard of in general rehabilitation circles, have been so strongly emphasized in facilities for head-injured clients that they have become the benchmarks of accreditation and other evaluation criteria.

Team Approach and Case Management Concepts

Working with a general rehabilitation population, a rehabilitation counselor would have to encounter a variety of severely disabled clients before he or she would experience all of the features that a single head-injured individual might present. For this reason, the NHIF and reputable providers in head injury rehabilitation insist that treatment services be provided by experienced, specialized *interdisciplinary* teams. Furthermore, the treatment team is often extended to include facility management, family members, third-party payers, and attending physicians. This is necessary because no one team member will have all the skills needed to serve the head-injured client whose treatment issues are many, variable, and in constant flux.

Jaques (1970) described the "team concept" as a democratic approach for providing coordinated services through the sharing of multidisciplinary knowledge. She also described the "stumbling blocks" to effective team functioning, including problems of trust and respect among professionals, the inherent danger of specialization, and poor communication.

Quality head injury programs have taken seriously the implementation of a true team approach and have implemented concrete measures to maximize its success. These include employee selection and evaluation on the basis of teamwork issues, organization of staff to preclude departmentalization, and ongoing team-building activities. Transcending the notion of *interdisciplinary* is the concept of the *transdisciplinary* approach, which requires that each professional is involved in the active instruction of discipline-specific theories and techniques to other team members. Each team member may provide input on any area of treatment programming, especially in the cognitive, social, and behavioral realms, input that cuts across all therapeutic endeavors. This notion is congruent with "Theory Z" management principles as described by Vogenthaler and Riggar (1985).

Particularly in post-acute treatment environments, but even in some acute programs, teams are lead by case managers who emerge as leaders from every conceivable discipline. Case managers are the architects of treatment plans synthesized from the written assessments of all team members. While monitoring costs, case managers drive the team toward the realization of progressively higher levels of client function. The case manager brings the idea of a team concept to reality by using all available data to develop, describe, and implement treatment objectives that represent the client as a unique, whole person (Cassell & Mulkey, 1985).

As a coordinator of medical, psychosocial, family, vocational, educational, cognitive, communication, and recreational services, the case manager is the single, unchanging, visible contact point for families and third-party payers. Given the traditional professional roles that rehabilitation counselors have performed, it is no coincidence that rehabilitation counselors are heavily recruited for these positions.

Behavioral Problems and Interventions

The behavioral consequences of traumatic brain injury have created the need for unique treatment environments. These behavioral consequences were often unfamiliar to staff members in hospitals or general rehabilitation environments. Usually the behavioral problems prevented the management of many medically stable head-injured individuals on an outpatient basis, creating the need for specialized community reentry and supervised living programs.

Traditional psychiatric interventions as applied to the problems of traumatic brain injury have generally failed. Such treatment approaches placed expectations on head-injured clients that failed to take into account, or that overestimated, their cognitive abilities (Malec, 1984). The placement and misplacement of head-injured persons in psychiatric inpatient settings is still a problem of epidemic proportions. More than 25% of the total hospital beds in this country are occupied by patients diagnosed with "organic psychosis" or "organic brain syndrome" (Alexander, 1982; Segal, Boomer, & Bouthelet, 1975). They are medicated with neuroleptics and antidepressants, some of which lower the seizure threshold.

Due to the history of head injury treatment options described earlier, there exists in current head injury rehabilitation a preference for non-psychiatric, behaviorally oriented treatment approaches for the development of prosocial behaviors. Often, these behavioral problems appear in direct relation to improvement in other (typically cognitive) areas. For example, a client whose memory is improving becomes more capable of comparing his or her pre- and postinjury status. Greater awareness of deficits ensues. When accompanied by disinhibition and a tendency toward impulsivity, the resulting emotion is often one of extreme frustration, manifested in terms of abusive, assaultive, or threatening behavior (Fordyce, Roueche, & Prigatano, 1983).

Prigatano (in press) categorizes behavioral problems in head injury into four broad classes. These problems manifest themselves in varying degrees and do not necessarily occur sequentially. The first is the *anxiety and catastrophic reaction.* In this situation, head-injured individuals are calm and cooperative as long as they feel capable of performing required tasks. If they cannot or perceive that they cannot, they may become agitated, rude, evasive, and sometimes aggressive as a means of releasing performance anxiety (Goldstein, 1952). Others attribute this phenomenon to a loss of linguistic abilities, or to left hemisphere dysfunction (Gianotti, 1972).

The second behavioral problem area involves *denial of the disorder.* Probably a consequence of both organic and psychological defense mechanisms, denial may appear as a minimizing of the client's deficits, underestimating the amount of hard work required during the rehabilitation process, or outright repression of the horror surrounding the traumatic event itself. Since denial is one of the most primitive ego defense mechanisms, it is also (regrettably) likely to be the first to reappear in the process of cognitive restoration. Only by understanding that head-injured persons absolutely require this denial (on an interim basis) for their own psychological survival, will the rehabilitation counselor be able to contend with the client's anger and frustration, emotions that often become misdirected at the professional.

The third area of behavioral problems, *paranoia and psychomotor agitation,* may be related to temporal lobe damage, premorbid personality problems, or both. Brief trials of anti-psychotic medication are sometimes required in problem management, especially when impulsivity, restlessness, impatience, and intimidation are present.

The final area, *depression, social withdrawal, and amotivational states,* describes difficulties most head-injured persons experience, albeit at different levels. In addition to the areas of concern described by Prigatano (in press), still other areas of behavioral problems include the client's egocentrism or childlike immaturity, lack of initiative and a sense of responsibility, and a generally lowered tolerance for alcohol.

These psychological and behavioral problems, coupled with cognitive deficits, are the most formidable barriers to employment, social adjustment, and independent living (Jennett & Bond, 1975; Oddy, Humphrey, & Uttley, 1978). They also cause the greatest stress (Oddy et al., 1978), depression (Rosenbaum & Najenson, 1976), and general disruption to cohesion among family members (Bond & Brooks, 1976).

Generally speaking, applied behavior analysis principles and techniques appear to be effective in the behavior management of head-injured individuals (Hall & Hall, 1982). These rely heavily upon social praise as a primary reinforcer. Intensive teaching, positive reinforcement, reinforcing approximations of desired behavior, contingency contracting, and the simplicity of this approach are all effective aspects of applied behavior analysis with this population. Point systems or token economies are less effective since they tend to treat clients as children and are often offensive to the already sensitive head-injured client. Philosophical underpinnings of both applied behavior analysis and rehabilitation emphasize the positive in dealings with clients, while building upon known areas of client proficiency. In post-acute treatment environments, in which physical and chemical restraints are not permissible, applied behavior analysis provides a variety of progressive methods for teaching clients to monitor, regulate, and control their behaviors.

Family Education and Therapy

The families are often seen as the true victims by counselors who work with head-injured clients. One can readily appreciate the shock families experience when a member is suddenly and severely disabled. During the client's period of coma, which may last for weeks or even months, families typically spend long hours in either bedside vigils, prayer, or both. Little information is available to them, since prognostic indicators are crude and not always used. Lack of feedback greatly exacerbates the family's level of stress. Most family members believe (and some are led to believe) that if and when the client regains consciousness, everything will be fine (Lezak, 1978).

An alternate use of at least some of the time during the coma period involves family participation in a program of family education (Rosenthal, 1984). Many quality head injury rehabilitation programs, as well as state and local chapters of the NHIF, offer educational services designed to answer such questions as:

1. What is a head injury?
2. What has happened to my family member?
3. How does the brain work?
4. What are the typical stages of recovery from a head injury?
5. What ultimate outcome can I expect with my family member?
6. What is a coma?
7. What are seizures, post-traumatic amnesia, spasticity, contractures, hematomas, contusions, etc.?
8. What happens in the rehabilitation process?
9. Who are the members of the treatment team and what are their jobs?
10. How can I be helpful?

Throughout the rehabilitation process, particularly in the first 2 years, clients and their families will often have shared denial systems, sometimes guised as "faith" or "hope." In the midst of all that has occurred, family members need to deny the inevitable reality that a complete return to premorbid function is extremely unlikely, and that a number of permanent impairments requiring lifelong intervention are probable. Regrettably, this single dynamic often leads to conflict between families and professionals. Perhaps the words of Bond (1975) can help many professionals contain their frustration: ". . . denial usually alternates with periods of insight . . . . a process which is shared with relatives . . . . a process designed to abolish anxiety about matters which are potentially overwhelming emotionally" (p. 129). Accordingly, the family's receptiveness to education and therapy is highly variable, and the timing of these interventions is critical.

Because most head-injured individuals are young adults, the changes in the family constellation after injury have become predictable. If the head-injured individual is married, divorce is highly likely in a matter of months. Parents, often elderly or in ill health, are recalled as the primary caregivers or responsible parties. After a number of months of attempting to manage their loved one at home, families become more amenable to professional assistance. The major barriers to effective "family reentry" for head-injured individuals are identical to the major barriers to reemployment. It is not the physical, seizure, or communication problems that are paramount, but the cognitive, behavioral, and personality problems.

Among the primary cognitive problems are deficits in thinking and reasoning, memory, concentration and attention, and speed of information processing. Personality and/or behavioral problems include major depressive episodes, lack of initiative and responsibility, childlike immaturity, social isolation, denial, impulsivity, and a lowered tolerance for alcohol. These are the specific problems that can disrupt and dissolve normal family functioning.

Since an intact, supportive, and cooperative family is a correlate of success in head injury rehabilitation (Fowler, 1981), the treatment team should anticipate these problems and assist the family in their management. Involving the family as an integral part of the treatment team will go a long way toward maximizing the probabilities of treatment goal attainment. Personal adjustment counseling for family members should also be prescribed as a routine ingredient in treatment regardless of the family's initial reaction. Finally, regular attendance at the local head injury association support group is strongly encouraged.

In some instances, the rehabilitation counselor will be involved with a completely dysfunctional family unit in which no family member emerges as an involved partner with the treatment team. These situations will involve considerably more case management and/or cooperative work with other community health/human services agencies and professionals.

Issues in Community Reentry

Community reentry programs for head-injured adults strive to maximize behavioral self-regulation, independent living skills, and vocational restoration of the resident toward the ultimate goal of returning to the home community and to a least restrictive environment. Community reentry programs are achieving amazing success with some clients several years after their injury. This is surprising since the prevailing medical opinion is that most of the spontaneous neurological recovery occurs within the first 2 years after injury. Even if this were the case, there are often a number of life areas in need of restoration, in which further gains are achievable. These include the behavioral, self-care, vocational, physical restoration, recreational, family, and psychological domains. Given these possibilities, and the interactions among these areas, it is not surprising that many clients can significantly improve their overall level of functioning given adequate levels of appropriate services.

Pancsofar and Blackwell (1986) enumerated the essential characteristics of a true community reentry program for severely disabled persons. First, a quality program has an overall guiding principle for its operation, such as normalization, competence/deviance, dignity of risk, or least restrictive environment. Second, a quality program seeks to assist its residents in developing a sequence of competencies in at least one of four areas: community mobility, domestic living, recreation/leisure, and vocational experience.

Third, the facility programs for generalization by conducting most of its training in community environments where the behaviors are likely to be performed, and in interaction with nonhandicapped peers and neighbors. Fourth, community reentry training is a systematic, instructional process with data-based assessment and decision procedures. Ethical guidelines are established to decrease aberrant behaviors, using the least intrusive, yet most effective, interventions available.

Additional hallmarks of quality programs include regular scheduling of staff in-service training, utilization of generic medical and community services, and development of a detailed daily schedule for each resident. These considerations should prove helpful for the rehabilitation counselor asked to recommend or evaluate a community reentry program for head-injured individuals.

Standards for Evaluation of Head Injury Rehabilitation Programs

Rehabilitation counselors in all service environments will be confronted routinely with requests for information regarding quality rehabilitation facilities that offer services to head-injured individuals. Similarly, many rehabilitation counselors will need to arrange for services with a facility that specializes in this area. When this occurs, it is helpful to remember that guidelines have been developed that can assist the rehabilitation counselor in determining quality.

First, in 1985 the Commission on the Accreditation of Rehabilitation Facilities (CARF) established standards specific to head injury rehabilitation at the *acute care* level (CARF, 1985). To achieve accreditation in this area, a program must first meet all of the standards pertaining to comprehensive inpatient rehabilitation. Beyond these, there exist 13 additional standards specific to head injury, seven of which follow:

> 1. a comprehensive, categorically designated program of services (not just designated beds);
> 2. a sufficient volume of head injury admissions with whom the staff can develop the necessary specialized skills (at least 30 new patients per year);
> 3. treatment and discharge planning must address not only medical but cognitive and behavioral issues as well;
> 4. a core, interdisciplinary team of professionals must exist whose primary involvement and expertise is in head injury;
> 5. designated, safe, and secure treatment space must exist;
> 6. services to families must be provided;
> 7. there must be a designated administrator, physician, and quality assurance individual for the program. (CARF, 1985, pp. 46–50)

Because the development of these standards is relatively recent, the rehabilitation counselor may have to make a determination whether these standards are met by a program which has not completed the full accreditation process. Additionally, at the time of this writing, similar standards were developed for CARF approval that are intended to apply to community reentry and outpatient head injury rehabilitation programs.

Not coincidentally, the National Head Injury Foundation has offered the following guidelines that evolved from a study, conducted by the Santa Clara Medical Center, of "model program characteristics" in a medical rehabilitation environment (Cervelli, 1984):

1. A comprehensive team should be organized and readily available to meet the specialized needs of the head-injured individual. There should be representatives on the team from each of the following disciplines: physical medicine, rehabilitation medicine, nursing, dietary, occupational therapy, speech and language, outpatient service coordinator, psychology, neuropsychology, special education, recreation, social services, vocational counseling, liaison nursing, and public health nursing.
2. There needs to be an identifiable bed allocation, in a specially structured environment. Safety precautions that allow for freedom of movement yet that will not allow the individual to leave the premises, and place/person-orienting materials are examples of modifications that create such an environment.
3. There should be a sufficient volume of head injury patients (30–50 a year) to allow the treatment staff the opportunity to develop expertise in the care of head-injured patients.
4. An interdisciplinary team approach should be employed. This calls for the treatment team to define goals relative to the patient's care, and to concentrate all its energies on finding the best solutions for the unique needs of each individual case. The interdisciplinary team defines itself as a group, plans and manages the patient's goals together and makes every effort to reinforce each discipline's therapy goals.
5. An integrated treatment philosophy should be applied that attacks problems simultaneously and comprehensively, rather than a singular treatment method that deals with psychological problems and ignores cognitive and behavioral problems.
6. Utilization of admission, treatment, and discharge criteria based on widely known and predictable factors of recovery is needed in order to achieve a common language and understanding (e.g., the Glasgow Outcome Scale or the Rappaport Disability Scale). (Even existing measures could benefit from further refinement in order to establish their reliability across treatment centers.)

7. A predetermined method of evaluation and progress reporting fosters interagency and intrateam communication. This includes a reporting system to insurance carriers.
8. Essential to maintaining the gains of a rehabilitation program is the commitment to long-term follow-up care. The family and the patient will feel they are receiving support and that the program is "on call" for them.
9. There should be a commitment to cooperation and communication with community agencies to aid in recovering independence and promoting vocational opportunity, awareness of the availability of transitional living facilities, vocational training programs, community colleges, and other agencies. This commitment is the bridge between the rehabilitation setting and the desired goal of reentry into a productive life.
10. A funding and administrative organization that allows patients to participate in all program activities should be in place.

Between CARF standards and NHIF guidelines, the rehabilitation counselor not only has a basis for referral, but can also develop a feel for the unique spirit and philosophy of head injury rehabilitation. Additional features that have become trademarks of quality head injury rehabilitation programs include the aforementioned family education and therapy, behaviorally anchored programming, the team concept, and case management.

FEASIBILITY FOR EMPLOYMENT

Whether the purpose is to determine eligibility for services in the state-federal program, prepare expert witness testimony, or advise insurance carriers on the value of a return on their rehabilitation investment, the question of feasibility for a client's employment following head injury is a matter of major importance. From a strict cost-analysis perspective, significant expenditures may well be required to return the head-injured person to gainful employment—a matter of valid concern to insurance carriers, attorneys, and service providers.

There are additional noneconomic reasons why resolution of the feasibility question is desirable. First, the realization of a concrete vocational direction, and the acceptance or rejection of this direction by the client, provides a valuable means of gauging the overall psychological adjustment to head injury. Second, family members often have urgent needs to plan for necessary short- and long-term levels of economic, supervisory, and environmental assistance.

Since several individuals involved with the head-injured client might have a vested interest in a feasibility decision, opinions will often vary widely with little regard to scientific methods of inquiry or objective findings. Accordingly, a feasibility decision that builds upon what is known about head injury and return to work, in the absence of political or financial exigencies, is the preferred if not ideal occurrence.

These varied interests in the client's employability are important because they relate directly to the sources of information selected by the rehabilitation counselor as a basis for the feasibility decision. For example, a decision maker who is confronted by a client who has mastered illness behavior, besieged by a cost-conscious supervisor, and closely monitored by an aggressive plaintiff attorney is likely to perceive the application of pressures to arrive at a pessimistic vocational prognosis. The rehabilitation counselor in such a situation might respond to such pressure by choosing the following sources of information:

1. The reports or opinions of the neurosurgeon, who engages clients at the time of trauma (when they are medically at their worst) and who rarely follows clients on a long-term basis
2. The reports of the neuropsychologist designed to pinpoint and describe the nature and extent of cognitive deficits, with little attention to assets or compensatory mechanisms
3. Standardized work sample approaches, the parameters of which defy successful performance by most head-injured individuals
4. Strict medical indices, such as the length and depth of coma, in isolation from other factors

However, if the decision maker relied upon the results of situational assessments, on-the-job evaluations, or the reports of experienced work evaluators—evaluations that seek to identify residual assets, compensatory mechanisms, and opportunities for environmental restructuring—a more realistic and optimistic prognostication would likely ensue. Still, unduly optimistic vocational projections might result if based solely upon functional data, the aspirations of family members, client self-appraisals, or the assessments of professionals inexperienced in the area of head injury.

What are the facts? Are severely head-injured persons likely to return to work? Are they "good investments" for our vocational rehabilitation dollar?

Answers to these questions are not entirely clear, but this much is known. First, it is currently impossible to determine definitively which head-injured individuals will or will not return to work, at which level of employment, and/or when. Second, a significant minority (believed to be between 25% and 33% of even severely head-injured persons) have returned to work at a reduced level of functioning without the benefit of formalized vocational rehabilitation assistance (Kay, Ezrachi, & Cavallo, 1984). Third, there exist some comprehensive rehabilitation programs in which vocational rehabilitation services are provided to all head-injured clients without regard to feasibility prognostications. Under these circumstances, there are instances of even very severely head-injured individuals returning to work, albeit at reduced levels of functioning.

It is therefore recommended that in the absence of certainty, feasibility decisions might be avoided altogether, or at least designed to maximize rather than restrict access to vocational rehabilitation services. As this applies to the state-federal vocational rehabilitation system, no client population will so test this program's commitment to establish priorities in services to severely disabled persons. (For additional related discussion, see the "Job Readiness/Rehabilitation Potential" section in Chapter 12.)

CAREER OPPORTUNITIES FOR REHABILITATION COUNSELORS

Career opportunities in head injury rehabilitation for rehabilitation counselors with graduate-level training are very promising for a number of reasons. Any rehabilitation field that experiences the extremes of growth described earlier is likely to expand the opportunity structure for all rehabilitation professions. But beyond this, it also appears likely that rehabilitation counselors are qualified for a greater number of occupations within this field. One large organization that provides services to head-injured clients, for example, employs graduate-trained rehabilitation counselors as life skills counselors, behavior specialists, vocational specialists, personal adjustment counselors, and case managers.

The life skills counselor is a primary provider of instructional services for clients, to facilitate their movement toward individually determined behavioral self-management, independent living, and/or vocational goals.

The behavior specialist directs and supports the behavioral emphasis of the program across all aspects of program activities and services. The behavior specialist designs, implements, and trains staff to implement programs that increase the client's prosocial behavior and decrease behaviors that interfere with the client's movement to the least restrictive environment.

The vocational specialist provides vocational evaluation, counseling, training, job coaching, placement, and follow-up services to assist clients in attaining their maximum level of vocational functioning.

The personal adjustment counselor works closely with the psychosocial adjustment issues of the client and family to clarify goals and expectations, provide counseling and support, and advocate for the client and family when needed. The maximization of personal, emotional, and interpersonal growth to assist the client to reintegrate successfully into the community is the primary responsibility of this team member.

The case manager occupies a position of leadership. This professional performs case management functions involving the design, monitoring, and evaluation of individually written treatment plans, client advocacy, liaison to the family and to the funding source, and staff supervision.

The attractiveness of the well-trained rehabilitation counselor to recruiters of head injury rehabilitation professionals lies in the perception of members of this discipline as good "team players" who are oriented toward working with severely disabled persons. By virtue of their training, rehabilitation counselors endorse the "whole person" approach that is absolutely necessary in working with multiply disabled clients. Indeed, the basic philosophy of rehabilitation, to which all rehabilitation counselors are introduced, is essential to the characteristics of successful head injury rehabilitation. This philosophy, as summarized by Jaques (1970, p. 5), focuses upon:

1. The holistic nature of humans
2. The assets or residual capacity of the individual
3. The development of coping behaviors
4. The unified effort of professionals directed toward client goals
5. The active participation of the client in implementing rehabilitation goals (often difficult to achieve with clients who have significant cognitive impairment)

It is not surprising, therefore, that rehabilitation counselors are heavily recruited not only into direct services positions but into management positions as well. But generic rehabilitation counseling skills, while necessary, will not be sufficient for the rehabilitation counselor to succeed in the highly competitive field of head injury rehabilitation. Beyond the content areas required in the typical curriculum approved by the Council on Rehabilitation Education, the head injury rehabilitation counselor will also need exposure to the following:

1. The realities of private sector rehabilitation, including insurance policies and practices
2. A basic familiarity with and commitment to fundamental health care marketing issues and techniques
3. A basic knowledge of the physical, psychosocial, cognitive, and communication consequences of head injury (as summarized in Chapter 12)
4. A basic, working knowledge of neurology, neuropsychology, physiological psychology, and applied behavior analysis
5. Familiarity with those rehabilitation counseling considerations that are specific to working with head-injured persons
6. Roles and functions of allied health professionals

SUMMARY

The intention of this chapter is to provide the practicing rehabilitation counselor with an appreciation for the scope and uniqueness of the head injury rehabilitation movement, as well as an idea of where and how rehabilitation counselors fit into this movement. Head injury rehabilitation, in its emphasis upon complex brain-behavior relationships, is presently one of the true "pioneering" areas for vocational rehabilitation counselors and their allied health and human service colleagues. It is a field that presents an exciting professional challenge that is not likely to wane quickly. Chapter 12 deals with more specific, treatment-related considerations.

REFERENCES

Alexander, M. P. (1982). Traumatic brain injury. In D. Benson & D. Blumer (Eds.), *Psychiatric aspects of neurological disease* (Vol. II, pp. 219–245). New York: Grune & Stratton.

Bond, M. R. (1975). Assessment of the psychosocial outcome after severe head injury. *Ciba Foundation Symposium, 34,* 141–153.

Bond, M. R., & Brooks, D. N. (1976). Understanding the process of recovery as a basis for the investigation of rehabilitation for the brain injured. *Scandanavian Journal of Rehabilitation Medicine, 8,* 127–133.

Cassell, J. L., & Mulkey, S. W. (1985). *Rehabilitation caseload management: Concepts and practice.* Austin, TX: PRO-ED.

Cervelli, L. (1984). Head injury rehabilitation: A model for choice. *Rehabilitation Forum, 11*(2).

Commission on Accreditation of Rehabilitation Facilities. (1985). *Standards manual for facilities serving people with disabilities.* Tucson, AZ: Author.

Fordyce, D. L., Roueche, J. R., & Prigatano, G. P. (1983). Enhanced emotional reactions in chronic head trauma patients. *Journal of Neurology, Neurosurgery, and Psychiatry, 46,* 620–624.

Fowler, R. S. (1981). Stroke and cerebral trauma: Psychosocial and vocational aspects. In W. C. Stolov & M. R. Clowers (Eds.), *Handbook of severe disability* (pp. 127–135). Washington, DC: U.S. Department of Education, Rehabilitation Services Administration.

Goldstein, H. (1952). The effect of brain damage on the personality. *Psychiatry, 15,* 245–260.

Gianotti, G. (1972). Emotional behavior and hemispheric side of lesion. *Cortex, 8,* 41–55.

Hackler, E., & Tobis, J. (1983). Reintegration into the community. In M. Rosenthal (Ed.), *Rehabilitation of the head injured adult* (pp. 421–434). Philadelphia: F. A. Davis.

Hall, R. V., & Hall, M. C. (1982). *How to use systematic attention and approval (social reinforcement).* Austin, TX: PRO-ED.

Jaques, M. E. (1970). *Rehabilitation counseling: Scope and services.* Boston: Houghton Mifflin.

Jennett, B. (1975). Who cares for head injuries? *British Medical Journal, 3,* 267–270.

Jennett, B., & Bond, M. (1975). Assessment of outcome of severe brain damage: A practical scale. *Lancet, 1,* 480–484.

Kay, T., Ezrachi, O., & Cavallo, M. (1984). *Annotated bibliography of research on vocational outcome following head trauma.* New York: NYU Medical Center Research and Training Center on Head Trauma and Stroke.

Lasden, M. (1982, June 27). Coming out of coma. *The New York Times Magazine,* pp. 31–36.

Lezak, M. D. (1978). Living with the characterologically altered brain injured patient. *Journal of Clinical Psychiatry, 29,* 592–598.

Malec, J. (1984). Training the brain injured client in behavioral self-management skills. In B. A. Edelstein & E. T. Couture (Eds.), *Behavioral assessment and rehabilitation of the traumatically brain injured* (pp. 121–150). New York: Plenum.

National Head Injury Foundation (1982). *The silent epidemic.* Framingham, MA: Author.

National Head Injury Foundation (1985a). *Cooperative agreement (A memorandum of understanding): National Head Injury Foundation with OSERS, RSA, OSEP, NIHR, CSAVR, and NASDSE.* Framingham, MA: Author.

National Head Injury Foundation (1985b). *National directory of head injury rehabilitation services* (2nd ed.). Framingham, MA: Author.

Oddy, M., Humphrey, M., & Uttley, D. (1978). Stresses upon relatives of head-injured patients. *British Journal of Psychiatry, 133,* 507–513.

Pancsofar, E., & Blackwell, R. (1986). *A user's guide to community re-entry for the severely handicapped.* Albany: State University of New York Press.

Prigatano, G. (in press). Personality and psychosocial consequences after brain injury. In M. Meir, L. Diller, & A. Benton (Eds.), *Neuropsychological Rehabilitation.* London: Churchill Livingston.

Prigatano, G., & Fordyce, D. (in press). Neuropsychological rehabilitation program. In B. Caplan & G. Bray (Eds.), *Handbook of contemporary rehabilitation psychology.* Rockville, MD: Aspen Systems.

Rosenbaum, M., & Najenson, T. (1976). Changes in life patterns and symptoms of low mood as reported by wives of severely brain injured soldiers. *Journal of Consulting and Clinical Psychiatry, 44,* 881–888.

Rosenthal, M. (1984). Strategies for intervention with families of brain-injured patients. In B. A. Edelstein & E. T. Couture (Eds.), *Behavioral assessment and rehabilitation of the traumatically brain-damaged* (pp. 227–246). New York: Plenum.

Segal, J., Boomer, D. S., & Bouthelet, L. (Eds.). (1975). *Research in the service of mental health* (Publication No. [ADM] 75-236). Washington, DC: DHEW, National Institute of Mental Health.

Smith, R. K. (1983). Prevocational programming in the rehabilitation of the head injured patient: A summary. *Physical Therapy, 63,* 2026–2069.

Twelfth Institute on Rehabilitation Issues (1985). *Rehabilitation on TBI (traumatic brain injury).* Menomonie: University of Wisconsin–Stout, Vocational Rehabilitation Institute, Research and Training Center.

Vogenthaler, D. R., & Riggar, T. F. (1985). Theory Z in rehabilitation administration. *Journal of Rehabilitation, 51*(1), 42–45, 79.

Wehman, P. (1981). *Competitive employment: New horizons for severely disabled individuals.* Baltimore: Paul H. Brookes Publishing Co.

Wood, R. L. (1984). Behavior disorders following severe brain injury: Their presentation and psychological management. In N. Brooks (Ed.), *Closed head injury: Psychological, social and family consequences* (pp. 195–219). London: Oxford University Press.

12

Vocational Rehabilitation Counseling with Head-Injured Persons

Robert T. Fraser, Brian T. McMahon, and Donald R. Vogenthaler

EACH YEAR MORE than 422,000 Americans sustain head injuries (Anderson & McLaurin, 1980). While over 100,000 of these persons die as a result of the injury, more than 50,000 of them incur physical, cognitive, psychosocial, and communicative impairments so severe that a return to premorbid levels of independence and productivity are impossible.

In spite of mandatory seat belt laws and drinking/driving reforms, head injuries resulting from motor vehicle accidents continue to exceed the number resulting from home and industrial accidents, falls, assaults, sporting accidents, and firearms combined. Medical advances result in increasing numbers of survivors, many of whom are the most severely injured. While 42% of all head injuries occur to persons under 20, 70% occur to persons under 30, with an additional 12% sustained by those between the ages of 30 and 39. Since head injury survivors tend to have a normal life span (Levin, Benton, & Grossman, 1982) the persisting disabilities have long-term implications for injured persons, their social support system, the rehabilitation profession, and society in general.

Head-injured persons and their families have become more assertive in requesting and securing optimal inpatient and outpatient rehabilitation services. Advocacy groups, legislative directives, and responses by the insurance industry have brought about an increased supply of targeted head injury rehabilitation and allied health services.

This chapter presents some vocational rehabilitation approaches currently being used with head-injured persons. The early sections briefly review the biomechanics of head injury and provide an overview of the types of permanent disability that result. This is followed by a brief section on rehabilitation staffing practices and an overview of cognitive remediation practices in head injury rehabilitation. The bulk of the chapter, however, covers: 1) eligibility determination, 2) elements of the vocational evaluation, 3) considerations relative to planning and counseling, 4) job placement, and 5) case examples.

BIOMECHANICS AND EARLY ASSESSMENT OF HEAD INJURY SEVERITY

Head injuries can be broadly classified as either *penetrating* injuries or *closed head* injuries. In penetrating injuries, an object such as a bullet lacerates the scalp, fractures the skull, and rips the soft tissue in its path, killing nerve cells in the process. In a closed head injury, the initial damage is caused by the collision of the head with another surface (e.g., a car windshield), which results in the brain smashing against the inner surface of the skull. In addition to the nerve damage caused by the brain's impact on the skull (especially when this involves several bony protrusions near the temporal and frontal lobes), even more widespread damage can occur when the brain mass rotates severely within the cranial vault ("shearing"). Because the brain floats in cerebrospinal fluid and is anchored at its base by the spinal cord and the pairs of cranial nerves, a violent twisting action causes the upper mass of the brain to rotate while its lower end is securely anchored in a stationary position. Thus, while the whole brain may be induced to rotate within the skull, its movement may tear the nerve tissue that acts as its anchor. The ascending nature (i.e., these nerves rise to higher levels in the brain) of many of these damaged nerve tracts results in a rather diffuse effect upon widespread areas of the brain that may, themselves, not have been damaged. Additional, often widespread damage can result from secondary factors such as increased intracranial pressure (caused by edema or hemorrhage) and lack of oxygen (caused by respiratory failure or hemorrhage).

The distinction between a penetrating and closed head injury is an important one. Penetrating injuries tend to result in more localized damage and relatively more predictable and discrete disabilities than do closed head injuries. In closed head injury, the nature of the diffuse brain damage results in a mosaic of disabilities that are highly variable, necessitating special awareness and skill among those concerned with the injured person's posttrauma recovery.

Fortunately, it is possible to make at least a crude estimate of the severity of the injury soon after the initial insult. The Glasgow Coma Scale (GCS) (Teasdale & Jennett, 1974) is a 15-point standardized instrument for assessing overall neurological response (i.e., the initial severity of the injury). The scale assesses patients' abilities in three areas: 1) eye-opening ability (i.e., spontaneously, to speech, to pain, none at all), 2) motor responsiveness, and 3) verbal responsiveness (i.e., oriented, confused, incomprehensible, none at all). Several researchers have indicated that a GCS score of 13–15 can be classified as a mild injury, while a score from 9–12 is a moderate injury, and a score of 8 or below is a severe head injury.

Correlational research has shown that Glasgow Coma Scale scores and various other neurological indices are significantly related to various measures of eventual outcome (Brooks, Aughton, Bond, Jones, & Rizvi, 1980; Vogenthaler, 1987). While this is true, it is only possible to gauge the ultimate severity of head injury by assessing its eventual long-term outcome. The Glasgow Outcome Scale is an instrument that has been widely used for assessing global outcome after head injury.

DISABILITY RESULTING FROM HEAD INJURY

The amount of disability resulting from head injury may be significantly affected by the degree of expertise and aggressiveness present during the period of acute medical care. Swift resolution of increased intracranial pressure, hemorrhaging, and lack of oxygen can help minimize the damage to brain tissue. Once medically stabilized, the patient enters the period of acute rehabilitation. During this period some patients will remain in prolonged coma (1–9 months). For many patients, this period is characterized by gradual, steady improvement in various functions (e.g., physical, cognitive, behavioral). While some persons seem to fully recover all functions, for many others the extent of recovery across functions varies, with some functions showing no recovery whatsoever (Jennett, 1983). Ideally, the acute rehabilitation period ends with the client recovering sufficiently to resume most previous activities.

For many, however, the process of recovery may take years and never be fully complete. It is these persons who receive the bulk of postacute rehabilitation services, of which vocational rehabilitation counseling is but one. Other postacute rehabilitation services include, but are not limited to, speech and language rehabilitation, cognitive remediation, physical therapy, psychotherapy, behavior therapy, activities of daily living training, independent living rehabilitation, and therapeutic recreation. For many of these patients, the period of postacute rehabilitation can begin about 6 months after injury (depending upon length of coma, availability of services, etc.) and can last from a few months to several years (depending upon financial resources, level of insurance benefits, etc.). A brief overview of some of the postinjury symptoms in three major categories of injury severity is presented below. More detailed descriptions can be found in Vogenthaler (1987), Rosenthal, Griffith, Bond, and Miller (1983), and Lishman (1973).

Mild Head Injury

Mild head injury constitutes 85% of all head injuries. Persons with such injuries may have a brief (usually less than 20 minutes) or no loss of consciousness, posttraumatic amnesia of less than 1 hour, and/or a GCS score of 13–15. While neurological exams (including CAT scans and EEG) are often normal, permanent structural microscopic nerve damage often results from mild head injury. Many of the disabilities resulting from mild head injury are subtle and are neither easily recognized nor understood by the patient or those around him or her. Some deficits (termed the *postconcussive syndrome*) can persist for months, years or indefinitely. These deficits may include fatigue, headache, dizziness, lethargy, irritability, personality changes, cognitive deficits, decreased information-processing speed, and perceptual difficulties.

Impairments in mental functioning can lead to feelings of incompetence, guilt, and frustration. Family members can become impatient and frustrated when the patient outwardly appears normal but continues to perform subnormally in many areas. The reasons for the subnormal performance are difficult for rehabilitationists without head injury training or experience to recognize and understand. Vocational counselors typically become involved with such persons with mild head injuries after they have returned to work and failed.

Moderate Head Injury

Moderate head injury accounts for roughly 10% of all head injuries and is characterized by a period of unconsciousness, by post-traumatic amnesia ranging from 1 to 24 hours, and/or by Glasgow Coma Scale scores of 9–12. There is wide variability among these individuals in the extent of permanent physical and cognitive impairment experienced. Muscle spasticity, poor coordination, paralysis, seizures, and sensory communication problems are all common. Cognitive impairments in the areas of planning, sequencing, judgment, reasoning, functional language, and computation skills are also possible. Psychosocial problems can include self-centeredness, denial, mood swings, agitation, depression, lethargy, sexual dysfunction, emotional lability, low frustration tolerance, disinhibition, poor judgment, impulsivity, and behavioral outbursts. The Twelfth Institute on Rehabilitation Issues (TIRI) (1985) reported that it is usually 6–12 months before many of these patients think about returning or attempt to return to work. Studies have reported that 66% of these patients are unable to work for a year or more after the injury (TIRI, 1985).

Severe Head Injury

Roughly 5% of all head injuries can be categorized as severe. Persons with severe head injury experience a period of unconsciousness or posttrauma amnesia in excess of 8 days, and score 8 or less on the Glasgow Coma Scale. In addition to the cognitive, psychological, and behavioral disabilities noted under the other severity levels, these individuals are likely to have brain stem damage resulting in severe, permanent physical disabilities such as paralysis, weakness, spasticity, and tremors. Oftentimes, the speech apparatus is affected. Persons with severe head injury can spend up to a year or more in a rehabilitation hospital setting, followed by a sequence of treatment in residential, transitional, supervised living, or day treatment centers. Progress can be slow, extended courses of recovery are routine, and it may be several months or years before any attempt is made to return to work. If a return to work is achieved, it is usually in a reduced capacity, and often with a benevolent employer. Most of these patients remain very dependent upon families and social agencies for a substantial amount of care.

Catastrophic Head Injury

Catastrophic head injury, a subcategory of severe head injury, is characterized by coma of several months duration, after which a coma-like state (the persistent vegetative state) emerges. Persons with catastrophic head injuries may appear to be awake in the sense that they have sleep/wake cycles and allow themselves to be fed. However, they never regain any meaningful communication with their environment and usually remain institutionalized for life.

It is important to note, however, that exceedingly long periods of true coma do not automatically lead to persistent vegetative state. There are reports of head-injured adults being comatose for as long as 5–9 months who, after regaining consciousness, were able to participate in meaningful rehabilitation activities (although all would be classified as severely disabled on the Glasgow Outcome Scale).

STANDARD PROBLEM CHECKLISTS

A rehabilitation counselor who is seeing a number of head-injured clients should utilize one of the available standard problem checklists for assessing the array of symptoms and areas of difficulty experienced by those with head injury (Lynch & Mauss, 1981; TIRI, 1985). While it is beyond the scope of this chapter to discuss these problem checklists in any detail, it should be noted that they include assessment of such areas as physical status and accompanying medical conditions, disturbance of oral functions and communication, inappropriate social behavior and changes in emotional response, disorientation to time and place, self-centeredness, nonacceptance of the disability, fixation on memory of previous normal state, changes in intellectual functioning, impairments in activities of daily living, sensory and motor problems, and other effects of the trauma. Depending upon the client's postinjury stage of recovery, different types of assessment tools and strategies must be employed (Long, Gouvier, & Cole, 1984).

REHABILITATION STAFFING PATTERNS

The professional approaches used in the management and rehabilitation of the head-injured person are dependent upon the stage of postinjury adjustment. Initially, the acute medical nature of the injury requires the involvement of the neurosurgeon and allied medical personnel. By noting clinical signs such as Glasgow Coma Scale score, amount of time needed to follow a command, or length of posttrauma amnesia, the neurosurgeon's report can provide information regarding the initial severity of the injury. This information can help establish some initial parameters and expectations for rehabilitation practitioners who will be involved with the patient later in the recovery course.

Once a patient is medically stable, a neurologist will review neurosurgical data and determine if the patient is to be given anti-seizure medication. The work of Jennett (1975) has provided neurologists with a method for determining the likelihood that seizures will develop. Depending upon the combination of these factors, the risk of seizures ranges from 3% to 70%. A complete discussion of this topic is provided by Fraser (1985).

The physiatrist is a medical doctor who is the rehabilitation team leader in the hospital setting, and who has the skills to develop a comprehensive picture of the patient's range of neurological assets and deficits. The physiatrist directs the physical therapist, speech and language pathologist, occupational therapist, neuropsychologist, nurses, and other staff in the assessment and treatment of the patient. As the patient improves medically, a neuropsychologist, a clinical or counseling psychologist, or a speech and language pathologist will often assume leadership of the treatment team.

When medical concerns have substantially decreased and the patient moves from the hospital, concerns in other areas such as emotion, behavior, and cognition emerge more forcefully. The variety of treatment strategies and programming designed to ameliorate these problems has increased greatly over the last decade (even though it is recognized that the supply of head injury rehabilitation services remains inadequate to meet demand).

Because so wide a variety of postinjury deficits emerge (and in varying levels of intensity), and because each individual head-injured person's environment (e.g., premorbid socioeconomic status; strength of their social support system) is unique, a wide variety of program models is needed to provide optimal treatment for these clients. These program models include "day care programs, learning disability programs, transitional living programs, specialized vocational training programs, behavioral modification programs, long-term maintenance programs, sheltered living facilities'' (Santa Clara Valley Medical Center, 1982, p. *i*-2). Several books and articles have been written describing various program models and their constituent elements (Long et al., 1984; Rosenthal et al., 1983; TIRI, 1985; Vogenthaler, in press).

When an outpatient rehabilitation case management approach is used, treatment supervision and case management responsibilities should be handled by experienced head injury rehabilitation professionals, whether they be a neurologist, clinical or counseling psychologist, speech pathologist, rehabilitation counselor, social worker, or nurse. It is essential that the case manager be knowledgeable about head injury deficit patterns and the multitude of treatment strategies that are available.

Effective case managers, using an interdisciplinary approach, should evaluate treatment efficacy by involving the treatment team and other relevant professionals. For example, when cognitive remediation efforts or independent living training are done in isolation of other professional input, useful information about the client's level of cognitive, psychodynamic, and behavioral functioning are missed. In such a situation, providing cognitive training without an adequate neuropsychological conceptualization of the clients' abilities can prove to be fruitless, frustrating, and expensive. It is dismaying that professional territoriality or economic concerns can prevent a client from getting coordinated advice on a cognitive remediation or other rehabilitation program. The Twelfth Institute on Rehabilitation Issues (1985) recommended that the rehabilitation case manager always try to seek services from an ''integrated rehabilitation team'' with experience in this area. Because cognitive retraining is such an important part of head injury rehabilitation, the following section is presented as a basic orientation to this specialization.

COGNITIVE RETRAINING

Cognitive deficits clearly overshadow physical deficits as the primary cause of difficulties experienced by head-injured individuals in independent living, social readaptation, family life, and vocational pursuits (Ben-Yishay & Diller, 1983). As a result, much activity is presently being devoted to developing new cognitive remediation strategies. The interested reader is referred to Gianutsos (1980) for a brief overview of the developments in cognitive remediation and Trexler (1982) for an in-depth orientation.

In general, cognitive retraining is a set of interventions designed to ameliorate the sensory/perceptual, language-related, and central processing deficits of head-injured patients. Ben-Yishay and Diller (1983) have developed a carefully structured and sequenced treatment protocol for the retraining of attention, orientation, control of impulsivity, visual and auditory perception, language, and simple to complex problem solving.

The advent of the microcomputer has spurred a dramatic rise in the number and variety of computer-based cognitive remediation strategies. Whether computer-based or not, cognitive remediation treatment plans are often presented to the rehabilitation counselor or case manager as a well-organized, detailed set of procedures that result in specific, discrete gains for the client. A careful review of these interventions nationally would probably indicate that there is a paucity of empirical data regarding the effectiveness of these strategies. Oftentimes the computer software used is not well keyed to a client's age, preinjury level of functioning, or location and extent of cerebral damage (and the client's resultant neuropsychological strengths and weaknesses).

Two of the more empirically developed and researched cognitive retraining systems are those of Ben-Yishay and Diller (1983) and the REHABIT system of Reitan (1982). The REHABIT system addresses the areas of language, visual-spatial perception, and higher order analytic skills as distinct areas for cognitive retraining. This system allows for sequential building upon previously learned skills, and also provides a presentation of tasks that demand the utilization of skills within all three areas simultaneously. Reitan (1986) indicates that initial reports of REHABIT'S utility in cognitive rehabilitation are still somewhat conflicting.

It is unclear which head-injured patients will profit from the various cognitive retraining procedures. Likewise, the maintenance of gains made through the various cognitive remediation interventions and the extent of generalizability to areas of vocational functioning and activities for daily living are unclear (Diller & Gordon, 1981).

It is likely that cognitive retraining will be more valuable to the client if it closely relates to specific job-related skills or adaptive abilities that assist in independent living. This approach should have more face validity to the client, and should also allow the rehabilitation counselor to assess more closely progress and treatment effectiveness.

Mikula (1984) has established some basic guidelines for the provision of services in cognitive remediation. These guidelines include: 1) the necessity for assessing the cognitive strengths and weaknesses of the client; 2) the development of a written treatment plan with specific, functionally stated goals and objectives; 3) a description of the cognitive remediation methods to be used; 4) criteria for advancing to more difficult levels of the program; 5) expected duration of the program; and 6) established criteria for completion of cognitive remediation services.

The TIRI (1985) provides an excellent review of cognitive rehabilitation. The interested reader is also referred to the reviews by Blanton and Gouvier (1986), Diller and Gordon (1981), and Miller (1980). While the literature indicates that cognitive remediation programs seldom specify their criteria for accepting or rejecting patients for treatment (Diller & Gordon, 1981), the rehabilitation counselor should use the above-mentioned guidelines when assessing the sophistication of the treatment program. A consulting neuropsychologist can also be of help to the rehabilitation counselor in determining the appropriateness of available cognitive remediation programs for head-injured clients.

THE VOCATIONAL REHABILITATION PROCESS WITH HEAD-INJURED PERSONS

Many referrals for state vocational rehabilitation services are individuals with mild and moderate degrees of injury severity. In many cases, the person who is referred with a mild or moderate head injury will be someone who returned to work after the injury, failed to perform adequately, and was fired or put on medical leave. Persons with moderate injuries are frequently referred by physicians or other allied health professionals. Because of their very short involvement in the medical setting (a few hours to a day or so) and apparent lack of disabling sequelae, persons with mild injuries are usually self-referred. Referrals of severely injured persons will also occur, but normally after a period of stabilization that can last anywhere from 6 months to 2 years after injury.

In some cases, the disabling consequences that prompt the referral are fairly evident (e.g., epilepsy). When probing beyond the client's "presenting condition," the clinician may find that the other consequences of head injury (of which epilepsy is but one) are actually more vocationally disabling. Head-injured persons who continue to experience memory deficits, problem-solving difficulties, mental inflexibility, and lack of insight into their limitations may lose several jobs without clearly knowing the reasons. For example, an individual may have a seizure condition as a result of a head injury received in a car accident. While the presenting disability might be the seizure disorder, in fact it is the subtle difficulties related to a mild, or even a more severe, head injury (e.g., memory deficits, marginal problem-solving difficulties, or mental inflexibility) that are more vocationally disabling. An astute rehabilitation counselor will probe beyond the presenting condition and perhaps find a history of minor head injury. It is possible that a client's job history can give clues about the presence of brain injury sequelae. Head injury–related disabilities can be subtle and difficult to recognize and conceptualize for both client and counselor. Some of the clients with head injury will be unrealistic in their vocational goals, and the agency counselor may have to work with or around that difficulty for a period of time (see the counseling section in this chapter for further suggestions).

Because of the wide variety and severity of deficits resulting from head injury, a rehabilitation counselor may find the vocational evaluation process to be especially complex and demanding. In addition to an awareness of the somewhat obvious deficits, the counselor, particularly when serving as case manager, needs to possess a knowledge of and appreciation for the many subtle and even obscure deficits that may be present (e.g., marginal memory problems, deficits in executive thinking, difficulty in learning new material). The disruption of perceptual, cognitive, and emotional functioning can result in a subtle mosaic of deficit patterns that are, many times, much less than obvious.

The report from the TIRI (1985) identified four criteria that should be considered in most cases before a client is accepted for vocational rehabilitation services. They are: 1) the client's ability to participate in the evaluation process, 2) the client's stage of recovery, 3) the appropriateness of the services being requested, and 4) the existence of alternative sources of funding. These four criteria are briefly reviewed below.

First, an assessment must be made of the client's ability to participate actively in the evaluation process. A valid vocational evaluation can only be undertaken with clients who are awake, alert, and oriented. Second, the vocational rehabilitation counselor will want to determine the client's stage of recovery. Because much spontaneous neurological recovery occurs in the first 6–12 months after injury, particularly for the moderate to severely injured, it may be wise to delay an assessment of vocational potential until later in the recovery course, when it appears that the client's period of rapid progress has leveled off somewhat. When the assessment occurs at an optimal period in time, the evaluator will be able to draw a more valid picture of that client's ultimate vocational potential.

Third, the vocational rehabilitation counselor must determine the appropriateness of the services being requested. Generally, requests made relatively soon after injury tend to be medically related, while later requests tend to be more vocationally or prevocationally related. While each case is unique and decisions must be made on a case-by-case basis, a general rule of thumb for state vocational rehabilitation counselors is "vocational rehabilitation funding is most appropriate for services that *specifically further the process of vocational placement*" (TIRI, 1985, p. 38). One could argue that the need for a wheelchair, while facilitative of vocational activities, is a general need and not specifically related to the vocational process. Cognitive retraining may be a vocationally relevant service for a client who has difficulty remaining alert and attentive. However, it may not be vocationally relevant for a client with cognitive deficits who has lost jobs due to temper outbursts. Because of the nature of this client's job, the cognitive deficits may not be a handicap while the inability to control one's anger is a handicap. Elaborating on this issue, the TIRI stated:

> It is a mistake to narrowly define what services are "specific" to vocational return. For example, virtually *all* traumatically brain injured clients are unrealistic and at least partially unaware of their deficits. To go through a profes-

> sionally guided process of becoming aware of one's deficits, coming to terms with them, and redefining one's life and vocational goals, may be absolutely crucial if the client stands a chance of returning to work. To provide such professional services in fact becomes *specific* to the vocational process, and thus an appropriate service for the vocational rehabilitation counselor to fund. (1985, p. 39)

Therefore, individual psychotherapy or group therapy emphasizing self- and social awareness may be very appropriate. Fourth, the person managing the case must be aware of all existing sources of funding for the purchase of services and products for the client (e.g., worker's compensation insurance, personal liability insurance). Many private head trauma rehabilitation centers (residential and nonresidential) have been recently created, and many more are likely to be developed. These programs may be the best source of services for a given client, and if the state vocational rehabilitation counselor is aware of third-party funding, he or she should inform the client and significant others of these facts.

It is a difficult task to assess employability in the head-injured population. Sbordone and Howard (1985) reviewed the various demographic, neurological, behavioral, and environmental factors that may positively or negatively affect rehabilitation outcome. The factors identified are based upon professional opinion rather than research. They simply present a framework in which the counselor can weigh the merits of a client's potential to benefit from vocational rehabilitation services. No studies to date have comprehensively considered these factors in relation to predicting rehabilitation outcome.

In many cases, the vocational evaluation of persons with head injuries is more complicated and time consuming than evaluations of persons with other disabilities. Regardless of the amount of time elapsed since the injury, if an appropriate referral has been received, then the following categories of evaluation information should be collected.

Sociodemographic History

A thorough history for the preinjury period, emphasizing vocational information, should include: 1) demographics; 2) preinjury job or job goal with work values/interests; 3) relevant work history, including chronological work history (levels of productivity, work quality, and salary level can be particularly helpful); 4) educational history or specific vocational training; 5) premorbid health background (to include alcohol, drug, or psychiatric history); and 6) social history and behavioral predispositions (e.g., how they dealt with adversity).

The history of the client for the postinjury period should include: 1) level of independence at home, including activities of daily living (ADLs) and household chores (this information can provide very valuable clues about ability to function on a job); 2) financial status and support sources; 3) level of independence in travel; 4) existence of unsettled lawsuits; 5) how free time is spent; and 6) in what organizations the client is involved.

Medical History

Medical history should include history since injury, indices of the injury severity (GCS score, length of coma, period of posttraumatic amnesia, or time to command), results of diagnostic exams, other physical complications, and the course of hospital treatment. Much of this information can be secured from a discharge summary.

It is important to review the course of treatment. If an individual had brain surgery or developed a seizure condition, additional complications may be present. As a result of the surgery, an individual may have a shunt that must be medically monitored. Similarly, seizure conditions will require monitoring by the neurologist and medications should be assessed in relation to potential side effects. Finally, current medical status and needs are also required information.

Deficits

The range of deficits, levels of intensity, and the extraordinary variety of deficit combinations and interactions make assessment most challenging for the vocational rehabilitation counselor. The counselor must understand what deficits are possible and how they affect return to work. In most cases, the rehabilitation counselor will rely upon the reports of other professional specializations when determining a client's physical, cognitive, executive, and behavioral/psychosocial deficits. The counselor will want these professionals to specify how a given deficit will interfere with daily functioning. Additionally, the rehabilitation counselor will want to know the ways in which the deficit can be remediated (if at all) or compensated for (e.g., the use of a note system for memory impairment). Finally, the rehabilitation counselor must gauge the impact of the deficit upon vocational functioning. Is a given deficit a handicap to employment?

The report of the TIRI (1985) and Vogenthaler (1987) provides overviews of the myriad deficits possible after head injury. Very briefly these deficits can be categorized into: 1) physical deficits (e.g., weakness, incoordination, balance, speech, the five senses, fatigue); 2) cognitive deficits (e.g., arousal, attention/concentration, learning and memory, language, perception, constructional functions, reasoning and concept formation); 3) behavioral/psychosocial deficits (e.g., impulsivity, aggression, depression); and 4) executive deficits. It is, perhaps, the area of executive deficit that sets brain-injured clients apart from other disability groups. Examples include problems in goal formation, planning, executing plans, self-monitoring, awareness of others, and ability to anticipate. The TIRI stated:

> Executive functioning is difficult to measure in formal testing situations, precisely because it is called into play when the client . . . must provide the structure, planning, and organization. Clients with well developed skill areas may fail at a job because they cannot plan and anticipate, monitor their own performance, or take the needs of others into account. . . .Traumatically brain injured clients are notorious for ''talking a good game;'' i.e., impressing you with the descriptions of what they do, what they want, and what they are capable of. If the client has significant executive dysfunctions, this verbal self-description may bear scant resemblance to the reality of the person's life, much less their realistic potential. Probably thousands of traumatically brain injured clients have failed in return to work because counselors based vocational plans on what the client *appeared* to be capable of. It is extremely important to gather information on the executive deficits of traumatically brain injured clients, if a realistic vocational rehabilitation plan is to be effected. (1985, p. 59)

Family/Significant Other Support

While formal evaluation efforts can be very helpful, the best information may be provided by family members and allied health professionals in the individual's environment on a daily basis. In developing a rehabilitation plan for the head-injured client, it is definitely of value to review the individual's community support system. A good support system may enable the counselor to attempt service activities that would otherwise be impossible. Additionally, the counselor should know that some type of community services management will be necessary if there is no support system, or if the available support system is inadequate. Contracts with community agencies can be negotiated in this regard.

Neuropsychological Functioning

Psychologists with a neuropsychological specialty are invaluable in the rehabilitation process. In seeking a qualified neuropsychologist, the counselor should seek an individual who is a diplomate of the American Board of Clinical Neuropsychology, a board-eligible Ph.D. with 1 year of supervised experience, or a Ph.D. or Ed.D. with 2 or more years of supervised experience in clinical neuropsychology (TIRI, 1985). When difficulty in identifying such a professional occurs, the National Head Injury Foundation, a state psychological association, or local universities and hospitals can be contacted in order to secure these services.

Neuropsychological testing involves a comprehensive evaluation of intelligence, language, memory, and other higher cortical functions. These tests have proven to be sensitive to the presence, location, and severity of brain dysfunction. A test battery of this type provides basic information that enables the case manager and treatment team to conceptualize a client's neurological pattern of asset and deficit and develop a clearer understanding of specific brain-behavior relationships.

Neuropsychological testing is critical in brain injury rehabilitation and can be administered in a serial fashion to complement the client's stages of recovery. For example, Cripe (1985) proposed tests such as the Galveston Orientation and Amnesia Test, the Russell Administration of the Wechsler Memory Scale, and measures of speed of information processing such as the Trail Making Test or the Symbol Digit Modality Test for use during the posttrauma amnesia phase of recovery. Cripe recommended that standardized batteries not be used until a level of neuropsychological stabilization is reached. In most instances, after a 6-month period of recovery after injury, standardized neuropsychological batteries such as the Luria, the Luria-Nebraska, and Halstead-Reitan may be considered. Familiarity with these batteries can aid the rehabilitation counselor in developing vocational planning steps for individuals having a specific pattern (e.g., right versus left, or type of memory impairment) or level of disablement (e.g., mild, moderate, or severe).

Additional individualized testing can be added to a battery for assessing a client's upper limits or range of abilities, specifically as they relate to a job goal. Continued experience with a standardized, core battery enables the rehabilitation counselor to develop a context for understanding the type of rehabilitation plan that is likely to be successful with a client having certain neuropsychological impairments. It should be cautioned that to some degree, neuropsychological test battery results will underestimate an individual's capacity for functional daily activities. Nonetheless, if these measures are not considered and descriptions of the individual's everyday abilities solely relied upon, cognitive abilities will be overestimated (Williams, 1985). The most valid information for initial planning involves synthesizing data from the neuropsychological battery with the individual's observed functional abilities.

The standard referral questions that neuropsychologists are prepared to address are related to levels of impairment; individual abilities; pattern of abilities; differences in sensory, motor and reflex functioning on the two sides of the body; and the presence of pathognomonic signs (e.g., specific aphasic signs, visual field defects, auditory or visual-spatial deficits). The TIRI (1985) proposed that the neuropsychologist focus more on the client's specific functional capacities. These include:

1. Specific vocational and functional limitations
2. Whether formal training or educational programs are reasonable for the individual
3. Difficulties that may have been encountered in prior employment
4. Level of supervision necessary in present work activities
5. The individual's level of stamina
6. Level of insight into present neuropsychological functioning
7. The individual's ability to compensate for deficits

8. The individual's ability to identify and correct errors
9. The ability to initiate and remain focused on job tasks

It is the responsibility of the rehabilitation counselor to request this type of information from the neuropsychologist. The relevance of a neuropsychological report is generally based on its functional nature and the neuropsychologist's ability to respond to the relevant referral questions. Most rehabilitation counselors value the neuropsychological evaluation highly if it includes specific recommendations for treatment planning. For a more complete description of these issues, the reader is directed to Appendix C of the final report of the TIRI (1985).

Psychological Functioning

Emotional and personality functioning with head-injured populations has been assessed through use of the Minnesota Multiphasic Personality Inventory (MMPI). Dikmen and Reitan (1979) indicate that the profiles of head-injured patients with chronic dysfunction suggest depression, anxiety, somatic concerns, and the endorsement of more unusual experiences than other patient groups. During the course of recovery, these patients were found to improve on the inventory in regard to their emotional and personality functioning. A more recent study by Fordyce, Roueche, and Prigatano (1983), however, suggests that head-injured patients experience more difficulties over the course of time, and postulates that clients' psychosocial maladjustment is related to their awareness of the neuropsychological deficits that became obvious during the course of rehabilitation treatment.

The MMPI has been most helpful as a general indicator of adjustment following head injury and a rough indicator of vocational readiness. However, the MMPI is a relatively long inventory involving 566 items. Shorter inventories such as the Millon Clinical Multiaxial Inventory or rating forms that are completed by other observers (e.g., the Brief Psychiatric Rating Form or the Katz Adjustment Scale) may prove useful.

Vocational Functioning

A number of traditional aptitude, interest, personality, work sample, and other assessment tools can be utilized with head-injured clients. In a number of cases, however, administration may need to be modified. For example, a client with certain language deficits may no longer be able to read and comprehend a vocational interest inventory. The same inventory, however, might be reviewed with the client item by item.

Standardized work samples may have some vocational prognostic value with head-injured populations, but are probably more useful in assessing how these clients can best learn. Variations in the prescribed method of providing instructions and flexible time requirements are recommended, as the intent is often to maximize performance. When the samples are used in this manner, the norms become invalid and the results, although clinically relevant, should not be interpreted against the established norms. Often, failure in a simple task does not preclude success on a higher level task which was well learned premorbidly and is still maintained (e.g., driving, in some cases). Thus, aborting a sequence of work samples after several failures (as is often recommended by the manual) may not be wise. Given fatigue and other psychosocial sequelae associated with head injury, several short evaluation sessions are often recommended to establish an accurate range of the individual's performance. Isolated point-in-time evaluations may generate meaningless findings.

Weinberger (1984) provided an example of the use of work samples to gauge the learning capacities of a 19-year-old head-injured patient. The patient was unable to follow the multi-step directions related to the computing work sample of the JEVS system. This appeared to be the result of cognitive impairments including attention deficit, short-term memory deficit, and limited frustration tolerance. The evaluator assisted the patient by reading the instructions and by developing a flow chart. Each step of the task was then modeled for the patient, having the patient repeat each step on his own. In approximately 3 hours, the patient was able to follow the flow chart independently and successfully complete the task. By the third day he was completing the task independently. This case demonstrates how flexible and creative the skilled evaluator must be when assessing the vocational potential of persons with head injuries.

Generally speaking, situational assessments are often preferred to the use of standardized work samples. Occupational trials in the community, volunteer opportunities, or previous employment sites represent excellent on-the-job evaluation opportunities. Within the rehabilitation environment, work stations can be established around a variety of work or work-related situations such as cafeteria, building maintenance, business office, groundskeeping, laundry, or transportation. The most important ingredients are the availability of competent supervision and "real work" activities.

Cautions for the Vocational Evaluator

When a client is referred for vocational evaluation, it should be made clear to the referral sources or family members that the client is being observed, not trained. Avoiding the term "evaluation" with the head-injured client can often help minimize anxiety related to the experience. Particular focus should be placed on attention span, concentration, stamina, interpersonal skills, response to authority, and sense of production/task completion. The evaluator should also attempt to identify compensatory mechanisms that can maximize performance if used.

Anger and frustration, which may be expressed outwardly or through withdrawal, are likely to mirror the degree of perceived confrontation, competitiveness, or pressure in the environment. Vocational evaluation findings must be tied closely to the key psychological factors that can influence vocational adjustment for a specific client. The vocational evaluator should synthesize his or her findings with the neuropsychologist's in order to distinguish between organic/structural deficits and those which are treatable or modifiable given the proper instruction, conditions, or environment. The evaluator should identify the inefficient behaviors that may be amenable to change through training or behavioral management techniques. Family input regarding the vocational evaluator's findings can serve to refine recommendations and the anticipated barriers to employment.

Potentially helpful strategies for remediating unrealistic client expectations include further occupational exploration (especially involving key worker contacts), on-the-job evaluation, and planned failure. The latter is useful only in the context of a solid counseling relationship with a client whose expectations are uncompromising. This extreme approach calls for providing a full measure of professional assistance toward the expressed vocational choice, while pointing out alternative directions in related occupations along the way. If/when failure occurs, the rehabilitation counselor should adopt a supportive posture and request cooperation from the client in the pursuit of compromise objectives.

Planning and Counseling

Planning and counseling are critical functions in the determination of rehabilitation outcome. This section reviews these functions and gives specific attention to dealing with unrealistic client expectations and basic counseling interaction concerns.

Planning The rehabilitation counselor's planning function with head-injured persons usually involves a higher level of management and coordination skill than with other rehabilitation populations. The role of the counselor will vary with the resources available in the community. In some cases, the counselor must assume a primary role for counseling the client and family members. In other cases, these functions are assumed by a neuropsychologist, clinical psychologist, social worker, or other staff members within a specialized community program. The counselor should be informed about the case and work with interdisciplinary team members that are available in the community, such as the neuropsychologist, work evaluator, speech pathologist, or teacher, to develop the optimal program for the client. Some cases require a substantial amount of contractual work with community resource people such as specialized teachers, home health personnel, and special educators. In many instances, the actual case management function will be handled by another rehabilitation or health care agency due to the case's time demands and complexity.

With a gradual increase in day treatment and transitional living programs for head-injured persons, rehabilitation counselors will need to become more sophisticated in evaluating and referring to these programs. Since job placement remains a critical concern for the rehabilitation counselor, the vocational outcomes of these programs should be carefully assessed. In a review of the existing literature on vocational outcome following head trauma, Kay, Ezrachi, and Cavallo (1986) found that the rate of return to work varied from 25% to 97%, with the length of time from injury to return to employment ranging from 6 months to 5 years. Community-based head injury treatment programs report between 25% and 80% of their referrals being returned to competitive employment, although often in a part-time capacity and/or at reduced levels of employment. Unfortunately, it is often difficult to determine whether the individual's return to work is the result of such factors as the efforts of a very receptive former employer, spontaneous remission of difficulties (as in mild head injury), or the treatment effects of the community head injury program.

If the client is moderately to severely disabled by the head injury, it is desirable to discuss with community agency representatives their rehabilitation practices and record of vocational outcomes with clients having similar levels of impairment. For example, it would be helpful to review a program's vocational outcomes for those individuals with posttrauma amnesia of more than 2 weeks, a GCS of 10 and below, or Halstead-Reitan neuropsychological impairment indices in the moderate to severe ranges. The counselor should also determine the program's follow-up practices and the duration of employment for those clients placed. Through this review, the counselor can acquire a clearer picture of the performance of the community rehabilitation unit with more challenging clients. By approaching the purchase of services in this manner, the counselor will have a better understanding of both the agency's vocational rehabilitation practices and their ultimate value.

Counseling The counseling role of the vocational rehabilitation professional with the head-injured individual can require some significant shifts in focus depending on the client's stage of recovery. In the first few months following the head injury, much time should be spent educating family members and significant others about the disability and dealing with its by-products (e.g., emotional alterations, dependency, deficits in social awareness, or difficulties with learning and problem solving). As clients further recover from head trauma, more staff time should be spent helping them adjust to the disability, dealing with family members, and handling other problems faced in interacting with their environment. For a more complete review of working with family members, the reader is directed to Diehl (1983), Lezak (1978), and Rosenthal and Muir (1983).

Most family members will require some intensive counseling and advisement in relation to taking care of their own needs. It is important that significant individuals in the head-injured person's environment be able to maintain their own functional roles. Spouses and young children can have a particularly difficult time and need to understand clearly the ramifications of the disability.

There will be a number of persons referred for vocational rehabilitation services who have emotional and behavioral difficulties that can be positively altered through behavioral treatment interventions. In some cases, treatment should be provided within a residential treatment center. In many other cases, however, behaviorally trained psychologists and social workers in the community can be helpful in developing programs to deal with difficulties related to employment. The interested reader is referred to articles by Goodman-Smith and Turnbull (1983), MacNeill, Horton, and Howe (1981), and a "how to" manual by Olson and Henig (1983).

Much of the therapy with head-injured persons can be more effectively implemented within a group context. The group approach can assist in relieving isolation while at the same time improving social perception and social skills functioning. An encouraging report by Braunling-McMorrow, Lloyd, and Fralish (1986) suggests that social skills such as giving compliments, confrontation, and social dialogue do generalize outside the group setting in which the skills are taught.

Use of videotaping in individual and group therapy situations for the head-injured client is an effective adjunct to treatment. Given the poor self-awareness, problem-solving deficits, rigidity in thinking, and other difficulties experienced by the head-injured person, the use of videotape acts as a stimulus that facilitates interactions and the grasping of insights. Through direct feedback, this medium enables the client and/or family members to formulate a clearer understanding of the problem. It can enable the head-injured client to understand better the range of difficulties being experienced and to assess progress on a number of different adjustment tracks. Pre- and post-trauma changes in the individual's emotional and cognitive integration can be reviewed at therapy termination to reinforce the patient's awareness of what occurred during the intervention. Finally, the videotape can be stored and used to reorient the patient to the areas of difficulty; the relevant compensatory strategies; and prior gains made, in the event that patient or family members begin to function inadequately in the community.

The most frequently encountered issue in vocational counseling with head-injured individuals is unrealistic client vocational goals. Although there are several possible manifestations of this problem, the most common are overestimating career goals and underestimating the time and effort required to achieve them. It is important to realize that this is a perfectly normal consequence of head injury and that its management is within the purview of the rehabilitation counselor. As such, it should not be minimized, discounted, deferred, or dismissed. The following course of action is recommended.

First, consult with the psychologist or personal adjustment counselor who is following the case. Even brief collaboration will demonstrate that the degree of unrealism/overestimation of vocational goals occurs in direct proportion to the lack of awareness/acceptance regarding the disabling condition. Thus it is crucial that all professionals coordinate their respective approaches to the client during this phase of adjustment.

Second, all team members must be made aware that unrealistic expectations are often present in the adjustment process. Unrealistic client goals may provide a primary source of hope or directionality that is then responsible for compliance in other important areas of the client's rehabilitation program, such as physical restoration or social skills training. Accordingly, the rehabilitation counselor's timing for interventions designed to improve the client's realism, as well as the selection of intervention techniques, should be processed with the entire treatment team before proceeding.

Third, the unequivocal and active involvement of all family members, in addition to treatment team support, in an intervention strategy and the timing of its deployment is fundamental. Families are primary influences on career development for most young adults, whether disabled or not.

Basic Interactional Considerations

There are several interaction guidelines that may be helpful for the counselor working with the head-injured client. These include:

1. Be consistent with the client by modeling calm, controlled behavior
2. When locked into perseverative confrontation with an agitated client, redirect the topic and offer options, while reinforcing positive directions
3. Channel the client's attention by using relevant cues emphasizing an appropriate cognitive or sensory modality to engage the client
4. Review available information from medical records, family members, the neuropsychological report, or other consulting specialists to ensure the counseling interaction is emphasizing the client's cognitive or sensory assets: language related, visual-spatial, tactile, or auditory
5. Teach the client skills in more than one setting to maximize generalization
6. Focus on a specific vocational/avocational goal
7. Allow clients sufficient time for reframing their self-concept, or actual mourning time to absorb the implications of the impairments discussed in counseling sessions
8. Help modulate the amount of stress in the client's environment
9. Expect the unexpected
10. Accentuate positive gains

Job Placement Approaches

For some head-injured individuals, job placement can be related to prior work activity insofar as it utilizes their residual assets. For individuals who cannot return to a prior job, who do not have the immediate available abilities necessary to assume a specific new position, or who have never worked, the road to placement involves them in a progressive continuum of vocational adjustment and placement services.

Miller (1980) suggests that the technologies developed for training persons who are mentally retarded are a starting point for assessing the training and return-to-work issues for head-injured populations. It should be noted that the job placement process for a moderate to severely impaired head-injured client can reasonably last from 6 months to 2 years or more. This presupposes that the client is stabilized neuropsychologically and the goal is competitive employment. The application of behavior technologies and the use of supported employment models (Wehman, 1981) may shorten time lines considerably.

Having individuals involved with work-related materials and tools as soon as possible following the head trauma would probably reduce retraining or training time. Walls, Sienicki, and Crist (1981) were successful in reducing training time for a group of mentally retarded clients who were familiarized with basic mechanical operations and tool use before being involved in a more formalized training program. In an initial program, an individual might be involved in as little as 20–30 minutes of work activity a day. This occupational trial could involve general labor, clerical activities, assembly tasks, or other work activities specifically related to a prior job. Occupational trials can be gradually increased (based on the individual's ability to attend to the task and on physical stamina or capabilities) until a substantial part of the day is spent in work activity. For an individual without prior work activity or with difficulty identifying a job interest, several different types of work activities can be used in the trials for vocational interest assessment. Individuals unable to sustain work activity due to cognitive or physical limitations might still be involved in watching work-related films, having employers visit their vocational group, and similar activities to maintain a vocational orientation. As a client is discharged from a rehabilitation program, volunteer job tryouts or community work stations can be established within hospitals, universities, or federal agencies. Federal agency work-experience programs allow the individual the necessary time to adapt to the visual-spatial demands of the job, learn the work tasks, and perhaps to improve motor speed.

Training enclaves (semi-protected settings within the private sector with salary level keyed to productivity) can be another avenue to competitive employment. The supported employment model that has been used with developmentally disabled clients (Wehman, 1981) has promise for head-injured individuals. This model involves training at the work site by a job coach who has previously performed the job and clearly understands its tasks. Step-wise training procedures and other behavioral technologies (Bellamy, Horner, & Inman, 1979; Wehman, McLaughlin, Revell, Kriloff, & Sarkees, 1980) can then be utilized to train the client on the job site with the job coach gradually fading and providing fewer cues until the individual is functioning independently. While this model may be more widely utilized nationally and may become a standard job placement approach with head-injured clients, there is currently a lack of empirical research available on the value of this model for the head-injured population.

In some cases, the client's residual assets and compensatory strategies may enable him or her to return to the former job. In other cases, however, this may be impossible. It is very important to examine the individual's preinjury work values and interests so that the new work activity and environment are desirable for the client.

Postemployment Services

Postemployment services are critical to the adjustment of moderately and severely head-injured clients. In many cases, counseling assistance will be required to deal with the interpersonal demands of the job. Some clients may need a brief period of retraining in order to reestablish the task sequence or compensate for some new variations in the job task or environmental demands. Since head injury rehabilitation is a relatively new field, program evaluation of the newly developing centers and day programs can reveal the needed components of postemployment services. In any case, services of this nature appear to be critical, and staff expenditure of postemployment service efforts should be anticipated on an intermittent basis for many head-injured clients who are competitively placed. Service demands of this type will be reduced if a placement meshes well with the client's neuropsychological pattern of assets and deficits, if the work setting is congruent with the individual's orientations, and/or if the client has been trained on the job.

CASE EXAMPLES

To provide more insight into job placement strategies for the head injured, several case examples are offered. Reflecting the heterogeneity of the population, placement approaches are discussed with mildly, moderately, and severely brain-impaired individuals. In addition to offering a range of illustrative placement examples, this section emphasizes the importance of examining work-related values and interests.

K. H. is a 28-year-old male who suffered a head injury in a car accident at age 22. At the time, this young man was a quality control inspector for a computer manufacturing company. As a consequence of the accident, he developed a generalized tonic-clonic seizure disorder and lost the functional use of his right eye. At intake, he appeared very frustrated because he was unable to maintain work since the accident. He was very concerned about securing a good medical benefit program since his anticonvulsants and seizure-related trips to hospital emergency rooms could result in very costly medical bills. Neuropsychological testing indicated a mild level of impairment, but pointed to significant deficits in verbal and visual-spatial memory.

K. H. was placed as a ''permanent'' rotating clerical employee within a large air freight company. Although he rotated among several clerical jobs within the company, the positions tended to involve well-structured clerical activity that did not require a substantial amount of memory as a work activity component. K. H. was only assigned positions within his range of abilities. He enjoyed a reasonable salary in the position and was particularly pleased with the medical benefit program.

A. W. was a 27-year-old college graduate who presented herself on an outpatient basis seeking vocational assistance. She had failed in a series of jobs (e.g., fast food manager and hospital admitting clerk) and was desperate for some type of job security at a work level congruent with being a college graduate. Neuropsychological testing indicated severely impaired receptive language abilities, but exceptional visual-spatial problem-solving and motoric abilities. After comprehensive vocational interest assessment utilizing inventories and several reference texts, this young woman was delighted to begin on-the-job training as a prosthetics-orthotics technician. Although a physical ''hands-on'' work activity, it emphasized her strengths (visual-spatial problem solving and manual dexterity), and the hospital clinic setting met her prestige needs as a college graduate.

W. B. was a 37-year-old male who had difficulty maintaining jobs since sustaining a head injury while on a vacation camping trip. Prior to injury, he had earned a bachelor's degree in fine arts with considerable course work in landscape architecture. Neuropsychological testing indicated a moderate degree of impairment, with a number of test scores just outside normal limits. W. B. was able to work as a manager for landscape architects by using a number of compensatory techniques (e.g., taking sufficient time to strategize technical issues, not feeling pressed to respond quickly, and constantly noting all job-related needs on a pad and establishing priorities). Above all, he learned to set reasonable expectations for himself. His willingness to work overtime and his commitment to the job were more than adequate to compensate the employer for his neuropsychological inefficiency.

In a final case, R.Q. had worked as a window designer prior to being injured. Neuropsychological testing at hospital release and 2 years later suggested that this 28-year-old male had severe and diffuse neuropsychological impairment, prohibiting any return to his preinjury career. Stepwise training procedures were utilized by a job coach to aid him in functioning as a linen attendant at an attractive urban athletic club. Working in the club appealed to

R.Q. chiefly due to its aesthetic environment. The reasonable salary and benefit package were of secondary concern to him. This same individual would not have worked as a hospital custodian or as a counter attendant in an area restaurant. A luxurious work environment was the reinforcer that aided in this man's return to work.

CONCLUSION

This chapter summarizes rehabilitation counseling considerations specific to the needs of head-injured clients. This embryonic rehabilitation specialization is expected to develop rapidly, given the high priority of these issues, the growth of recent research activity, and the transfer of knowledge contained in the rehabilitation of related groups. These events suggest that head injury rehabilitation will be an exciting area of endeavor for years to come.

REFERENCES

Anderson, D., & McLaurin, R. (Eds). (1980). *Report on the national spinal cord injury survey*. Bethesda, MD: National Institute for Neurological and Communicative Disorders and Stroke.

Bellamy, G. T., Horner, R. H., & Inman, D. P. (1979). *Vocational habilitation of severely retarded adults*. Baltimore: University Park Press.

Ben-Yishay, Y., & Diller, L. (1983). Cognitive deficits. In M. Rosenthal, E. Griffith, M. Bond, & J. Miller (Eds.), *Rehabilitation of the head injured adult* (pp. 167–182). Philadelphia: Davis.

Blanton, P. D., & Gouvier, W. D. (1986). Cognitive retraining therapy for neurologically impaired patients. *The Behavior Therapist, 3,* 47–50.

Braunling-McMorrow, D., Lloyd, K., & Fralish, K. (1986). Teaching social skills to head injured adults. *Journal of Rehabilitation, 52,* 39–44.

Brooks, D., Aughton, M., Bond, M., Jones, P., & Rizvi, S. (1980). Cognitive sequelae in relationship to early indices of severity of brain damage after severe blunt head injury. *Journal of Neurology, Neurosurgery, and Psychiatry, 43,* 529–534.

Cripe, L. (1985, March). *The neurological assessments and management of closed head injury: General guideline*. Paper presented at the Biannual U.S. Army Medical Department Psychology Conference, San Francisco.

Diehl, L. (1983). Patient-family education. In M. Rosenthal, E. Griffith, M. Bond, & J. Miller (Eds.), *Rehabilitation of the head injured adult* (pp. 395–403). Philadelphia: Davis.

Dikmen, S., & Reitan, R. (1979). Emotional sequelae of head injury. *Annals of Neurology, 2,* 492–494.

Diller, L., & Gordon, W. A. (1981). Interventions for cognitive deficits in brain injured adults. *Journal of Consulting and Clinical Psychology, 49,* 822–834.

Fordyce, D. L., Roueche, J. R., & Prigatano, G. P. (1983). Enhanced emotional reactions in chronic head trauma patients. *Journal of Neurology, Neurosurgery, and Psychiatry, 46,* 620–624.

Fraser, R. T. (1985). Post-traumatic epilepsy. In P. M. Deutsch & H. W. Sawyer (Eds.), *Guide to rehabilitation*. New York: Matthew Bender.

Gianutsos, R. (1980). What is cognitive rehabilitation? *Journal of Rehabilitation, 46*(3), 37–40.

Goodman-Smith, A., & Turnbull, J. (1983). A behavioral approach to the rehabilitation of severely brain-injured adults. *Physiotherapy, 69,* 393–396.

Jennett, B. (1975). *Epilepsy after non-missile head injuries* (2nd ed.). London: Heinemann.

Jennett, B. (1983). Scale and scope of the problem. In M. Rosenthal, E. Griffith, M. Bond, & J. Miller (Eds.), *Rehabilitation of the head injured adult* (pp. 3–8). Philadelphia: Davis.

Kay, T., Ezrachi, O., & Cavallo, M. (1986). *Annotated bibliography of research on vocational outcome following head trauma.* New York: New York University Medical Center, Institute on Rehabilitation Medicine.

Levin, H. S., Benton, A. L., & Grossman, R. G. (1982). *Neurobehavioral consequences of closed head injury.* New York: Oxford University Press.

Lezak, M. D. (1978). Living with the characterologically altered brain injured patient. *Journal of Clinical Psychiatry, 39,* 592–598.

Lishman, W. (1973). The psychiatric sequelae of head injury: A review. *Psychological Medicine, 60,* 1208–1215.

Long, D. J., Gouvier, W. D., & Cole, J. C. (1984). A model of recovery for the total rehabilitation of individuals with head trauma. *Journal of Rehabilitation, 50*(1), 39–45, 70.

Lynch, W. J., & Mauss, N. K. (1981). Brain injury rehabilitation: Standard problem lists. *Archives of Physical Medicine and Rehabilitation, 62,* 223–227.

MacNeill, H., Jr., & Howe, N. R. (1981). Behavioral treatment of the traumatically brain injured: A case study. *Perceptual and Motor Skills, 53,* 349–350.

Mikula, J. (1984, December). Standards for cognitive rehabilitation. In J. Mikula (Chair), *Subcommittee on cognitive rehabilitation standards.* Proceedings of the meeting of the American Congress of Rehabilitation Medicine.

Miller, E. (1980). Psychological intervention in the management and rehabilitation of neuropsychological impairments. *Behavior Research and Therapy, 18,* 527–535.

Olson, D., & Henig, E. (1983). *A manual of behavior management strategies for traumatically brain injured adults.* Chicago: Rehabilitation Institute of Chicago.

Reitan, R. (1982). *REHABIT—Reitan evaluation of hemispheric abilities and brain improvement training.* Unpublished manuscript, University of Arizona, Tucson.

Reitan, A. (1986, May). *REHABIT: Review and update.* Paper presented in head injury rehabilitation course, Phoenix, AZ.

Rosenthal, M., Griffith, E., Bond, M., & Miller, J. (1983). *Rehabilitation of the head injured adult.* Philadelphia: Davis.

Rosenthal, M., & Muir, C. (1983). Methods of family intervention. In M. Rosenthal, E. Griffith, M. Bond, & J. Miller (Eds.), *Rehabilitation of the head injured adult* (pp. 407–418). Philadelphia: Davis.

Santa Clara Valley Medical Center. (1982). *Severe head trauma: A comprehensive medical approach* (National Institute for Handicapped Research Grant No. 13-P-59156/9). Santa Clara, CA: Author.

Sbordone, R. J., & Howard, N. E. (1985). Pre-injury predictors of rehabilitation potential and outcome from head trauma. In *Twelfth Institute on Rehabilitation Issues, Rehabilitation of the traumatic brain injured* (pp. 79–82). Menomonie: University of Wisconsin–Stout, Research and Training Center.

Teasdale, G., & Jennett, B. (1974). Assessment of coma and impaired consciousness: A practical scale. *Lancet, 2,* 81–84.

Trexler, L. E. (Ed.). (1982). *Cognitive rehabilitation: Conceptualization and intervention.* New York: Plenum.

Twelfth Institute on Rehabilitation Issues. (1985). *Rehabilitation of the traumatic brain injured.* Menomonie: University of Wisconsin–Stout, Research and Training Center.

Vogenthaler, D. R. (1987). *Head injury: Describing and predicting long-term outcomes.* Unpublished doctoral dissertation, Southern Illinois University, Carbondale.

Vogenthaler, D. R. (in press). Rehabilitation after closed head injury: A primer. *Journal of Rehabilitation.*

Walls, R. T., Sienicki, D. A., & Crist, K. (1981). Operations training in vocational skills. *American Journal of Mental Deficiency, 85,* 357–367.

Wehman, P. (1981). *Competitive employment: New horizons for severely disabled individuals.* Baltimore: Paul H. Brookes Publishing Co.

Wehman, P., McLaughlin, P. J., Revell, W. G., Jr., Kriloff, L. J., & Sarkees, M. D. (1980). *Vocational curriculum for developmentally disabled persons.* Baltimore: University Park Press.

Weinberger, J. (1984, September). *The vocational evaluation of head injured patients.* Paper presented at the National Forum on Issues in Vocational Assessment, Atlanta.

Williams, J. M. (1985, August). *The role of assessment, goal planning, and cognitive retraining in comprehensive rehabilitation.* Paper presented at the American Psychological Association Meeting, Los Angeles.

13

The Family and the Rehabilitation Process

Counselor Roles and Functions

Paul W. Power

SINCE THE ORIGIN in 1920 of the federal-state delivery system for vocational rehabilitation services, the client's family and the rehabilitation counselor have been infrequent partners. A report issued by the Rehabilitation Services Administration (Davis, 1985) stated that of all the persons rehabilitated during fiscal year 1983 in the federal-state vocational rehabilitation system, 97.8% received no family attention or services. This alarming statistic suggests that either the client's family is not regarded as a necessary component in the rehabilitation process, that clients can be successfully rehabilitated without family services, that rehabilitation counselors choose not to work with families, or that families do not wish to take part in the rehabilitation process. The report does not indicate how many clients who, after being referred, interviewed, and even evaluated for vocational rehabilitation services, dropped out of the process and have been termed "unsuccessful." One way to reduce the size of this unsuccessful client population is through the utilization of the client's family in the rehabilitation process.

In a national study of rehabilitation counselor roles, functions, and sources of role strain conducted in 1979, Emener and Rubin (1980) found that rehabilitation counselors in state rehabilitation agencies, private facilities, and private practice; administrators/supervisors; and educators all reported that they considered intervention with the client's family as a less than substantial part of the counselor's job. But they all expressed a desire to increase the extent to which family intervention constitutes part of their job. Today, with current emphases in vocational rehabilitation on serving severely disabled persons and enabling school-to-work transition, the apparent desire of rehabilitation personnel to engage in working with clients' families seems most appropriate. The reason that the wish has not been translated into action, and that the reported statistic is so low for service to families, may be a lack of awareness of the role and functions of the rehabilitation counselor and of the opportunities for working with families. This chapter explains these roles and functions, and identifies selected opportunities. To understand these dimensions of rehabilitation practice, two topics are discussed that bring into sharper focus the utilization of the family during the rehabilitation process. One is the identification of a socio-cultural conceptualization of disability; the other is a review of the recent literature that emphasizes the importance of and varied approaches to family involvement in rehabilitation.

A SOCIOCULTURAL CONCEPTUALIZATION OF DISABILITY

Gill (1985) states that since 1970 rehabilitation policy has reflected a growing concern with social factors that mediate a disabled person's likelihood of functioning successfully. One such factor is the family system.

The rehabilitation literature indicates progress toward a more comprehensive sociocultural conceptualization of disability. Hahn (1985) explains that there has been a shift of emphasis from a medical definition of disability and from an economic perspective that emphasizes vocational limitations, to a sociopolitical orientation that regards a handicap as a product of the interaction between the individual and the environment. Implied in the new orientation is a focusing of attention on external influences and a realization that the definition of disability is fundamentally determined by public policy. Consequently, the major problems associated with disability could be perceived as the result of a handicapping environment such as the family. Chronic stress within the available family group and low expectations from family members about the potential productivity of the client are examples of two problems that could prevent the client from achieving rehabilitation goals (Power & Dell Orto, 1980).

When one accepts the assumption that the client's family plays a part in the rehabilitation process, then the rehabilitation counselor-client relationship no longer remains a dyad. The disabled individual is viewed within the context of available family relationships and broader interactional networks. The core "helping services" then consist of the rehabilitation counselor, the client, and the client's family. Any of these participants can support or undermine the relationship among the others.

A REVIEW OF RECENT LITERATURE

Counselors have universally observed the apparent adverse affect of the home environment on the rehabilitation process of a client (Kerosky, 1984). Nau (1973) wrote that "when a disability strikes, every other member of the family is also adversely affected" (p. 14). Other authors have stated that "an illness in one member has a significant and individual impact on everyone else in the family" (Kramer, 1981, p. 155). Further, "unless the context of the family life is taken into account, the needs of the developmentally disabled cannot be dealt with completely" (O'Hara, Chaiklin, & Mosher, 1980, p. 88).

Livsey (1972) suggested that when working with families and the disabled person, attention should be given to the following factors: 1) family roles (who does what and when), 2) role intactness after disability impact, 3) the coping mechanisms used by the family and the client, 4) the interaction between the family and the system of care, 5) the feelings the family members have regarding the client's disability, and 6) whether a chronic or serious problem other than the disability or illness affects a family member. In addition, Livsey (1972) found that many families could be viewed as "severely disturbed" before the onset of disability, and the awareness of this disturbance can be of invaluable help to the counselor. It would be difficult for a family to be a resource for their member's rehabilitation if the family unit itself needs therapeutic attention.

Looking at family involvement from another perspective, Jacus (1981) explained that the inclusion of family counseling in rehabilitation hospitals is often an integral part of the team concept in patient care. Family reactions can profoundly affect family functioning and client adjustment. A family systems approach to problems of family and client adjustment is being used in rehabilitation settings, especially when family members are emotionally devastated by the impact of the severe illness or injury. Jacus emphasizes that rehabilitation professionals, when meeting with the family, should help family members assess personal support systems, assist families to set realistic expectations for rehabilitation, and show family members how to channel their time and energy. Further, an attempt should be made to involve all family members in the client's rehabilitation, with particular attention given to whether the nondisabled spouse tries to take over the mate's former home responsibilities (Jacus, 1981). Family members quickly can become tired and overwhelmed when trying to tackle many jobs simultaneously.

Jaffe (1978) states that family relationships, behavior patterns, and the family's manner of responding to stress are important factors to explore when assisting family members in suitable adjustment to chronic illness. "Family is the most central and potent external force not only in shaping the individual personally but also in the expression of physical illness" (Jaffe, 1978, p.

169). Jaffe also identifies characteristics of family relationships that can contribute to both illness and rehabilitation: 1) intervening variables of chronic stress; 2) secondary gain (the reality that disability, chronic pain, and illness can bring a family member benefits and excuse that person from many responsibilities, such as household chores or even returning to a previous occupation); and 3) lethal dyads (couples who escalate each other's potentiality for illness by the structure of their relationship and nature of their demands on each other). In his intervention program for families and the client, Jaffe emphasizes exploring the meaning of the disability/illness, educating family members about the relation of stress factors to the client's disability and rehabilitation, and encouraging both a family system change and involvement in a support group when possible.

Bray (1980) has argued that families can play a negative or positive role in the client's rehabilitation. He has developed programs involving multi-disciplinary rehabilitation teams for families who have a member who has had either a spinal cord injury or a stroke. Bray has pointed out that the rehabilitation counselor can play a major role in facilitating positive family involvement during the extended phase of the disability. During this phase, the counselor has a unique opportunity to involve the client and the available family in the rehabilitation process. For example, family members can be assisted to anticipate problems. Because of the emotional impact of disability on its members, the family may also need to improve communications skills. Family members usually are not accustomed to speaking to health and rehabilitation professionals about their concerns. Moreover, within the family the disabled person is frequently given less status than deserved. Consequently, it may become essential for both the client and family members to develop a more assertive level of communication with health care and rehabilitation professionals (Bray, 1980).

The above articles suggest that family dynamics can have a direct bearing on the attitudes and behaviors of disabled persons and that these influences may be related to the outcome of vocational rehabilitation. The reviewed literature also implies that an array of services may be needed by families to deal with the impact of physical disability. A survey of the literature indicates that when the issue of the role of the family in rehabilitation is addressed, physical disability is the usual focus of attention (Power & Dell Orto, 1980).

However, since 1978, families of mentally ill persons have received attention in the rehabilitation literature. Hatfield (1978) found that families of persons who are mentally ill risk the deterioration of their psychological and physical resources to the point that their personal efficiency may be reduced and the organization and stability of family life threatened. A mentally ill client's rehabilitation does not take place in a counselor's or therapist's office; it occurs in the situation in which he or she lives, and this situation can be of great benefit to the achievement of vocational rehabilitation goals (Hatfield, 1981). To be a valuable resource in rehabilitation efforts, family members need advice concerning appropriate expectations for the client, specific techniques for managing disturbed behavior in the home when necessary, and information on the availability of community resources. The morale of the client and family is contingent upon a reduction of their sense of futility and helplessness, the encouragement of their feelings of competence as they work on behalf of their family member's well-being, and the full recognition of the efforts they are making to assist the client's adjustment in the home and the community (Hatfield, 1984).

Through the research and practice of many helping professionals, awareness is growing of the factors that have a significant impact on rehabilitation outcome. Vocational rehabilitation is mushrooming to encompass diverse activities that improve the delivery of services. As yet, however, there are only a few rough theories and many clinical observations that move beyond the basic assumption that the family system is vital to the client's vocational rehabilitation (Power, 1985). Families can provide the client with much motivation to work toward the achievement of rehabilitation goals. Even in families with impaired or limited family function, available family members are support systems, and clients may be dependent upon them for a long time. In terms of the individual's rehabilitation outcome, the question can become not "How can I afford the time to work with families?" but "How can I *not* afford the time to work with families?" (Kneipp & Bender, 1981). In turn, family members should be afforded every opportunity to take part in the disabled member's vocational rehabilitation. Several approaches on how the rehabilitation counselor can work with families, and how the family can be involved in rehabilitation efforts, are discussed in the next section.

ROLES AND FUNCTIONS FOR WORKING WITH FAMILIES

For many rehabilitation counselors, time with the family can often be scheduled during office visits with the client. A family meeting may be initiated during the beginning interview when both eligibility for vocational rehabilitation and extent of services are being determined. The counselor may have doubts about the client's sincerity to pursue the rehabilitation process, or perceive barriers within the client's home environment to the achievement of rehabilitation goals.

When the client states that the family is seeking information on the vocational rehabilitation process or on resources that will assist them in their adjustment efforts, contact with the family would serve a beneficial purpose, and a meeting should be discussed. When a client is either living with the family, or when the family is easily accessible, the client's permission can be obtained to include family members in the next agency visit. If the family members show reluctance to come to this meeting, this reluctance should be explored and suggestions offered on how the family may be of assistance to both the client and the counselor. All the family members or significant others with whom the client lives should be invited, when possible, to this agency meeting. Each member can have an influence on the client's vocational rehabilitation. The purpose of the initial family visit is to help identify those persons who can facilitate or hinder the rehabilitation process.

In the first and succeeding meetings with the family, the counselor may assume as many as five counselor roles: assessor of family functions, provider of information, developer of support systems, challenger to the family to meet the need of further counseling assistance, and facilitator of the prevention of possible client problems during the rehabilitation process. Identification of these roles evolves both from the author's rehabilitation practice with families and the work of Doherty and Baird (1983). According to Doherty and Baird, the family physician has an opportunity to work with families on a counseling, not a family therapy, dimension. Doherty and Baird advocate short-term intervention with families, and recommend that the functions of the family physician include education, support, challenge, and prevention. With modifications, these roles have direct relevance to the rehabilitation counselor.

Assessor of Family Functioning

To understand the family dynamics that have an impact on the client, the following areas should be explored by the rehabilitation counselor.

What is the emotional reaction of the family to the disability, and at what point during this reaction can family members be most influential for rehabilitation outcomes? Bray (1977), Giacquinta (1977), and Epperson (1977) have identified specific stages of family reaction to disability and emphasized that families experience different phases of coping as they gradually move toward a continued definite mode of adjustment. This chapter also presents a conceptualization of a series of stages that families frequently experience emotionally as they react and attempt to adjust to the disability event. The information that follows is derived from 10-year experience in working with families during the rehabilitation process. Each stage represents a collective emotion of the family, though at any particular time during the reactive process a family member may harbor a different feeling than one felt by others. For example, on the one hand, the spouse of a disabled person may predominantly feel hope when the in-hospital rehabilitation phase is completed and the early signs of physical or mental restoration are evident. On the other hand, the adolescent siblings may be continually angry because they realize that family income and savings may dwindle, and with them, hopes for an education at the college of their choice.

Generally a counselor can recognize at a particular time one dominant emotional reaction phase in which family members are located. These phases are outlined in Figure 1.

During the *denial* phase, which may continue for a brief or a long period of time, the family clings to the belief that both the disabled member and family life will return to predisability functioning. This denial of the implications of the disability phase plays a functional role for most families, since it may give family members time to gather personal and family resources to cope with later adjustment demands. With input from health professionals and the family's own gradual realization that the spouse or child will not return to predisability functioning, family members slowly enter the *acknowledgment/search for meaning* phase in which they acknowledge the disability as permanent. This is a very vulnerable time for families as they begin to search for the meaning of the event for their family and personal lives. Family members may ask such questions as:

1. "Will the disability mean that I, as a spouse, must find a job?"
2. "Who will take my disabled family member for treatment appointments?"
3. "How will the bills be paid?"
4. "What family duties must change?"
5. "On whom can I rely for support?"
6. "Will it be possible for my disabled spouse to return, even on a part-time basis, to a former job?"
7. "Will taking care of my disabled family member take away all my free time?"
8. "Will my disabled spouse have any potential, physically or mentally, to generate future family income?"
9. "How will my friends react when they know that my spouse/parent/child is permanently disabled?"

The answers to many of these questions may well determine whether a family will encourage the disabled member to seek and to cooperate in vocational rehabilitation services. Families are frequently in a better financial position than before the disability, because disability compensation payments awarded may give the family more income than it had when the disabled person was employed. Also, many families enjoy the new-found attention from medical and allied health professionals. One spouse explained, "Why, as a family we were never special . . . we even felt isolated from our neighbors. But since my husband had his accident and has been at home, people are aware of us. This attention might change if my husband were to return to work."

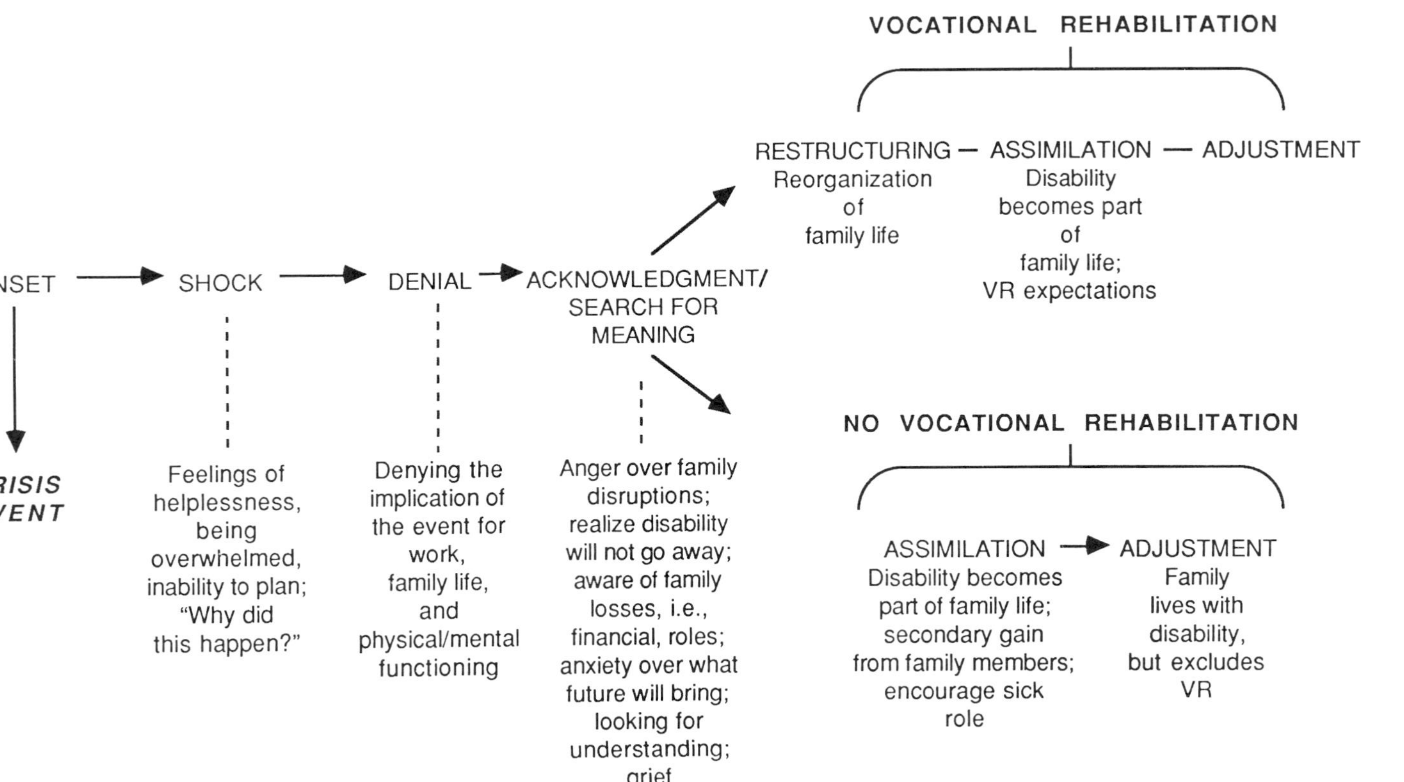

Figure 1. The emotional reaction of the family to disability.

During this *acknowledgment/search for meaning* phase, family members can recognize both the disabled person's remaining capabilities and the advantages to this person and to the family of a return to some kind of employment. A reorganization of family life may take place and selected family responsibilities may have to change, even if only temporarily. Disability is assimilated into the daily family routine, and there is the expectation that vocational rehabilitation, when feasible, will occur. The family adjusts, and the business of family living, though somewhat changed or modified, continues.

However, when family members perceive only what the disabled member cannot do, and realize that the reinforcements for not working are greater than for a return to employment, then the client often will not receive encouragement to participate in the vocational rehabilitation process. Family members may become a source of secondary gain and encourage client dependency. Or, chronic stress due to ongoing family problems may be so severe that vocational rehabilitation goals receive a low priority. Family adjustment to the disability can eventually take place, though some families live in a constant state of crisis. But this phase is a time of adjustment, characterized by general client inactivity and the assumption from family members that the disabled person will simply never be able to work.

What is the unique composition of the family and what are the strengths and weaknesses inherent in that structure that can influence the client's rehabilitation? To identify the family dynamics that may promote the client's vocational rehabilitation, the counselor should look for indicators during the initial visit, whether in the office or in the client's home, of warm and trusting attitudes shown in familial interactions, an open and mutual respect demonstrated toward each family member, whether family members speak honestly about any adjustment concerns, and whether they have assumed personal responsibility, when appropriate, for the client's treatment and rehabilitation needs. The family spokesperson and the principal caregivers for the client should also be identified (Doherty & Baird, 1983).

However, the meeting may reveal information and disagreement about events affecting family life, conflicts over the performance of family responsibilities, or family communication characterized by distorted or unrealistic views of one another. Family members may also be angry because the disability has interfered with their life-style, privacy, vacations, and future plans, and because it has diverted the spouse's time from other family members. If the anger existed prior to the disability, the disability itself may only have exacerbated long-standing family feelings.

What information does the family have about the disability or illness, and with this knowledge what expectations does the family have for their disabled family member? The counselor can also explore whether family members are aware of: 1) what the client can still do in the home, 2) what community resources may be utilized for respite care, 3) the various work options still available to the client, and 4) the different phases of the rehabilitation process. Information about the disability may already have been given to the family by health professionals; but family members, because of their anxieties, tend not to process information very well during their initial conferences with the physician (Polinko, 1985).

What services does the family need, such as financial, respite care, or family counseling? The family may be seeking information on how other families are coping with such disability-related circumstances as reduced family income, new restrictions on time and freedom, and the availability of needed resources.

What strengths exist in the family that will facilitate the family's involvement in the rehabilitation process? Identification of family strengths can become a guide for the rehabilitation counselor when suggesting family intervention strategies with the client. Such strengths also serve as reinforcements that can be expressed by the counselor to family members. Disability lowers family self-esteem; many family members feel stigmatized because of the presence of a disabling condition. When the counselor can indicate strengths that family members possess, such communication often results in a new-found family self-confidence (Power, 1985). These strengths may include:

1. The ability of the family members to listen to each other and to allied health professionals, including the rehabilitation counselor
2. The family members' realistic perception of the functioning of the client
3. The family's ability to clarify the issues related to disability, to render them more manageable and responsive to problem-solving efforts (e.g., can family members realize the importance of involving the disabled person, when feasible, in family activities, or maintaining their positive expectations for the productivity of the client?)
4. The family's ability to enjoy their leisure time
5. The family's ability to use community resources
6. The family's ability to talk with other family members and helping professionals about disability-related concerns
7. The family's capability to use everyday family life as an activity resource for the client (e.g., client's ability to perform the most basic functions of family living and the opportunity to relearn everyday living skills can be a prelude to involvement in the rehabilitation process)

When working with families, the rehabilitation counselor's role of "assessor" targets many areas. Information about each area can help the counselor assess the ability of family members to assist the client in the rehabilitation process. Effective assessment of family functioning can be just one of many steps that lead to the achievement of appropriate rehabilitation goals.

Provider of Information

Information given to families should focus primarily on an explanation of the different phases of the rehabilitation process, and the expected delays as the client progresses through this process. Questions about the rehabilitation process are the most frequently asked (Power & Dell Orto, 1980). Family members want to know what is involved in vocational rehabilitation and if the client has a realistic perspective of the future. These inquiries focus on particular questions, such as:

1. "Who will be responsible for my spouse's rehabilitation if he or she is being referred to many people for different services?"
2. "How long docs vocational evaluation take?"
3. "Are there jobs available if my spouse gets some training?"
4. "How different will it be for us when he or she starts to work again?"

Information can include offering suggestions to the family on how the client can get involved again in family life or explaining how, even with compensation-related payments, vocational rehabilitation can positively affect the client's life. The sharing of information implies, of course, responding to those family needs identified during the initial family meeting; that is, location of community resources and knowledge about the client's residual capabilities that can be utilized to achieve vocational rehabilitation goals. Family expectations for the client should also be discussed, and the counselor might consider, with the client's permission, providing information to the family on the client's emotional concerns resulting from the disability.

Developer of Support Systems

The family usually needs some informal support from the rehabilitation counselor and, when available, peer support as well. The rehabilitation counselor is often the only professional seen after hospital discharge who provides ongoing encouragement for the family concerning vocational rehabilitation (Spaniol, Zipple, & Fitzgerald, 1984). This support can be expressed by acknowledging what the family is doing to help the client to prepare for vocational rehabilitation; listening to the plans, anxieties, frustrations, and questions of family members; and encouraging family members to join a peer support group.

Family members also frequently need to learn how to provide support to a disabled family member. Unemployment and the loss of self-esteem, for example, can have a devastating effect. Family members may perceive the reality of these losses (Power, 1976). Loss of earning power or the diminution of physical capacities can be burdens borne alone by ill or disabled family members. Families can be encouraged to become aware of these losses, and the client can learn to seek support from the family. By listening to each other and accepting feedback from the rehabilitation counselor, the family can gradually appreciate the problems associated with disability adjustment.

Family support implies that the family member, despite physical or mental limitations, will receive reassurance of continued involvement in family life. With family support and acceptance, feelings of worth are partially achieved through a recrystallization of self in terms of acceptance of the problem. As the family provides the best opportunity for growth and fulfillment, so the home is the place where individuals can best express their natural potential and satisfy creative and emotional needs.

Informal support can be provided through the counselor's communication of his or her availability to answer phone calls when family members have questions about vocational rehabilitation. This type of availability may be all that the family really needs from the rehabilitation counselor, since it demonstrates that someone cares about their welfare. Families also appreciate having the counselor occasionally call, with the client's permission, to inform them of the client's progress in vocational evaluation or training. This communication acknowledges the family's involvement in the client's rehabilitation and conveys the message that vocational rehabilitation is important.

Challenger to the Family

The rehabilitation counselor must challenge unrealistic expectations about family life, challenge family members to work together for the benefit of the client and themselves, and challenge family members to be alert to opportunities within the home environment as an appropriate resource for the client's rehabilitation (Doherty & Baird, 1983). In the role of "challenger to the family," the rehabilitation counselor must not lose sight of the fact that one of the keys for coping with a disability is to make living with the disability as satisfying as it can be within the framework of the family's limitations and strengths (Power, 1976). This may necessitate urging the family to build successful experiences for the disabled person and themselves. For the disabled family member, it may imply encouraging him or her to maintain normal activities, and to seek appropriate new activities that will provide both a respite from providing care and a resource for enjoyment. Frequently the family needs to be confronted with the importance of this respite, so that family members may also satisfy their own needs. For a client to reach needed vocational rehabilitation goals often necessitates that the available family itself survive. Survival is facilitated by the maintenance of appropriate patterns of living for family members.

In the challenger role, the counselor may also help the family to realize, when necessary, the importance of family counseling services. Recognition that the disability is aggravating an existing family pathology may convince the counselor that the family needs to receive assistance if the client is to achieve rehabilitation goals. Resistance by family members to suggestions made concerning the value of extended family counseling is frequently encountered. Yet many families become at least more willing to explore this service when it is cogently indicated how counseling intervention can make a decided difference, not only in their family member's rehabilitation, but also in their own development of useful coping skills to deal with disruptions or crises related to disability (Schwartz, 1984).

Facilitator of Prevention

Anticipatory guidance to prevent potential problems can greatly assist many families confronted with a significant transition, not only immediately after the disability occurs, but also upon entering the rehabilitation process after many months of the in-hospital and then at-home environments. For recently disabled adults, getting involved in such steps as vocational evaluation, retraining, and associating for the first time with other disabled people may cause anxiety about one's rehabilitation future. When meeting with the family, the rehabilitation counselor can identify the areas of potential difficulty for the client in the rehabilitation process. Having the family member leave home each day for training and eventual employment may also present quite a change for the family. The counselor can explore those areas within a family that may cause adjustment problems because of the client's transition.

To adjust adequately to transition means that the client and the family must respond to the requirements of the situation and to their feelings about the change (Moss, 1977). In communicating with the family, the rehabilitation counselor may assist family members to break down problems into manageable parts that can be handled one at a time, help them to be optimistic about their ability to handle whatever eventualities arise, and prepare them for stresses by discussing them in advance.

IMPLEMENTATION OF ROLES

The implementation of all these roles implies counselor willingness to contact and to work briefly with families. Even when the rehabilitation counselor perceives that a family will significantly affect the vocational rehabilitation of the client, the counselor who is employed in an agency, particularly a state vocational rehabilitation (VR) office, may not have the opportunity for extended family involvement. The suggested roles are for short-term interventions, possibly for two or three family meetings. Not every family needs more than one interview. However, it is important for the rehabilitation counselor to have the opportunity for at least an initial meeting with the client's family.

There seems to be a ''system failure'' with respect to services to family members that is similar to that reported by Smits and Emener (1980) with respect to job placement. Factors such as strict adherence to traditional individual modes of treatment, perception of the client as a freestanding entity rather than as a member of a larger interacting system, bureaucratic pressures, and the lack of administrative policies and incentives can all contribute to the lack of attention to the family (Lindenberg, 1977). The author has also found from continued feedback in national and regional workshops on the family and rehabilitation that many counselors point to their rehabilitation counselor training program as deficient in emphasis on the client's family. They indicate that most academic programs emphasize both the one-to-one counseling relationship and group counseling as the preferred modes of counseling intervention. When electives are offered in family dynamics and family counseling, there is seldom an integration of these methods with the job functions of the rehabilitation counselor.

In addition to the need for advocacy and the practical motivations to meet the client's family, a third ingredient is necessary for effective practice of these suggested roles. This factor is the counselor's own helping attitude toward families and their part in the rehabilitation process. Rehabilitation counselors both claim authority and have it thrust upon them. Part of the exercise of authority and expertise is determining what people need and, sometimes, convincing them that they need it (Ryglewicz, 1985). This determination becomes particularly challenging when working with families. At the initial meeting with the family, the counselor may be seen as intruding into their daily life and most intimate relationships. This initial meeting will be more strained if counselors have attitudes toward the family such as, "I feel sorry for you . . . I know what's best for you . . . all that matters is the disability of your family member." Family members can detect these attitudes by how counselors speak to them and from the manner in which questions are asked and information communicated. These attitudes inhibit counselors from recognizing that family members need help. Fortunately, the growing trend for working with families involves close attention and responsiveness to families, but in forms that acknowledge their expertise, strengths, everyday needs, and complementary caregiving role (Ryglewicz, 1985). In other words, families must not be forced to fit the counselor's own helping model. Implementation of these suggested roles depends on the ability and willingness of the rehabilitation counselor to learn how family members can be a resource to the client's rehabilitation. The counselor's roles suggested in this chapter can act as guidelines for possible intervention. Each role offers a stimulus to the family to play an important part in the rehabilitation process.

CONCLUSION

Rehabilitation professionals are beginning to express an interest in re-evaluating the nature of their relationships with families (Spaniol et al., 1984). Family members are also demanding new responses from professionals (Ryglewicz, 1985). New approaches to working with families are emerging;

the growing trend is a responsiveness to families who are involved, because of a disabled family member, in the vocational rehabilitation process. This responsiveness should take a form that acknowledges the family's strengths, needs, and complementary roles. It is in the best interests of the client for the rehabilitation counselor to seek the family's help and, by working with the family, to improve the effectiveness of the services offered.

REFERENCES

Bray, G. P. (1977). Reactive patterns in families of the severely disabled. *Rehabilitation Counseling Bulletin, 20,* 236–239.

Bray, G. P. (1980). Team strategies for family involvement in rehabilitation. *Journal of Rehabilitation, 46,* 20–23.

Davis, R. L. (1985). *Information memorandum: Transmittal of tabulations: Characteristics of clients whose cases were closed in fiscal year 1983.* Washington, DC: Rehabilitation Services Administration.

Doherty, W., & Baird, M. (1983). *Family therapy and family medicine.* New York: Guilford Press.

Emener, W. G., & Rubin, S. E. (1980). Rehabilitation counselor roles and functions and sources of role strain. *Journal of Applied Rehabilitation Counseling, 44,* 29–42.

Epperson, M. (1977). Families in sudden crisis. *Social Work in Health Care, 2,* 265–273.

Giacquinta, B. (1977). Helping families face the crisis of cancer. *American Journal of Nursing, 77,* 1585–1588.

Gill, C. J. (1985). The family/professional alliance in rehabilitation viewed from a minority perspective. *American Behavioral Scientist, 28,* 424–428.

Hahn, H. (1985). Changing perceptions of disability and the future of rehabilitation. In L. Perlman (Ed.), *Social influences in rehabilitation planning: Blueprint for the 21st Century* (pp. 53–66) (Mary E. Switzer Memorial Seminar). Alexandria, VA: National Rehabilitation Association.

Hatfield, A. B. (1978). Psychological costs of schizophrenia to the family. *Social Work, 23,* 355–359.

Hatfield, A. B. (1981). Coping effectiveness in families of the mentally ill: An exploratory study. *Journal of Psychiatric Treatment and Evaluation, 3,* 11–19.

Hatfield, A. B. (1984). The family. In J. A. Talbott (Ed.), *The chronic mental patient* (pp. 307–323). New York: Grune & Stratton.

Jacus, C. M. (1981). Working with families in a rehabilitation setting. *Rehabilitation Nursing, 6,* 10–14.

Jaffe, D. T. (1978). The role of family therapy in treating physical illnesses. *Hospital and Community Psychiatry, 29,* 170–174.

Kerosky, M. (1984). Services to family members by the state vocational rehabilitation agencies. *Journal of Applied Rehabilitation Counseling, 15,* 50–51.

Kneipp, S., & Bender, F. (1981). Services to family members by the state vocational rehabilitation agencies. *Journal of Applied Rehabilitation Counseling, 12,* 130–134.

Kramer, R. F. (1981). Living with childhood cancer: Healthy siblings' perspective. *Issues in Comprehensive Pediatric Nursing,* 5, 155–165.

Lindenberg, R. E. (1977). Work with families in rehabilitation. *Rehabilitation Counseling Bulletin, 21,* 67–76.

Livsey, C. G. (1972). Physical illness and family dynamics. *Advances in Psychosomatic Medicine, 8,* 237–251.

Moss, H. (1977). *Coping with physical illness.* New York: Plenum Medical Book Co.

Nau, L. (1973). *Family rehabilitation: A viable human service delivery approach.* Paper presented at the American Psychological Association Convention, Montreal, Canada.

O'Hara, D., Chaiklin, H., & Mosher, B. (1980). A family life cycle plan for delivering services to the developmentally handicapped. *Child Welfare, 59,* 80–90.

Polinko, P. (1985). Working with the family: The acute phase. In M. Ylvisaker (Ed.), *Head injury rehabilitation* (pp. 94–101). San Diego: College-Hill Press.

Power, P. (1976, Spring). The utilization of the family in the rehabilitation of the chronically ill patient: Some new perspectives for the allied health professional. *Journal of Allied Health, 5,* 42–51.

Power, P. (1985). Family coping behaviors in chronic illness—A rehabilitation perspective. *Rehabilitation Literature, 46,* 78–83.

Power, P., & Dell Orto, A. (1980). *Role of the family in the rehabilitation of the physically disabled.* Austin, TX: PRO-ED.

Ryglewicz, H. (1985). How can professionals help families and patients?: Issues and approaches. *The Lines, II,* 1–4.

Schwartz, R. (1984). Enriching your role as a referral agent. *Employee Assistance Digest,* 1, 27–30.

Smits, S. J., & Emener, W. G. (1980). Insufficient/ineffective counselor involvement in job placement activities: A system failure. *Journal of Rehabilitation Administration, 4,* 147–155.

Spaniol, L., Zipple, A., & Fitzgerald, S. (1984). How professionals can share power with families: A new approach to working with families of the mentally ill. *Monograph of the Rehabilitation and Training Center, Boston University,* 1–13.

14

Computer Applications and Issues Related to Their Use in Rehabilitation Counseling

Fong Chan, Ralph E. Matkin, Harry J. Parker, and Paul S. McCollum

THE RAPID DEVELOPMENT of integrated circuit technology in the past decade has enabled computer manufacturers to condense the main component of the computer, the central processing unit (CPU), into a very inexpensive silicon chip smaller than a postage stamp (Restak, 1980). This technological breakthrough has resulted in a proliferation of low-cost but powerful mini- and microcomputer systems that can perform complex electronic computing functions that once required costly and large mainframe computer systems.

The same technology also has facilitated the development of super performance mainframe computers. These computers have made possible telecommunications, computer networks, office automation, and distributed processing systems (Synnott & Gruber, 1981). The widespread availability of computer telecommunication technology to the public is changing the way American workers prepare for and perform their jobs. Naisbitt (1982) already has observed that the United States is moving rapidly from a manufacture-based to an information- and service-based economy.

The field of rehabilitation counseling is not insulated from these developments, and for this reason, rehabilitation counselors must learn to take advantage of, and adapt to, this new information technology. Descriptions and discussions of computer applications in rehabilitation counseling, vocational evaluation, work adjustment, and job placement began to emerge in the 1980s (Burkhead & Sampson, 1985; Chan, McCollum, & Parker, 1985; Chan & Questad, 1981; Crimando & Sawyer, 1983; McCollum & Chan, 1985a; Sampson, 1983). The purpose of this chapter is to review this topical area and discuss critical issues involving the use of computer technology by rehabilitation counselors.

COMPUTER APPLICATIONS IN REHABILITATION COUNSELING

As computer technology continues to redesign and restructure the world of work, the delivery of rehabilitation services will be affected (Herr, 1985; Schmitt & Growick, 1985). Both the rehabilitation counselor and the disabled client can benefit from these technological changes. In order to take full advantage of current technological developments, however, rehabilitation counselors will have to expand greatly their knowledge of specific computer applications (Herr, 1985). These include computerized systems designed to aid rehabilitation counselors in professional practices, such as office automation, as well as applications that are designed to enhance the independent living and vocational functioning of clients with disabilities (e.g., electronic assistive devices).

Counselor-Oriented Applications

Computers can be used to facilitate caseload management and counseling functions. For example, computer-managed counseling can use word processing, data management, and electronic spreadsheet/budgeting to facilitate management of resources (Crimando & Sawyer, 1983; Schmitt & Growick, 1985). This can assist rehabilitation counselors by providing timely and essential information for clinical decision making and program planning, and by reducing the amount of clerical and administrative time associated with the rehabilitation process.

Counseling functions can be assisted by computer applications as well. For example, computer-assisted counseling can be used to facilitate client behavior change by correcting maladaptive behavior through client-directed computer exercises (Schmitt & Growick, 1985).

Computer-Managed Counseling On the one hand, rehabilitation counselors generally prefer to spend the majority of their time performing counseling/therapy functions (Emener & Rubin, 1980; Rubin et al., 1984). On the other hand, less time can be spent in counseling because caseload management activities tend to consume disproportionate amounts of counselors' time. Specifically, rehabilitation counselors spend considerable amounts of time in handling paperwork such as correspondence, case notes, and agency forms. Valuable time frequently is spent completing duplicate information and investigating procedural requirements for different services and funding sources. Documentation activities can be handled more efficiently by using microcomputers, printers, and word processing software. The major advantage of the word processing approach is that it allows pieces of information to be entered one time, after which modification or duplication requires minimal effort (Crimando & Sawyer, 1983).

Data management programs that allow easy access to and retrieval of case information also can be extremely helpful for rehabilitation counselors. Counselors can store community, employer, agency, and client information on the computer using data management software. Data management software often has utility programs for generating standard forms on a display screen. Information such as client demographic data, already available in the data base, will be displayed automatically on the appropriate space of the form on the screen; data entry is required only for new information. Form-generator utility programs can aid rehabilitation counselors to more efficiently process requisitions, vouchers, client statistical forms, mailing lists, and correspondence. Similarly, data management programs are ideal for manipulating client data for case processing, statistical reporting, and program evaluation purposes (Crimando & Sawyer, 1983).

Electronic spreadsheet/budgeting software can be an invaluable tool in case management (Crimando & Sawyer, 1983). Spreadsheet programs are useful for rehabilitation counselors when planning and budgeting case expenditures. Counselors can perform hypothetical scenarios in order to determine optimal use of funds when making various case service decisions.

Rehabilitation counselors also spend a large portion of time developing community contacts and coordinating services (e.g., services related to feasibility determination, rehabilitation treatment, job development/placement, and follow-up support) for clients with disabilities. Successful counselors have to manage time schedules systematically and optimally. In this regard, an electronic calendar program can be another valuable tool for counselors. For instance, counselors can assign priority and time blocks available to a list of activities (client contacts, employer contacts, and community agency contacts) and enter the information into their computers. Accordingly, a calendar program can help manage and distribute these appointments, reminding the counselor of upcoming events and contacts on a daily, weekly, or monthly basis (Chan, McCollum, & Parker, 1985).

Rehabilitation counseling is an information-oriented profession. Counselors routinely collect and make reference to massive volumes of data that pertain to the rehabilitation process. More specifically, rehabilitation counselors must be knowledgeable about: 1) everchanging rules and regulations required to manage rehabilitation case loads properly, 2) community resources, 3) medical and psychosocial aspects of disabilities, 4) vocational implications of different disabilities, 5) work demands and requirements of different occupations, 6) job trends and training opportunities in the local and national economy, and 7) development and availability of job accommodation methods and assistive devices for people who are disabled (Roessler & Rubin, 1982). The time and energy required to update and obtain access to these types of everchanging sources of information without the use of high-speed computing devices could be overwhelming. As a management tool, modern computers can assist rehabilitation counselors in intake interviews and in administering, scoring, and reporting psychological tests and questionnaires of a personal, medical, social, educational, and occupational nature (Sampson, 1983; Schmitt & Growick, 1985).

Rehabilitation counselors also can use computers to gain access to national data bases, such as the ABLEDATA and Job Accommodation Network (JAN), for assistive devices and job accommodation information, and national/local electronic job opening bulletin boards for job placement information (Chan, McCollum, & Parker, 1985; Chan, McCollum, & Pool, 1985). Computerized job-matching programs, such as the Computer Assisted Vocational Rehabilitation Counseling Technique (VOCOMP) and the Ability Information System (AIS), are particularly relevant when seeking information about physical capacity, transferable skills analysis, employment outlook, and employer identification. These information management systems can provide the means by which to match systematically and effectively clients' residual capabilities with appropriate jobs (Chan, McCollum, & Parker, 1985).

The ability to store and retrieve large quantities of information, construct reporting formats and simplify their completion, and develop system pathways for decision-making purposes with the use of computers could ultimately increase staff productivity, minimize training costs, and ensure that more comprehensive services would be provided in state and private sector rehabilitation agencies. Many state vocational rehabilitation agencies (e.g., New York, Texas, Wyoming) and rehabilitation research and training centers (e.g., West Virginia University) are currently exploring the feasibility of microcomputer applications and office automation (Chan, McCollum, & Pool, 1985).

Computer-Assisted Counseling One major distinction between computer-managed counseling and computer-assisted counseling is the degree of client involvement with the computer. Software developed for case management is designed for use by counselors. Computer-assisted counseling programs, used as a "counseling/therapy" tool, focus on client behavior change. This type of software is designed for direct interaction between clients and computers.

Computer-assisted vocational guidance systems, for example, can be used by clients for vocational exploration and career decision making. By interacting directly with the computer, clients can learn about occupations in the world of work, personal values, and vocational interests and abilities, and can explore vocational training and job placement options. All these activities can help clients develop realistic vocational decision-making and goal-setting behaviors, and plan appropriate action strategies for goal attainment (Sampson, McMahon, & Burkhead, 1985).

Computer-assisted counseling also can be used effectively in psychoeducational and behavioral counseling, particularly when the purpose is to remediate maladaptive behavior and cognitive distortions through self-directed exercises (Schmitt & Growick, 1985). Presently, there is a range of computer-assisted counseling software that may be appropriate for rehabilitation counseling (Berven, 1985; Schmitt & Growick, 1985). Examples include ELIZA, which conducts computer-assisted counseling in the affective domain using an indirect counseling approach (Weizenbaum, 1965); MORTON, which conducts cognitive behavioral counseling to manage depression (Selmi, Klein, Greist, Johnson, & Harris, 1982); and the Dilemma Counseling System (DCS), which applies systematic problem-solving strategies for resolving avoidance-avoidance conflicts (Wagman, 1980; Wagman & Kerber, 1984).

The major advantages of the computer-assisted counseling approaches appear to be their step-by-step instructional technique, immediate access, and the unlimited time and interaction that a computer can provide to people with disabilities. The missing elements in computer counseling processes are human-to-human attention and a sense of caring. Careful selection of computer software, however, can augment counselor efforts by facilitating client behavior change in self-directed exercises of vocational, psychoeducational, and behavioral counseling (Schmitt & Growick, 1985).

Client-Oriented Computer Applications

With the advent of microelectronic and computer technology, increasingly sophisticated assistive devices are being developed to enhance the functional capacities of people with disabilities in their activities of daily living and in the workplace. In addition, special adaptations of both software and hardware of general purpose computers have been developed to provide persons with disabilities with equal access to the same commercial computer software available to the general population (Cook, Leins, & Woodall, 1985; Crimando & Godley, 1985; Office of Technology Assessment, 1983). Gaining equal access to computer use is critical for effective integration into present and future societies.

To rehabilitate clients to their fullest extent possible, counselors must assist clients to achieve optimal functional autonomy in the areas of both community living and work. According to Irons (1985), microcomputers and microprocessor-based assistive devices have tremenduous potential to help individuals with disabilities to achieve optimal functioning in five major areas: communication, education, environment control, recreation, and employment.

When a person is unable to communicate in a conventional manner because of an inability to verbalize and limited motor skills (e.g., a person with severe cerebral palsy), a computer can be used as an augmentative communication device. By using a head stick, a mouth stick, or a sensor (typically, the client will learn to activate a particular key on the keyboard using an eye-fixation technique), a person with virtually no manual dexterity can learn to use a computer keyboard. The typed message can be displayed on the computer screen to communicate with other people in the room, or broadcast through a computer network to communicate with others in remote sites. A person with limited manual dexterity can use key guards, enlarged keyboards, or, in some cases, single-switch entry devices to communicate through the computer (Cook et al., 1985; Irons, 1985; Restak, 1980; Vanderheiden, 1982).

The computer, especially the hand-held or ''notebook'' computer (Ahl, 1984), can be used by persons with disabilities in educational settings for numerous activities. It can be used to communicate in class, take notes, complete homework and class assignments, and interact with others (Cook et al., 1985; Irons, 1985). Computer-aided instruction (e.g., tutorial programs) can be particularly helpful to students with severe motor problems who may have difficulty taking notes and keeping pace with classroom instruction. Computer-aided instruction can be utilized as a ''private tutor'' to augment classroom learning experiences. The microcomputer with a modem can be used to link with mainframe computers and/or form microcomputer networks and communicate with instructors and fellow students (e.g., submitting and discussing homework assignments, respectively).

Perhaps the most important benefit from a computer for people with disabilities is acquiring control of one's environment (Irons, 1985; Vanderheiden, 1982). Computers can have a significant positive impact on the psychological well-being of a disabled client in terms of self-esteem, increasing opportunities for social interaction, and self-sufficiency. For example, a major concern for an individual with limited or no functional motor ability is a diminished sense of security (Irons, 1985). With the aid of a computerized emergency call system (security monitoring system), the individual can gain greater control of the environment and minimize feelings of insecurity to an extent not previously possible (Dahmke, 1982; Vanderheiden, 1982). Other similar applications include monitoring the home environment for safety, climate control, and programming home applicances (Apple Computer Inc., 1981; Irons, 1985).

Recreational computer games can represent a substantive socializing and educational tool as well. Playing popular electronic games provides opportunities for people with disabilities to interact and compete with others. This mainstream experience could greatly aid a person's social development. Game playing can also develop psychomotor and cognitive skills (Irons, 1985). For example, experts in cognitive rehabilitation have been using computer games extensively to provide cognitive restoration/retraining for head injury patients in areas of verbal skills, coordination skills, perception, memory, and visual field acuity (Schmitt & Growick, 1985). Many cognitive, psychomotor, and affective skills can be learned from game programs specifically designed to stimulate educational and social development (Trexler, 1982).

Finally, computers can be tremendously useful for vocational development and job placement of individuals (Bowe, 1985; Crimando & Godley, 1985; Irons, 1985). Although computer applications related to career exploration and decision making in rehabilitation already have been discussed, the computer can be used to improve job acquisition and job retention skills. More specifically, computer-aided instruction programs can be used to teach specific job skills, on-the-job social skills, and job-finding and job-seeking skills (Crimando & Godley, 1985). Many computer adaptations (electronic assistive devices and job-site modifications) developed to accomodate disabling conditions at work are now commercially available. If rehabilitation counselors and employers are aware of these computer-related innovations, many jobs typically deemed inappropriate or not feasible would be opened to persons with disabilities (Vanderheiden, 1981).

COMPUTER TECHNOLOGY APPLICATION ISSUES IN REHABILITATION COUNSELING

Computer technology can contribute significantly to the practice of rehabilitation counseling by enhancing rehabilitation counselor performance in daily practice and by improving rehabilitation client outcome. However, as with any other technology, the appropriate use of computers in rehabilitation counseling raises other issues as well.

Ethical Considerations

Rehabilitation is an information-based field (Miller, 1984; Perlman & Austin, 1984), in which the computer is being used increasingly. The ability of counselors to effectively utilize computers to obtain useful information (e.g., availability of specific electronic devices, job accommodation techniques, job openings) could ultimately affect outcome goals achieved in the rehabilitation process. It is crucial for rehabilitation counselors to become conversant with computer/information technology from ethical and technological perspectives (Chan, McCollum, & Pool, 1985).

Rehabilitation counselors must take an active role in designing and developing computer systems to be used in service delivery. Because those knowledgeable about computer system design and analysis may be unfamiliar with the field of rehabilitation and the work of counselors, participation of rehabilitation counselors in the design of software for use by people with disabling conditions is essential to ensure accuracy of the system logic, sound human-factor engineering principles, and human sensitivity (McCollum & Chan, 1985b).

Because rehabilitation counselors routinely collect client demographic information that may be confidential in nature, there are potential problems associated with maintaining the privacy of client data stored on a computer (Sampson & Pyle, 1983). For example, the widespread availability of microcomputers, computer networks, and communication links between microcomputers and large mainframe computers using telephone lines may increase the possibility for unauthorized access to confidential information (Sampson & Pyle, 1983). Thus, unwarranted electronic requests for release of confidential information among government agencies may increase. Rehabilitation counselors must be aware of these potential threats to confidentiality and develop appropriate procedures to safeguard the security of client files stored in their computers (Sampson & Pyle, 1983).

Information generated by computers generally is perceived by the public to be highly reliable and valid (Lister, 1970; Sampson & Pyle, 1983). In rehabilitation counseling, the computer is being increasingly used for testing, counseling, and job matching. Computer software used for these purposes generates printouts that may look impressive. However, rehabilitation counselors must be cautious when relying on these systems. The appropriateness of computer output largely depends on the reliability of the data input and the integrity of the program itself.

Many potential sources of error exist: data entry error, programming bugs, poor conceptualization of the system, lack of research efforts that go into the development of the program, and the like. For example, when appealing to a broad base of customers, some computerized job-matching programs sacrifice accuracy for flexibility of input data (Botterbusch, 1983). There are significant differences between using input data obtained as a result of a week of vocational evaluation, however, and the result of crude estimates based on little more than guessing. Even the substitution of test results obtained from one particular test (e.g., the General Aptitude Test Battery) with another similar test (e.g., the Differential Aptitude Test) may confound the outcome of computer results (Botterbusch, 1983). Rehabilitation counselors must develop the necessary skills for selecting appropriate computer hardware and software, and for interpreting computer output generated from these electronic aids, to the same degree that they are responsible for determining appropriate service programs (McCollum & Chan, 1985b).

Issues Related to Employment Preparation and Job Placement of Disabled Persons in the Information Age

The United States is moving rapidly from a manufacture-based to an information- and service-based economy. These changes will have a significant impact on the job placement of people with disabilities. For example, in an electronic society, the physical confines of work can depart from the traditional model (Martin, 1978). The HOMEBOUND program, sponsored by the Control Data Corporation, gives disabled workers the flexibility of working at home by using a computer terminal (Eighth Institute on Rehabilitation Issues, 1981). This movement toward telecommuting and flexible work places could lead to expanded employment opportunities for clients served by rehabilitation counselors (Bowe, 1985; Chan, McCollum, & Parker, 1985).

As consumer advocates, rehabilitation counselors should monitor technological changes closely. Counselors need to make certain these changes will not adversely affect employment opportunities of otherwise qualified job applicants. One critical issue is the accessibility of technologies used in information jobs (Bowe, 1985). It is essential for people with disabilities to have access to computers and computer software developed for the general population (Bowe, 1985). Many software programs developed for the general populations, however, are not accessible to selected disability groups. For example, a blind reporter who could write articles using synthesized speech output on a word processor may not be able to use some of the newer word processing programs that depend extensively upon icons, windows, and other graphics as part of their "user-friendly" assists (Bowe, 1985). A person may lose a job if an employer switches to a new technology that is inaccessible.

Rehabilitation counselors may wish to work closely with rehabilitation engineers and clients to explore innovative ways to create special computer adaptations to ensure that accessibility keeps pace with modern information technology.

Rehabilitation Education and Training Issues

Computers are being used with increasing frequency in virtually every function performed by rehabilitation counselors, including case management, counseling, assessment, career exploration, job placement, and job skills training (Berven, 1985). Like other professionals in the information world, rehabilitation counselors must be adequately prepared to use computer technology to meet the demands of contemporary professional practices (Berven, 1985). Universities and training units of rehabilitation agencies must consider the incorporation of "computer literacy" into their training curricula. Nevertheless, the definition of computer literacy for rehabilitation counseling may be different from other fields. Master's-level rehabilitation counselors may only need to become sophisticated users of the computer systems and related software. At the doctoral level, the computer literacy requirements could be more stringent (Nave & Browning, 1983). Doctoral-level trainees may need to develop a basic knowledge of computer operations, applications, limitations, and impact on society (Berven, 1985). In addition, in accordance with the standard definition of computer literacy, working knowledge of one or more computer programming languages may be required (Seidel, Anderson, & Hunter, 1982). More sophisticated and highly trained doctoral-level professionals may have to assume a leadership role to help shape the future directions of rehabilitation counseling. They must be creative and innovative and have a thorough understanding of the information world.

Research Issues

The extensive use of computer technology in rehabilitation counseling is still a very new phenonomen. The quality of computer technology and the relative efficacy of its utilization in rehabilitation is still unknown. Further programmatic research must be conducted to expand the existing knowledge base on the use of computer technology in rehabilitation services.

Research may be needed to identify: 1) potential or existing ethical dilemmas (and possible methods of resolution) that could emanate from abuses of computer technology; 2) methods by which the use of specific types of computer technology could improve delivery of rehabilitation counseling services; 3) whether computer technology increases the range, quality, and quantity of services available for rehabilitation counselors to use for/with persons with disabilities; 4) instructional methods for preparing future rehabilitation counselors to use specific types of computer technologies; 5) the necessary knowledge, skills, and abilities required presently (and optimally) by rehabilitation counselors to use computer technology effectively; 6) variables that can potentially affect attitudes toward and subsequent use of technologies by rehabilitation counselors; 7) employment settings currently providing resources and/or support for rehabilitation counselors in technological areas; and 8) specific computer and microelectronic technologies currently utilized by rehabilitation counselors.

Research may also be needed to develop methods to: 1) promote dialogue among rehabilitation counselors concerning issues pertaining to technology; 2) assess the degree of awareness possessed by rehabilitation counselors in various areas of technology; 3) identify and assess the nature of potential benefits and cautions emanating from the use of various technologies in daily practice by rehabilitation counselors; 4) assess current and projected attitudes among rehabilitation counselors regarding their use of technologies; 5) assess current and projected attitudes among rehabilitation administrators regarding counselor use of technologies; and 6) assess the actual use of such technologies by rehabilitation counselors, as compared to their hypothetical applications.

SUMMARY

The use of advanced computer and microelectronic technology may improve the performance of rehabilitation counselors and provide enhanced independent living and employment opportunities for people with disabilities. The advent of this technology also adds to the knowledge base required by rehabilitation counselors (Crimando & Godley, 1985). Rehabilitation counselors must become conversant with computer hardware and software available to professionals and electronic assistive devices for persons with disabilities. Also, counselors may have to give more attention to the changing labor market (i.e., the change from the manufacture-based to service/information-based economy) in the plan development and job placement phases of the rehabilitation process. Researchers need to advance beyond speculation and descriptions of the potential use of the computer to the actual validation of the effectiveness of computer applications in rehabilitation.

REFERENCES

Ahl, D. H. (1984). Choosing a notebook computer. *Creative Computing, 10,* 18–32.

Apple Computer Inc. (1981). *Personal computers for the physically disabled.* Cupertino, CA: Author.

Berven, N. L. (1985). Computer technology in professional education. *Rehabilitation Counseling Bulletin, 29,* 26–41.

Botterbusch, K. F. (1983). *A comparison of commercial vocational evaluation systems.* Menomonie: University of Wisconsin–Stout, Materials Development Center.

Bowe, F. G. (1985). Employment trends in the information age. *Rehabilitation Counseling Bulletin, 29,* 19–25.

Burkhead, E. J., & Sampson, J. P. (1985). Computer-assisted assessment in support of the rehabilitation process. *Rehabilitation Counseling Bulletin, 28,* 262–274.

Chan, F., McCollum, P. S., & Parker, H. J. (1985). Computer-assisted job placement: Selected applications. *American Rehabilitation, 11,* 18–21.

Chan, F., McCollum, P. S., & Pool, D. A. (1985). Computer assisted rehabilitation services: A preliminary draft of the Texas casework model. *Rehabilitation Counseling Bulletin, 28,* 219–232.

Chan, F., & Questad, K. (1981). Microcomputers in vocational evaluation: An application for staff training. *Vocational Evaluation and Work Adjustment Bulletin, 14,* 153–158.

Cook, A. M., Leins, J. D., & Woodall, H. E. (1985). Use of microcomputers by disabled persons: A rehabilitation engineering perspective. *Rehabilitation Counseling Bulletin, 28,* 283–292.

Crimando, W., & Godley, S. H. (1985). The computer's potential in enhancing employment opportunities of persons with disabilities. *Rehabilitation Counseling Bulletin, 28,* 275–282.

Crimando, W., & Sawyer, H. W. (1983). Microcomputers in private sector rehabilitation. *Rehabilitation Counseling Bulletin, 27,* 26–31.

Dahmke, M. (Ed.). (1982). Computers and the disabled [Special issue]. *Byte, 7*(9).

Eighth Institute on Rehabilitation Issues. (1981). *Computer-assisted rehabilitation service delivery.* Washington, DC: National Institute of Handicapped Research.

Emener, W. G., & Rubin, S. E. (1980). Rehabilitation counselor roles and functions and sources of role strain. *Journal of Applied Rehabilitation Counseling, 11,* 57–69.

Herr, E. L. (1985). Advanced technology, theory, and rehabilitation counseling. *Rehabilitation Counseling Bulletin, 29,* 6–18.

Irons, T. R. (1985). Microcomputer usage for the person with a disability. *Journal of Rehabilitation, 51,* 31–34.

Lister, C. (1970). Privacy and large-scale personal data systems. *Personal and Guidance Journal, 49,* 207–211.

Martin, J. (1978). *The wired society.* Englewood Cliffs, NJ: Prentice-Hall.

McCollum, P. S., & Chan, F. (Eds.). (1985a). Implementing computer technology in the rehabilitation process [Special issue]. *Rehabilitation Counseling Bulletin, 28*(4).

McCollum, P. S., & Chan, F. (1985b). Rehabilitation in the information age: Prologue to the future. *Rehabilitation Counseling Bulletin, 28,* 211–216.

Miller, D. (1984). What do computers have to do with rehabilitation (and vice versa)? *On-Line, 1,* 2–4.

Naisbitt, J. (1982). *Megatrends.* New York: Warner Books.

Nave, G., & Browning, P. (1983). Preparing rehabilitation leaders for the computer age. *Rehabilitation Counseling Bulletin, 26,* 364–367.

Office of Technology Assessment. (1983). *Technology and handicapped people.* New York: Springer-Verlag.

Perlman, L. G., & Austin, G. (Eds.). (1984). *Technology and rehabilitation of disabled persons in the information age.* Alexandria, VA: National Rehabilitation Association Press.

Restak, M. R. (1980, March). Smart machines learn to see, listen, and even think for us. *Smithsonian,* pp. 48–56.

Roessler, R. T., & Rubin, S. E. (1982). *Case management and rehabilitation counseling.* Austin, TX: PRO-ED.

Rubin, S. E., Matkin, R. E., Ashley, J. M., Beardsley, M. M., May, V. R., Onstott, K. L., & Puckett, F. D. (1984). Roles and functions of certified rehabilitation counselors. *Rehabilitation Counseling Bulletin, 27,* 199–224, 238–245.

Sampson, J. P. (1983). An integrated approach to computer applications in counseling psychology. *Counseling Psychologist, 11,* 65–74.

Sampson, J. P., McMahon, B. T., & Burkhead, E. J. (1985). Using computers for career exploration and decision making in vocational rehabilitation. *Rehabilitation Counseling Bulletin, 28,* 242–261.

Sampson, J. P., & Pyle, K. R. (1983). Ethical issues involved with the use of computer-assisted counseling, testing, and guidance systems. *Personnel and Guidance Journal, 61,* 283–286.

Schmitt, P., & Growick, B. (1985). Computer technology in rehabilitation counseling. *Rehabilitation Counseling Bulletin, 28,* 233–241.

Seidel, R. J., Anderson, R. E., & Hunter, B. (Eds.). (1982). *Computer literacy: Issues and directions for 1985.* New York: Academic Press.

Selmi, P. M., Klein, M. H., Greist, J. H., Johnson, J. H., & Harris, W. G. (1982). An investigation of computer-assisted cognitive-behavior therapy in the treatment of depression. *Behavioral Research Methods and Instrumentation, 14,* 181–185.

Synnott, W. R., & Gruber, W. H. (1981). *Information resources management.* New York: John Wiley & Sons.

Trexler, L. (Ed.). (1982). *Cognitive rehabilitation: Conceptualization and intervention.* New York: Plenum.

Vanderheiden, G. C. (1981). Practical application of microcomputers to aid the handicapped. *Computer, 14,* 54–61.

Vanderheiden, G. C. (1982). Computers can play a dual role for disabled individuals. *Byte, 1,* 136–140.

Wagman, M. (1980). PLATO DCS, an interactive computer system for personal counseling. *Journal of Counseling Psychology, 27,* 16–30.

Wagman, M., & Kerber, K. W. (1984). Computer-assisted counseling: Problems and prospects. *Counselor Education and Supervision, 24,* 142–154.

Weizenbaum, J. (1965). ELIZA—A computer program for the study of natural language communication between man and machine. *Communication of the Association for Computing Machinery, 9,* 36–45.

15

Challenges for Rehabilitation Counselor Education

Marvin D. Kuehn, Ralph M. Crystal, and Alex Ursprung

Many rehabilitation educators consider professional graduate preparation of rehabilitation counselors, called rehabilitation counselor education (RCE), to be at a pivotal stage in its evolutionary development. The complexity of administrative reorganization and funding trends in higher education, along with professional identification issues, creates additional obstacles for the continuing development of rehabilitation counselor education programs. This chapter reviews the factors influencing the image, growth, and development of RCE programs. Some significant challenges are proposed that must be addressed if RCE programs are to remain responsive to the expanding employment market for graduates through the improvement and provision of relevant curricula offerings.

Four broad areas of major importance for RCE programs are identified in this chapter. The first area relates to the influence of an always-changing federal policy in regard to priorities and client populations to be served and the types of personnel that may be most needed to respond to various client constituencies. The second segment of this chapter focuses on the establishment of a professional identity for rehabilitation counselors, the growth and changes in professional education, trends in specialization, and problems with

For her assistance in the conceptualization of and research for this chapter, gratitude is extended to Mary Brady, Supervisor in the Division of Operations, New York State Department of Education, Office of Vocational Rehabilitation, Albany, NY. Her comments in reading the chapter were relevant, encouraging, and sincerely appreciated.

expectations related to counselor roles and responsibilities. The third addresses external factors influencing RCE, such as certification, accreditation, professional organizations, conflicting perceptions of the profession, the meaning of the term *disability,* and funding and student recruitment concerns. The last section examines employment trends and the change in employment settings selected by graduates.

INFLUENCE OF FEDERAL LEGISLATION

Unlike some of the other established human service professions, the emergence of the rehabilitation counseling profession has been tied to federal legislative mandates, and its development has been closely related to the expansion of the state-federal system of vocational rehabilitation (Thomas, 1985).

Early rehabilitation legislation, such as the Smith-Fess Act of 1920 (PL 66-236), provided no federal funds to prepare trained personnel to deliver rehabilitation services. Even though the Barden-LaFollette Act of 1943 (PL 78-113) allowed administrators of state vocational rehabilitation programs the option to train or pay for training personnel, federal dollars were not appropriated for this purpose (Scalia & Wolfe, 1984). As the state-federal rehabilitation program grew and the rehabilitation counseling profession expanded to serve new populations, a clear need emerged for qualified personnel to deliver quality services to persons with disabling conditions.

In 1954, the federal government through the Rehabilitation Services Administration (RSA) awarded grants to public and nonprofit agencies and organizations, including institutions of higher education, to establish master's- and doctoral-level rehabilitation counseling programs. The purpose was to improve the quality of professional practice and increase the number of personnel trained to provide vocational rehabilitation services resulting in the employment of persons with disabilities. Early funding was earmarked for "training" personnel who desired to work in the state-federal rehabilitation program; training was, therefore, job specific. During the last 30 years, however, the use of the term "training" has been replaced by the concept of "education," which generally refers to preparation for a professional career.

In 1965, a federal appropriation of $19.8 million for rehabilitation training was distributed among 38 educational institutions. By 1970, 72 educational programs were receiving funding. By 1979, total federal funding for rehabilitation education had increased to $30.5 million (RSA, 1984). In 1983, 229 rehabilitation education programs and 76 state in-service programs were being partially supported by significantly reduced appropriations for rehabilitation education of $19.2 million. By funding a growing number of rehabilitation education programs, representing over 20 separate disciplines, with substantially lower resources, the issue becomes one centering on what "types of personnel" are most desirable to address the complex needs of diverse client populations.

Since the federal rehabilitation agency has supported education activities commensurate with professional development, rehabilitation counselor education has primarily been attached to the mandates of the federal rehabilitation program. The profession of rehabilitation counseling was essentially born out of the state-federal rehabilitation program (Brubaker, 1981; RSA, 1984).

The major focus of manpower development in the 1960s was employment of graduates of master's-level RCE programs in state rehabilitation agencies. In the last 15 years, various types of training programs have been created or expanded to include training in several rehabilitation subspecialties and disciplines. This expansion has included the development of bachelor's- and doctoral-level rehabilitation education programs, as well as continuing education programs.

Changing Service Populations

During the last 20 years, rehabilitation services have been provided to increasingly diverse client populations. By the end of the 1960s, rehabilitation counselors were providing comprehensive services to industrially injured workers, mentally retarded persons, public offenders, alcohol and drug abusers, severely physically disabled persons, and mentally ill persons (Wright, 1980).

The Rehabilitation Act of 1973 mandated that RCE programs give priority in training counselors to work with severely physically disabled persons. In addition, increased emphasis was placed on serving mentally retarded persons and those having other developmental disabilities as well as persons with severe neurotic and psychotic conditions. Thus, RCE programs have felt the pressure to expand coursework offerings; however, the feasibility of continually adding courses has emerged as a major concern.

With the increased legislative emphasis on the previously mentioned populations, the need for additional abilities and expertise emerged. Faced with the challenge of preparing rehabilitation counselors for a complex job role, individuals involved in RCE programs began conducting research on the minimal preparation required, the types or content of training needed, and the competencies necessary to provide services (Wright, 1980).

RCE programs recognized the necessity of specialized education (curriculum electives) that would address new federal priority areas such as supported work, job development and placement, transition services, learning disabilities, and independent living. Today's rehabilitation counselors must relate to and explain services to consumers and advocacy groups, workers' compensation agencies, and the legal system. Increased emphasis on serving special client groups, combined with the need for a larger body of knowledge and skills, has resulted in new challenges and frequent significant curriculum revision by RCE programs.

Politics and Bureaucracy

From 1965 through the mid-1970s, there was rapid and sustained growth in government-sponsored programs and public sector involvement in the provision of services to persons with disabilities. Rehabilitation services and income support expanded under SSI and SSDI programs. Additional services were provided through Medicaid, Medicare, and Title XX Social Service programs (Wright, 1980).

In the late 1970s, increases in funding for social and rehabilitation services were replaced by policies of fiscal restraint (Emener, 1985; National Rehabilitation Counseling Association [NRCA], 1985; Thomas, 1985). State-federal rehabilitation program funding stabilized and even began declining slightly after 1976. With the emphasis on serving the client who is severely physically disabled, state rehabilitation agency caseload size began declining due to the complexity of services and the length of time often necessary to meet client needs. The economic prognosis was for tighter restrictions on public funding of rehabilitation-related programs (The Urban Institute, 1981). As funding levels have declined, rehabilitation manpower issues have emerged. Concerns now seem to have shifted from management of staff growth to more efficient utilization of the manpower resources available (The Urban Institute, 1981).

The Reagan administration has attempted to reduce the federal government's role in terms of funding programs and providing direction and leadership. This administration has curtailed or reexamined social programs in every area, recently attacking Social Security, Medicare, the school lunch program, and various special education programs. As the federal government reduced funding for programs, it also lessened its control of these programs, resulting in a decreasing federal bureaucracy. Many disabled persons, however, still depend upon federal programs for needed services (Luck & Rothrock, 1984).

Changing governmental/bureaucratic priorities is not a new situation or tendency with which rehabilitation service delivery or education programs must deal. Bowe (1985) illustrated the challenge for RCE programs when he articulated the problems that result when there is no clear, rational federal disability policy:

> In the United States, we have created piecemeal programs that in turn have a piecemeal effect on meeting the needs of disabled people. First, we created a disability insurance program. Then, we created a rehabilitation program. We created a special education program and a supplemental security income program. These programs were all created to meet a different need at a different point in time, without thought for their interrelation. (p. 197)

The debilitating effects of modern governmental bureaucracy on rehabilitation counseling programs can be vividly seen in the ever-changing federal training priorities and guidelines calling for new program "emphases." The challenge for RCE programs has been to respond to these changes in a timely manner and to understand the rationale for changes in priorities, and for shifts or reductions in funding allocations. Frustrations arise when the expectations from funding sources appear unrealistic relative to how quickly RCE programs and service providers can respond, and relative to what education and training curricula should be emphasized or modified (RSA, 1984).

PROFESSIONAL IDENTITY

Rehabilitation counseling has had a comparatively short history of professional growth. Its professional status and impact continue to grow; however, several issues and historical influences have prevented a clear professional identity from emerging.

A major issue that pervaded the literature of the 1960s focused on the identity, role, and function of the rehabilitation counselor: "Is this professional a rehabilitation counselor, a coordinator, or a clinician?" Patterson (1967) suggested that state rehabilitation agencies could employ both rehabilitation counselors and rehabilitation coordinators. Counselors would function as psychological counselors with those clients needing to resolve personal adjustment concerns; coordinators would find cases, do intake interviews, manage cases, do public relations work, and place clients. Others, such as Whitehouse (1975), referred to the rehabilitation counselor as a rehabilitation clinician whose skills include those of a therapist, guidance counselor, case manager, psychometrician, educator, evaluator, advocate, and placement specialist.

These differences in functions, titles, and philosophical orientations illustrate what some perceive as the current identity problem of the profession. Recent research on rehabilitation counselor roles and functions suggests that the employment setting is a major determiner in defining and shaping professional identity (Emener & Rubin, 1980; Feinberg & McFarlane, 1979; Matkin, 1983; Rubin & Emener, 1979; Rubin & Puckett, 1984). Identification of the unique responsibilities of a rehabilitation counselor has become more complex in recent years due to a substantial increase in the different types of settings in which counselors work (Feinberg & McFarlane, 1979). The increase of different types of work settings has contributed to the difficulty of identifying the specific responsibilities and educational preparation necessary for a rehabilitation counselor.

Professional identity is also influenced by major methodological problems existing in the measurement and evaluation of rehabilitation counselor performance (Emener, 1985). Criticisms of current evaluation practices of rehabilitation counselor performance include marginal relevance of performance standards, minimal contribution to or facilitation of individual counselor development and improvement, and cosmetic use of evaluation data by agencies to make themselves "look good" statistically (Emener, 1985).

Emener (1985) pointed out a reason for this identity problem when he stated:

> The earlier job tasks of the rehabilitation counselor tended to be more finite and simplistic compared to those of recent years. Also, while the job tasks of the rehabilitation counselor were expanding . . . specific areas of specialization emerged . . . At the same time, specialty associations and corresponding journals and texts emerged. (pp. 61–62)

Since the early 1970s, new federal mandates that emphasize different client populations and priorities and expanding employment opportunities beyond the traditional state-federal rehabilitation agency, have resulted in mild "schizophrenia" for RCE programs, and given rise to the question, "Is the rehabilitation counselor a counselor specializing in rehabilitation, a generic rehabilitation professional with expertise in counseling, or a combination of both?" (NRCA, 1985).

Perhaps the time has come to discard arguments about "counselor versus coordinator" and accept the notion that both identities are necessary. Adopting the concept of the generic rehabilitation counselor who embraces both aspects of "service function" and "work setting" may be a major challenge for RCE programs in the future. Until there is a definite concensus as to what the rehabilitation counseling profession specifically encompasses, clear articulation of the "core competencies" and skills that RCE program graduates should possess will be controversial. RCE programs must prepare graduates with skills and "identities" that are desired in the human service marketplace. More attention to the practical, economic needs of persons with disabilities may be an appropriate focus that will assist RCE programs in addressing the professional identity issue.

Professional Education

National preparation standards and tasks required of graduates of RCE programs reflect various functions necessary to assist rehabilitation counselors in meeting client needs. Direction for preservice, master's-level rehabilitation counselor education curriculum content, and criteria for university program accreditation has been provided by the Council on Rehabilitation Education, Inc. (CORE). Assessment of rehabilitation counselor competencies in order to determine the "right" to practice are provided by the Commission on Rehabilitation Counseling Certification (CRCC). Both CORE and CRCC were established in the 1970s to assure program standards and practitioner qualifications. The activities and credibility of both organizations are extremely important because of their direct and indirect influence on RCE programs.

A standardized curriculum for the master's degree in rehabilitation counseling was developed in 1954. A meeting of national authorities on rehabilitation and graduate education provided the initial guidelines for curriculum planning (Wright, 1984). Rehabilitation education matured in the 1960s with assistance from the so-called Joint Liaison Committee that represented both educators and state-federal rehabilitation program administrators. This opportunity for educators and agency administrators to discuss the actual duties and demands of rehabilitation employment helped shape a practical curriculum based upon client needs.

In the 1960s, there was a general perception among some educators that RCE should be directed specifically toward preparing counselors to work in state agencies. Traditionally, state agencies have been a major employer of rehabilitation counselors; today, professional rehabilitation counselor education prepares individuals to work with diverse client populations. The objective of preparation has always been to provide services needed by individual consumers rather than training for a specific job or work setting.

While RSA recognizes the master's degree as the educational preparation necessary for entry-level rehabilitation counselors, state vocational rehabilitation (VR) agencies and civil service commissions generally have never fully accepted it, and many do not require it as the minimum educational requirement for employment (Luck & Rothrock, 1984). Even though a large percentage of RCE program graduates have traditionally entered professional employment with state vocational rehabilitation agencies, this policy/attitude still persists. The basic difference between the RSA's and the state agency's preferred educational preparation for entry-level rehabilitation counselors gives rise to several issues discussed later in this chapter.

In many respects, the long-standing program of providing federal monies, particularly for students in RCE programs, has been highly successful. Thousands of rehabilitation counselors have been educated over the years under the auspices of the federal rehabilitation training program, and nearly 100 colleges and universities now offer graduate training in rehabilitation counseling (Wright, 1980). RCE programs have also indirectly facilitated the production of considerable research and scholarship in areas relevant to rehabilitation counseling and to serving disabled persons (Farkas & Anthony, 1980; Geist & Emener, 1981; Kuehn, 1984; Parker & Hansen, 1981; Smits & Ledbetter, 1979; Thomas, 1985).

Organizations such as CORE, the National Council on Rehabilitation Education (NCRE), NCRA, the American Rehabilitation Counseling Association (ARCA), and RSA have proposed regulations and policies and supported state and federal certification to advance minimum standards of practice and preparation for rehabilitation counselors.

Even though there have been significant changes in technology, new employment opportunities in private sector rehabilitation, and criticism about curricula, the basic curricular core in RCE programs has remained intact; recent studies (Matkin, 1983; Rubin et al., 1984) consistently confirm the validity of the basic core curriculum. Still, RCE program curricula have not remained static. More courses and instructional units on unique populations, special services (group and family counseling), vocational assessment, job development and job placement, independent living rehabilitation, private for-profit rehabilitation, legal aspects, and workers' compensation rehabilitation have been incorporated into curricula (Kuehn, 1984).

Specialization

As a profession, rehabilitation counseling is composed of an extensive body of knowledge and technology. However, the expanding accumulation of information has grown beyond the scope of the typical curriculum of the traditionally prepared rehabilitation counselor (Wright, 1980).

The literature of the rehabilitation counseling profession is filled with discussions about whether counselors should be generalists, specialists, or both. Probably the most visible critic of the specialization concept has been C. H. Patterson (1967). Patterson contended that while specialization in rehabilitation counseling was probably inevitable, it risks focusing on the client's individual limitations and characteristics, rather than on the individual as a whole. He also pointed out several logistical problems in terms of training and the roles he felt would have to be carefully dealt with as the movement toward specialization became more widespread (Thomas, 1982).

Specialization in RCE was almost nonexistent when Patterson authored his 1967 article on the subject. Since that time, several graduate training programs offering different types of specialization in rehabilitation counseling have developed. The implications of responding to the movement toward specialization by RCE programs become obvious; the fragmentation which has occurred often creates major curriculum problems as programs try to respond to the complex needs of client populations.

The advantage of specialization allows the professional to exercise his or her particular pattern of interests, aptitudes, and abilities, thus making each counselor unique in the agency or office as its consulting authority on problems within a particular area. The advent of specialization affords an opportunity for a continuing, lifelong challenge of professional enrichment by expanding or even shifting one's specialty (Wright, 1980). Finally, a "specialist system" could help the whole profession of rehabilitation counseling move toward recommitment to professionalism and excellence in client service.

Specialization in rehabilitation counseling may be based on any one of the following criteria: 1) employment setting, such as public or voluntary agency, facility, or proprietary business; 2) type of disability, such as mental illness, retardation, or blindness; or 3) function or task, such as vocational or personal adjustment counseling, employee assistance programs, vocational expert consultancy, independent living, client assessment, or job placement (Wright, 1984).

Students may be prepared for employment in particular work settings; this type of specialization results primarily from the orientation of the faculty and the types of university and community resources available. Thomas (1982) pointed out that this orientation invariably results in giving students a narrow, unrealistic perspective of the profession and may limit the range of employment opportunities available after graduation.

The second and most common model of specialization would probably be preparation to work with a specific client population, such as persons who are blind, deaf, or mentally retarded. Thomas (1982) suggested that "specialized" university programs are usually offered either because special monies have been provided for this purpose by the federal government or because the strengths of the faculty and community resources naturally facilitate the development of expertise with a particular disability group. According to Thomas (1982), however, "There is also little research evidence to suggest that different client groups require different competencies or rehabilitation methods" (p. 50). Whether a large enough body of rehabilitation-related knowledge exists about any particular disability group to require more than one or two additional courses of study is questionable. By offering specialization options at the master's level, educators may unnecessarily limit the employment opportunities of students by focusing on a client group with little legislative or administrative priority in the future (Thomas, 1982).

The third type of specialization in RCE programs emphasizes remediating particular aspects of the client's adjustment problems. This type of specialization refers to the relative importance RCE programs place on preparing students to deal with vocational, personal, or social adjustment. It typically results from a bias on the part of the faculty; rehabilitation counselor educators sometimes feel some moral obligation to commit either for or against the relative importance of personal counseling versus vocational adjustment. However, an approach to counseling that treats vocational and personal adjustment as autonomous entities is likely to be ineffective (Thomas, 1982).

Patterson (1967) pointed out that specializing would fragment the perception of the client and the total rehabilitation process. He suggested that "specialized training must be in addition to the present two years of graduate preparation for rehabilitation counselors" (Patterson, 1967, p. 153); if this occurred, the choice of electives necessary for a specialization area would not preempt "core" coursework.

Each of the dimensions or models discussed has strengths and weaknesses, as well as potentially significant implications for RCE programs. Specialization poses several questions that can be summarized as follows: 1) Can the advantages of service coordination be preserved and the benefits that derive from specialization of function still be obtained? 2) Is the need for expanded areas of knowledge and skill by practitioners justification for developing new "professions" and changing the present RCE core standards? 3) Can there be subspecialities under the profession of rehabilitation counseling where a "core" body of knowledge and skill exists—is this not what gives the fields of social work and medicine a single professional identification? The issue is not whether specialization is needed, but how the three criteria of setting, disability type, and job task can be "tied together" under the "profession" of rehabilitation counseling.

In RCE, the challenge of keeping abreast of technical knowledge and the literature and services relevant to rehabilitation counseling practice is a reality. RCE programs are challenged to decide if or how curricula should be revised to reflect mandated programs for independent living, supported work, and transition services for the severely disabled population; increased emphases on accountability currently being used to evaluate counselor performance; the challenge to maintain a viable reputation for innovation; and flexibility to accommodate expanding needs, services, and cost-effectiveness.

Programs accredited by CORE must, appropriately, focus on a "core" curriculum that research shows to be common for all rehabilitation counselors regardless of the client population being served. The challenges arise in offering relevant electives and revising present courses with limited faculty and related resources. RCE programs are reassessing curricula emphases to better prepare graduates to become highly skilled and knowledgeable in working with diverse client populations. RCE programs must maintain flexibility in their curricula to respond to varying client needs in individual states. The problem for RCE programs becomes one of fragmentation and the potential loss of professional identification that can have an impact on recruitment, image, and sometimes funding allocations; funding reductions for RCE can result from cuts within the university itself, as well as from cuts occurring in external sources, such as federal and state grants.

The issue can be vividly seen in job titles of personnel in rehabilitation facilities where "specializations" have developed outside of the rehabilitation counseling profession; often, personnel are not identified as rehabilitation counselors performing specific duties (subspecialties of the "profession"), but under different titles as they have sought to establish unique, independent status as specialists. In certain settings, a rehabilitation counselor may function as a vocational counselor, psychotherapist, placement specialist, case coordinator, psychometrist, administrator, or various combinations thereof. In addition, a wide variation in job titles exists—vocational rehabilitation counselor, vocational counselor, counselor, psychologist, rehabilitation specialist, and coordinator. Because of the differences in job duties, training, and experience requirements, attempts to solidify the professional identify of a rehabilitation counselor are inherently more difficult than in other more homogeneous occupations.

Most specialists operate within the confines of an established discipline or institution to which they owe allegiance. Moreover, specialists are generally employed to perform functions that are unique to and consistent with a given discipline; they do not overlap with other fields of endeavor. Social work and psychology retain single professional identifications despite multifaceted specialization; for example, there are the subspecialties of medical, child, school, public, and psychiatric social work. Wright (1982) proposed that RCE could benefit from the prototype of the medical profession for which there is uniform initial preparation (the M.D. degree with an internship) that is generally followed by further training for specialization. The best structure or model to be followed for rehabilitation counseling specialization is not yet clear, but the idea of adopting a model or at least examining options is certainly worthy of consideration and discussion.

An Urban Institute study (1981) showed that "there do exist serious shortages of highly specialized counselors" (p. 44). The growth and development in the 1970s of baccalaureate programs in rehabilitation education might help solve the problem of training rehabilitation counselors as specialists. Could a 2-year master's degree program in rehabilitation counseling (on top of 2 years of undergraduate rehabilitation foundation courses) now accommodate some specialized knowledge and skills in the counseling area as well as in other rehabilitation subspecialities? Review of the curricular content of undergraduate rehabilitation education programs listed in the NCRE membership directory indicates that some coursework typically offered only at the master's level is now being offered in undergraduate programs (Kuehn, 1984). The result of these curricular offerings may, in fact, be the creation of more opportunities for "specialization" at the graduate level.

Roles and Functions

A major concern in the professional preparation of rehabilitation counselors has been changing roles and functions (Emener & Rubin, 1980). Historically, it has been difficult to trace changes across time in the role and function of the rehabilitation counselor due to methodological variability among studies.

Differing population samples and differences in perceived, reported, and preferred roles and functions of rehabilitation counselors have been the reasons for numerous problems in explaining rehabilitation counselor performance. The implications of these varying factors have been directly and indirectly related to ineffective client services (counselor performance) and negative image problems for RCE programs.

A study by Muthard and Salomone (1969) provided strong evidence supporting the importance of role and function research. It should be noted, however, that the primary subject groups examined in this study comprised only state agency rehabilitation counselors.

Rubin and Emener (1979) observed high variability across five rehabilitation counselor role and function studies "in regard to the number of role categories used as well as the labels of those categories" (p. 145). Evidence of significant role changes has been provided in several recent studies (Emener & Rubin, 1980; Rubin & Emener, 1979; Rubin & Puckett, 1984). Collectively, these studies suggest that, compared to their time allocations across job tasks in the middle 1960s, rehabilitation counselors are currently spending less time on counseling and guidance activities, more time on case recording, and more time on arranging and coordinating services.

Progress has been made in articulating a clear description of the typical role and functions of the rehabilitation counselor (Graves, 1979; Hershenson, 1982; Lynch & McSweeney, 1981; Matkin, 1983; Parker & Hansen, 1981; Rubin & Roessler, 1983; Rubin et al., 1984; Wright, 1982).

While at one time rehabilitation counselors were "jacks of all trades," they are now, as a result of many factors such as increasing technology, expected to be experts/specialists (Wright, 1980). Rubin and Roessler (1983) suggested that a more inclusive role for the rehabilitation counselor is needed. Following the "multifaceted viewpoint" model, the rehabilitation counselor may become a skilled professional working at the "hub" of an interdisciplinary program requiring the coordination of many professionals.

To avoid catering to the differing perceptions of counselor roles as seen by professional organizations and employers, RCE programs have tried to focus upon the needs of the client population. In the early years of RCE programs, much emphasis was put on counseling (skill development) rather than on other aspects of student preparation, such as knowledge of job placement techniques (Fraser & Clowers, 1978). The focus upon the client as a consumer of services rather than as an individual who needs "counseling" has led to substantial curricular changes in RCE programs (Brubaker, 1981; Finnerty-Fried, 1985; Luck & Rothrock, 1984).

A major result of an ambiguous professional role is seen in the differing perceptions and expectations of the rehabilitation counselor by clients (consumers). In order to make sound curricular decisions, RCE program faculties have to constantly examine the needs and expectations of employers and service recipients.

Often, the perceived value and competence of a professionally prepared rehabilitation counselor are determined by the personal experience of the client or the employer. Occasionally, the expectations of both the provider and client, relative to what should be "delivered" and how, are incongruent and create considerable dissatisfaction and resentment. Another debilitating consequence of this role conflict may be that the provider or the limited services of an agency/program are deemed ''incompetent'' or ''ridiculous'' by clients (consumers). Failure to meet role expectations is frustrating to both employer and employee. The end result of this frustration, however, is that frequently a perception persists that the individual counselor was inadequately ''trained.'' The conflict may eventually develop into mutual lack of respect, resulting in assumptions and opinions that may be unjustified or illogical in regard to the academic preparation of counselors (Kuehn, 1984). The preservice preparation of rehabilitation counselors has occasionally been blamed for their failure to meet client needs/expectations. However, in such a case it is important to ask whether the client is reacting to the counselor and his or her performance, or to the program and its policies? Does ''incompetent'' mean the rehabilitation counselor does not know something, or does it refer to the policies or procedures utilized by the agency/program? Answers to these questions are not ''black and white,'' and blame/fault may not be attributable solely to either party. Understanding why a role expectation is not met or why a role conflict develops requires a careful examination of the circumstances and perceptions of everyone involved.

A U.S. Department of Education committee report (1985) further illustrates the confusion of role and identity that develops when service goals and priorities are not congruent with rehabilitation counselor responsibilities. The confusion may rest with management's inability to clearly articulate policy and program direction. Regardless of the cause, there frequently appears to be little effort by employers to establish priorities in terms of counselor functions and services to be provided. Agencies should continually assess the relationship between their missions and client characteristics, counselor roles, and need for change. Trainers, educators, and agency management staff need to be unified when role priorities are identified and implemented.

A current role model that some RCE programs now promote suggests that the role identification of rehabilitation counselors should be modified to be more compatible with that of a consultant. Trainers of rehabilitation personnel are encouraged to train practicing counselors as well as those persons preparing to enter the rehabilitation field as service consultants. Just as state rehabilitation agencies purchase evaluation, placement, and training services, they might also be encouraged to experiment with purchasing counseling (U.S. Department of Education, 1985).

Rehabilitation counselor educators generally recognize that the effective rehabilitation counselor must be qualified for a variety of professional functions including, but not limited to, vocational and personal-social adjustment counseling. Some rehabilitation educators, however, believe that the only professional function of the rehabilitation counselor is counseling (therapy), and that placement and the like should be assigned to a ''subprofessional'' salesperson or aide with something less than master's-level preparation.

> To say that agency employers have made a counselor's work routine with such unchallenging tasks as report-writing and job placement reflects the older RCE notion that counseling is psychotherapy and that only this counselor function and goal is professionally appropriate and challenging in rehabilitation. (Wright, 1982, p. 156)

However, contemporary educators do see counseling as a basic responsibility that facilitates other critically important functions, such as job placement, which is viewed now as a professional rehabilitation counseling function involving a detailed knowledge of both the client and the world of work (Emener, 1985; Wright, 1982).

Emerging Concerns

Recently RCE programs have been criticized by state rehabilitation agency directors for their failure to significantly increase the percentage of master's-level (trained) counselors employed by state rehabilitation agencies. This concern may not be the fault of RCE programs, since they prepare individuals for the "profession" and do not determine salaries and dictate job responsibilities (Thomas, 1985). Another difficulty has been the tendency for some rehabilitation educators to be "inordinately deferential and acquiescent to those RSA personnel who control the training monies" (Thomas, 1985, p. 19). A consequence of this attitude is the perpetuation of unclear professional roles by RCE programs because they are responding to "financial issues" rather than client needs and the marketplace. Third, in some states it is often difficult, if not impossible, to document that a critical shortage of rehabilitation counselors exists in agencies of the state-federal rehabilitation program. The employment success of RCE program graduates has been much easier to document in other agencies and work settings than in the state-federal programs (Thomas, 1985).

There is considerable debate among professional organization leaders in rehabilitation counseling regarding the influence of government (NRCA, 1985; Thomas, 1985). Some believe government has usurped the power of the profession to define, control, and regulate itself, rendering it a relatively impotent, subservient, and highly unstable occupation. Conversely, others argue that rehabilitation counseling's ability to work cooperatively with federal and state government, while still maintaining a high degree of professional integrity, is evidence of the field's broad-based history, development, and relevance (Parker & Hansen, 1981).

An indirect criticism of RCE implies that rehabilitation counselors may not assume a leadership role in the identification and development of services or referral sources.

> Counselors are apparently inclined to match the client with services available through the agency's resources rather than identify client needs and sources where they can best be met. If there is not an appropriate resource for a client's

> need(s), the process usually breaks down. Often a client will be sent to a particular program not because it is best suited for that client but because the counselor has not been able to identify or arrange an appropriate program of services. Again, the client is being expected to conform to the process or system. (U.S. Department of Education, 1985, p. 13)

Another concern beginning to influence the curricula of RCE programs is the population of disabled aging persons. America now has more people over 65 than it has teenagers; according to Bowe (1984), in the 1980 election, fully one-third of all votes cast were those of people age 55 or over. Additionally, according to the U.S. Bureau of Census, about one in three over-65 persons has a physical, sensory, mental, or other disability (Bowe, 1984). Older persons may experience a number of life transitions that entail a series of losses. An individual's ability to negotiate a life transition successfully depends on available resources, and rehabilitation counselors can be critical in assisting older persons in transition to augment or replace psychosocial losses. Rehabilitation counselors will need to learn more about the problems of aging and the services that best meet this population's needs, and to be aware of their own feelings and attitudes about aging and older persons (Finnerty-Fried, 1985).

A final challenge for RCE programs requires an assessment of the training implications of the independent living (IL) movement and the new initiatives in transition and supported employment. Nosek (Chapter 3, this volume) pointed out many different settings in which IL services can be provided and where professionals can be employed. She also illustrated philosophical differences in job responsibilities as reflected in the comparison between a rehabilitation paradigm and an IL paradigm. However, a major concern for RCE programs is the reluctance of some programs to integrate "IL counseling and services" in RCE curricula, since IL philosophy is perceived as diluting the vocational focus of traditional rehabilitation counseling.

Tooman (Chapter 5, this volume) and Szymanski et al. (Chapter 7, this volume) also discuss recent initiatives of transition and supported work within the rehabilitation field, and they suggest expanded roles and new training emphases for RCE programs. A key question in evaluating the merits of the suggestions offered is whether adequate research exists to show the importance or appropriateness of the functions outlined for master's-level training programs. The need for knowledge and understanding of these initiatives and programs by graduates of RCE programs is not disputed; whether master's-level trained graduates will accept and retain employment in work settings requiring expertise in these new initiatives is another issue.

The issues discussed, particularly in Chapters 3, 5, and 7 in this volume, foster the spiraling confusion about the appropriate role/identity of the rehabilitation counselor. The result of these dilemmas and criticisms has stimulated the reassessment and sometimes modification of RCE curricula. New elective courses are being offered, such as adult development and aging, introduction to independent living, and issues in private rehabilitation. Changing and updating RCE program curricula is a continual process that is recognized as necessary and desirable. The challenge comes when faculty expertise is limited, opportunities for continuing education for faculty are minimal, and financial resources to purchase or obtain materials or hire part-time faculty are nonexistent because of funding cutbacks in higher education.

EXTERNAL INFLUENCES

Current professional literature clearly reflects the numerous related rehabilitation issues that presently have an impact on the professionalism of rehabilitation counseling and the curricula of RCE programs (Graves, 1979; Lynch & McSweeney, 1981; NRCA, 1985; Parker & Hansen, 1981; Szymanski, 1985; Wright, 1982). Though certification and accreditation are two separate processes controlled by organizations external to RCE programs, both are critical to the integrity and maintenance of RCE as a viable academic discipline. It is imperative that they both demand the same body of knowledge as the basis for their "stamp of approval."

The movement toward certification and accreditation in rehabilitation counseling began in the early 1970s with the creation of CRCC and CORE (Livingston, 1979; McAlees & Schumacher, 1975; Wright, 1980). There was belief on the part of the CRCC and CORE founders that certification and accreditation would be good for the profession; they perceived that a major advantage of credentialing would be to enhance the securing of RSA training monies. Support for these professional movements was evidenced by the fact that the purposes and concepts of both received the endorsement of ARCA and NRCA.

Certification

The initial establishment of certification standards for a rehabilitation counselor did not require a master's degree. In 1984, however, NCRE and other professional organizations, mainly ARCA and NRCA, urged CRCC to adopt the master's degree from an accredited university program in rehabilitation counseling as the major educational requirement. CRCC did agree to implement the requirement of a master's degree, which will go into effect at the end of 1992 (Commission on Rehabilitation Counselor Certification, 1985).

Certification is generally supported by educators and opposed by state rehabilitation agencies. State agencies argue that there is no empirical basis for certification and that the major force behind the movement is the counselors' drive for professional recognition and higher salaries (The Urban Institute, 1981). According to state rehabilitation administrators, requirements for counselor certification, if enacted, are likely to restrict the supply of counseling staff, and could drive up the cost to employ certified counselors. Proponents of certification believe it would enhance the quality of services provided (The Urban Institute, 1981). Rehabilitation counselor educators claim to have demonstrated that rehabilitation counselors with master's-level training have unique and identifiable abilities that are necessary for timely, high-quality rehabilitation of persons who are disabled.

A major research study funded in 1984 by the National Institute of Handicapped Research and awarded to NCRE is currently in progress; it indirectly addresses some of the issues related to the value and importance of certification.

Accreditation

When the concept of RCE program accreditation was first developed at the University of Wisconsin–Madison in the early 1970s, the hope was that it would set reasonable standards of competence and performance as well as encourage innovation and positive program development. CORE, in its introductory statement, "Accreditation of Rehabilitation Counselor Education Programs," states that: "A rehabilitation counselor education program has an ultimate goal of assuring that individuals with disabilities receive the high quality services to which they are entitled" (Council on Rehabilitation Education, Inc., 1983, p. 2). Even though the goals and purposes seem clear, fostering innovation and creativity in RCE programs has been difficult and not always easy to evaluate or observe. Some educators believe accreditation has encouraged uniformity and conformity, instead of enhancing positive program development. Essentially, accreditation should insure that minimal performance standards are being met by a training program; however, some critics state that nearly all programs are given the same "seal of approval." Instead of promoting excellence and competence, CORE has been accused of rewarding mediocrity and fostering stagnation and complacency (Kuehn, 1984).

To date, there are only two bodies that accredit counselor training programs: CORE and the Council for the Accreditation of Counseling and Related Educational Programs (CACREP). CORE has been involved in accrediting master's degree programs in RCE since 1975, and is nationally recognized by the Council on Post-Secondary Accreditation (COPA). CACREP is developing accreditation procedures for master's and educational specialist programs in community counseling, school counseling, student personnel services, and Ph.D. and Ed.D. programs in counselor education; it received official recognition by COPA in the summer of 1987.

An emerging problem for RCE programs, particularly those located in academic units with other counselor education programs, involves the potential cost of accreditation of more than one program within one department or division. When a certification or accreditation body establishes standards or competencies related to specific areas of practice, the professional training program within a department is locked into a prescribed academic curriculum. Coursework requirements frequently limit the ability of RCE programs to respond to new initiatives in the profession. In addition, faculty are often overloaded with the teaching of "required" courses, and are simply unable to offer new or innovative courses. This perceived lack of control by RCE programs themselves and the resultant inability to be more flexible and innovative is particularly frustrating for educators in RCE programs that have limited resources for part-time faculty or are located within large departments and colleges with other priorities.

Certification and accreditation also have political and survival implications for RCE programs. A significant issue seems to be who will influence and determine the development of rehabilitation counseling as a profession, and who will determine the education necessary to practice (Thomas, 1985). The real issue appears to relate to curriculum control. An examination of the structure of CRCC and CORE confirms that mechanisms for input and involvement from rehabilitation counselor educators are present; however, the respective member organizations may not be adequately monitoring individual representatives. Until this issue is resolved, a lack of commitment and a general skepticism on the part of RCE faculty in regard to the processes of certification and accreditation will remain.

The fear that special interest groups or "new federal initiatives" will mandate standards that could dictate significant curricula changes or modifications is also a concern (NRCA, 1985). Professional associations, practitioners, and rehabilitation educators and students are encouraged to evaluate their endorsement of and/or involvement in certification and accreditation processes.

Professional Organizations

The image of the rehabilitation counselor and the profession seems to be partially, if not almost completely, created by the strength and visibility of professional organizations. The ARCA and the NRCA were both established at about the same time (1956–1957) but with different constituencies, purposes, and parent organizations. NRCA and ARCA both bring great strength to the profession, in part because they have support from different parent associations. For years, the leaders of these two groups have talked of merger, but a single rehabilitation counseling organization may never be possible because of the legal and other problems connected with the dissolution of a division of a larger association (Field, 1981; Rasch, 1979).

In other professions such as medicine, psychology, and social work, universities and professional organizations appear to have a significant influence on the standards, competencies, and qualifications necessary for professional practice; in rehabilitation counseling, it is sometimes unclear who or what is influencing credential standards for the profession. Professional association representatives may be becoming more loyal to the certification bodies than to the associations they are supposed to represent or, ultimately, to the consumer. Certification bodies may not necessarily represent the viewpoints of their respective professional organizations and may, in some cases, have an almost adversarial relationship with them (Lynch, 1984; Lynch & Herbert, 1984).

Perceptions of Profession

A rehabilitation counselor's perceptions and attitudes are strongly and closely interwoven with work setting, history, and the current climate of consumer involvement (Brubaker, 1981; Emener, 1985; Wright, 1982).

The rehabilitation counselor's public image today seems to be a "thorn in the side" to gaining professional recognition and acceptance by other human service disciplines and society in general. Until 1954, when funding was poured into counselor education programs to assist them in training rehabilitation counselors, not much attention was paid to counselor preparation; therefore, perceptions were neither positive or negative. This is, in some measure, a reflection of policy makers' attitudes toward rehabilitation counselors (NRCA, 1985). Attitudes are often the result of the perceptions of the rehabilitation counselor's duties; sometimes the perceptions of duties are based on myths, inaccurate information, or unclear definitions of roles.

Early educators of rehabilitation counselors obtained their preparation in related disciplines and were often associated with psychology training programs or other counselor education programs. Some rehabilitation counselors, because of their "clinical training," have not until fairly recently felt a need to explain who they are and what they do (NRCA, 1985, p. 9).

Brinkman et al. (1982), in an article on models of helping, further suggested that the theoretical frame of reference that influences the professional training of a counselor has significant consequences for that person's perceived competency, status, and well-being. If training philosophies are not congruent with the objectives and goals of an agency/program, the result can undermine the effectiveness of the counselor and ultimately of service delivery itself. The philosophical orientation of RCE programs will influence a counselor's attitudes and job performance and, therefore, it may become either an ally or a detractor in fostering positive perceptions of the rehabilitation counseling profession.

The perceptions of consumers and providers often reflect the perception of society in general, which in turn influences policy makers. In addition, attitudes of rehabilitation counselors are affected by the RCE programs that provide them with preservice education. Rehabilitation counselors are also affected by administrators of rehabilitation programs who frequently tell them what to do and how to do it.

If service providers and clients are dissatisfied with a counselor's actions or attitudes, it is usually easier to criticize the counselor than to attack directly the agency or the administration that establish the policies the counselor is trying to carry out. This projected criticism toward an individual counselor therefore does not usually jeopardize future services from an agency/program; however, the dissatisfaction perceived and attributed to a rehabilitation counselor is sometimes also generalized to the education of the counselor (Kuehn, 1984).

An important question for RCE is what can be done to maintain and create a positive perception and image of the rehabilitation counselor. Many educators believe it can only happen if counselors are willing to take on the burden of affecting agency/program administration, legislation, and the policies that will enable improved perceptions to develop and grow. The probability of resolving the image problem or identity crisis may perhaps be dependent on the ability of educators from all rehabilitation disciplines to rise above "political/turf protection," jealousy between "professional organizations," and "academic" survival issues.

Meaning of Disability

Not only have the laws authorizing disability services changed, but the terminology that interprets and defines disability has changed as well (Hahn, 1985; National Council on the Handicapped [NCH], 1986; Roth, 1985).

The terms *handicap* and *disability* are commonplace in both ordinary usage and legal circles; however, these words have subtle meanings that are seldom considered. The range of people to whom they apply and the implications of imposing these labels on individuals are frequently obscured and forgotten. Legal and governmental definitions of the term *disability* tend to be formal and specific, depending on legislative, regulatory, or judicial interpretation. A definition of disability may be based on only one perspective, and can create frustration and misunderstanding as society attempts to determine whether a person or a population is disabled. In addition, the number of federal programs affecting persons with disabilities creates confusion; in 1986, over 45 separate federal programs for disabled persons were described in federal publications (NCH, 1986).

One approach to defining disability is to enumerate a list of the conditions chosen for inclusion in the definition. Another is to tailor the definition to the governmental purpose of the particular statute or regulation under consideration. A final approach involves deferral to professionals who make determinations as to what does or does not constitute a handicap. Each of these approaches has its limitations. The first tends to be so specific that it may exclude some persons who cannot be neatly categorized. The second approach may be too vague for determining which persons were meant to be included, and the third approach avoids actually explaining the term and defers to professionals (U.S. Commission on Civil Rights, 1983).

These differing approaches can also be influenced by various views about the primary source of the handicap; that is, whether this term labels limitations imposed by the disabling condition itself, or limitations imposed by environmental barriers. One view concentrates primarily on functional limitations of the disabled individual, while the other view focuses attention on handicapping factors external to the person (Berkowitz, 1979). This is particularly troublesome for students who are preparing to become rehabilitation counselors but are unsure of what services are really needed by disabled persons, or the eligibility of such persons. RCE program faculty must constantly articulate what rehabilitation counselors do for their clients and why, and must explain the parameters that may narrowly define a population. This communication must be reinforced and often modified when legislative priorities, and hence defined client populations, change.

Funding and Student Recruitment

Until the mid- to late 1970s, most rehabilitation counselors and rehabilitation counselor educators were not concerned with the politics and funding aspects of the state-federal rehabilitation program. Nonetheless, the inflationary-recessionary era of the late 1970s attracted everyone's attention. More recently, the effects of Reaganomics, the New Federalism, the allocation of block grants to states, and declining federal support of human services in general, have found virtually all rehabilitation personnel concerned and involved in political and funding issues (Dietl, 1986). Many RCE programs foresee declining state-federal job opportunities for graduates, and severe reductions in federal assistance for traineeships and program support from the Rehabilitation Services Administration.

There now appears to be considerable hesitancy by colleges and universities to support professional academic programs when job opportunities and external grant support are in question. This situation has been experienced by some RCE programs in colleges and/or universities through reduction of support for travel and professional development activities. In addition, a hiring freeze of faculty and other support positions has, in some cases, resulted in the restructuring of programs; for example, former departments are now programs within other larger academic units (Emener, 1985). Recent reductions in government expenditures for nearly all human services have affected every segment of the rehabilitation community; as a result, the continued existence of some RCE programs has been seriously threatened. In some cases, there has been no new funding from the Rehabilitation Services Administration for an RCE program when a grant project period for a program has ended.

The fear of reduced funding and its impact on student recruitment is a significant concern to many RCE programs. Declining student enrollment in some RCE programs has been primarily attributed to a reduction in student training monies (traineeships and guaranteed student loans), and the decrease in employment opportunities in public rehabilitation service programs (Rasch, Hollingsworth, Saxon, & Thomas, 1984). The long-term result of recruitment problems could be "a severe shortage of qualified rehabilitation counselors in the near future and a subsequent gradual deterioration in the quality of rehabilitation services by all segments in the rehabilitation field" (The Urban Institute, 1981, p. 47). For some programs, however, recruitment concerns are minimal since recent research studies have predicted a growing need for trained personnel in rehabilitation facilities and the private rehabilitation sector (McMahon, Matkin, Growick, Mahaffey, & Gianforte, 1983).

EMPLOYMENT TRENDS

The professional opportunities for rehabilitation counselors have broadened into a variety of new, nontraditional employment settings in recent years. Most notably, there has been a dramatic increase in employment opportunities for rehabilitation counselors in insurance and hospital rehabilitation programs, alcoholism, and related mental health settings, as well as in other positions in the private for-profit sector. However, job openings have declined in the state-federal rehabilitation system (The Urban Institute, 1981). Because this trend is expected to continue, RCE programs appear to be seriously examining the adequacy of graduate-level curricula to prepare graduates for these new arenas of employment.

Several studies that have explored the contemporary practice of rehabilitation counseling attest to the multiplicity of skills which counselors must possess. Selected role and function studies (Berven, 1979; Emener & Rubin, 1980; Rubin & Puckett, 1984; Rubin et al., 1984) have shown that counselors with diverse skills have numerous career opportunities. It has become increasingly apparent that counselors can apply such skills in many nontraditional settings such as mental health centers, alcohol and drug abuse centers, and rehabilitation programs in hospitals (Lynch & Herbert, 1984).

Anderson and Parente (1982), in attempting to forecast the future of rehabilitation counseling, asked counselors to make predictions concerning the profession; they found that counselors anticipated an increased growth in job opportunities, especially in the private sector. The employment potential of rehabilitation counselors seems limited only by their willingness to consider expanding opportunities in both the public and private work sectors.

Historically, the majority of graduates of RCE programs have gone to work in the field of rehabilitation. Research by Ugland, Coffey, & Menz (1985) on the employment obtained by graduates of accredited RCE programs revealed that 88.8% were employed in a direct service, rehabilitation setting, while 12.9% were working for state rehabilitation agencies. Over the last 6 years, the employment of these graduates in the private rehabilitation sector has increased from 6.1% to 29.2%. The Urban Institute study (1981) also clearly indicated that employment patterns for rehabilitation counselors are shifting. ''The state vocational rehabilitation agency no longer employs the majority of graduates of master's programs and is expected to continue to decline in importance through 1985. . . . [T]he strongest growth sectors are the private counseling firms and the rehabilitation facilities'' (The Urban Institute, 1981, p. 58).

In the 1980s, there is an emerging and mushrooming curricular emphasis that is more relevant to ''private sector'' employment opportunities for graduates. Sales (1979) suggested that the recent growth and projected increase in opportunities in the private rehabilitation counseling sector provides new challenges for rehabilitation educators in terms of preparing individuals to work effectively in the private arena.

Proposed curricula and training models to meet specific employment opportunities that have been developed merit careful consideration (Matkin, 1983). In terms of educational preparation, the potential rehabilitation counselor may need to supplement coursework from a variety of disciplines such as business, psychology, medicine, or personnel administration.

In some states, more RCE program graduates appear to be accepting positions in private rehabilitation rather than the state agency work setting. Since state agencies assumed a certain collective ownership of the RSA training grant program, RCE program graduates were simply expected to seek employment in a public rehabilitation setting (RSA, 1984). This expectation was never challenged until the private for-profit sector began to rapidly emerge in the 1970s. Manpower studies have shown that state rehabilitation agency needs have steadily decreased while private sector manpower needs have steadily increased (Gutowski, 1979; The Urban Institute, 1981). Because of this trend, continuing support of students in RCE programs is being questioned by the federal government, since increasing numbers of graduates do not obtain employment in the state-federal rehabilitation program. It appears that some RCE programs will have to decide whether to prepare graduates to meet the expectations of the federal rehabilitation grant program or to obtain employment for the ''broader'' profession of rehabilitation counseling (Luck & Rothrock, 1984). The key questions are: What is the intent of the federal Rehabilitation Act and its amendments, relative to the training of qualified rehabilitation counselors and other personnel? Are these trained professionals to work in only the public rehabilitation sector?

Recent changes in the workers' compensation laws and the passage of counselor licensure laws in many states have led to private practice opportunities for rehabilitation counselors. There are also increasing opportunities through private insurance carriers and corporations. Currently, both nonprofit agencies and for-profit private rehabilitation companies constitute a very significant market for rehabilitation counselors and related personnel. This market includes organizations working on behalf of persons who are blind, deaf, mentally retarded, head injured, or otherwise disabled (Ugland, Coffey, & Menz, 1985).

A potential problem for RCE programs in training a "new breed of rehabilitation counselor" is, on the one hand, that many RCE program faculty have not been able to obtain needed continuing education, or do not possess sufficient expertise in the relatively new content areas such as workers' compensation, legal aspects of disability, computer applications, head injury, and insurance rehabilitation. On the other hand, the expansion of employment opportunities into new employment markets that often offer better remuneration levels may be an advantage for program graduates. To address these issues, RCE faculties have begun working cooperatively with other rehabilitation education programs, such as rehabilitation continuing education programs, in-service training, and private rehabilitation companies, to share expertise. The challenges of expanding employment opportunities for graduates and revising curricula to meet the needs of the profession will ensure a more multifaceted growth for RCE programs. Utilizing approaches such as "networking" will facilitate the relevance, continuing strength, and success of RCE programs (Danek, Linkowski, Power, & Mitra, 1985).

CONCLUSIONS

With an extensive research and relevant literature base, developed primarily through an investment of several hundred thousand dollars from the federal government, RCE rests upon a sturdy foundation of specialized knowledge. Recognition of the importance and unique contribution of RCE to the profession is demonstrated by the fact that there are currently 77 universities that have accredited master's degree programs in rehabilitation counseling. A number of journals are devoted exclusively to rehabilitation literature, and together with many other periodicals, publish articles directly related to RCE.

As an academic discipline, RCE has developed a sound reputation. Graduates of RCE programs function as members of a psychosocial and health-related professional team providing a broad range of services for persons with disabilities. Primarily community based, the rehabilitation counselor works within and through a number of different agencies, to facilitate, provide, or coordinate needed services. RCE now has an "expanded identity," extending beyond the public rehabilitation agency as graduates provide services throughout the human services system to individuals with all types of disabilities.

To resolve or reduce the negative impact of the challenges and questions pointed out in this chapter will require interested individuals to listen to and work with each other to understand the implications of the situations, and to develop change strategies, alternative approaches, goals, and solutions. These challenges are not simple and unidimensional, and in many cases resolution may be currently unfeasible. Many issues are not unique to RCE; often the concerns reflect the frustrations of other organizations, agencies, and groups. No attempt is made here to address all the issues faced by RCE programs, simply because issues are frequently influenced by individual perspectives, opinions, legislation, program policy, and regional and academic environmental factors.

Seven suggestions are proposed by the authors that, if addressed by RCE program coordinators and federal RSA representatives, might lead to more qualified graduates for the profession, more comprehensive curricula, greater recognition of the importance and contributions of the rehabilitation counseling profession, and stronger, more viable RCE programs.

1. Review training curricula and mechanisms to deliver quality education to counselors, so that they can better meet the needs of the increasing number of rehabilitation clients from the private sector, and can respond more effectively to changing priorities in the public sector, such as transition services, independent living, and supported work.
2. Explore alternative ways of funding RCE students—solicit scholarship support from private rehabilitation companies; develop cooperative work-study programs; and offer flexible, quality programs that address the expanding work roles graduates select.
3. Pursue federal support for, and/or develop, procedures to enhance continuing education opportunities for rehabilitation counselor educators (some university faculty employed to provide academic training for pre-service students lack relevant, recent, field-based experience from either the public or private sectors in rehabilitation).
4. Continue to evaluate the importance of the processes of licensing and certification and the values of accreditation (students in RCE programs may need more opportunities to discuss the values of these processes as they relate to private practice and recognition of professional competence and training).
5. Efforts to promote and publicize RCE and the expanding roles of RCE programs and counselors should be developed; assessment of how to influence nationally recognized publications that define rehabilitation counseling, such as the *Occupational Outlook Handbook,* should be encouraged.
6. Support efforts are needed to bring about closer coordination between existing rehabilitation information systems and national and regional pro-

jects to disseminate information, including findings of national research and demonstration studies. This might bring about improved materials utilization by practitioners in the field, including the effective use and application of computer technology in teaching and service delivery.
7. Rather than concentrating upon the deficits and limitations of persons with disabilities, program faculties may need to underscore the external, socioeconomic aspects of discrimination, such as Social Security disability benefits, attitudinal and environmental barriers, and transportation and housing issues, and the impact these have on the individual's capacities.

Accepting the challenge of self-analysis is an ongoing process to which faculty of RCE programs must continue to respond. As the value and need for master's-level RCE training programs and counselors have received considerable scrutiny in recent years, national accreditation data appear to support the contention that programs are comprehensive, and meet the educational needs of graduates.

A cursory review of research and journal articles indicates that perhaps more change and responsiveness to issues is occurring than some realize or want to believe. The real challenge for RCE is to develop more effective ways of communicating the issues being addressed and the changes being implemented as a result of self-study and internal review; faculty of RCE programs must more clearly articulate to appropriate individuals and groups the curricula changes and emphases that have been implemented in response to the issues.

Even though the academic structures supporting RCE programs are complex and diverse, and other human services program curricula appear to encroach on traditional RCE coursework, the overall health of RCE is excellent. With continued cooperative efforts by groups interested in the preparation of qualified personnel for direct rehabilitation counseling services work, RCE will grow and change to meet the expanding needs of the marketplace.

RCE is unique, dynamic, and holistic; it is a strong independent professional education program. Even though some rehabilitation educators and preservice education critics believe the rehabilitation counseling profession is characterized by dependence on the federal government, lethargy, and insecurity, RCE programs are striving to be responsive and relevant. The reactions of RCE program faculty and concerned practitioners will, in large measure, determine the future emphases and directions of master's-level RCE programs. Several studies refute a pessimistic future for the profession (Anderson & Parente, 1982; Bowe, 1984; Burkhead & Sampson, 1985; Danek, Linkowski, Power, & Mitra, 1985; Dickman & Emener, 1982; Engram, 1981; Goodwin, 1986; Hershenson, 1982; McCollum & Chan, 1985; Szymanski, 1985). Joint efforts among the major rehabilitation counseling associations and existing training programs suggest that a concerted effort is being made to address realistically a number of the concerns presented in this chapter.

Rather than becoming an "endangered species," RCE may be experiencing an "awakening" of the sort that comes from positive self-examination. Resolution of the issues and challenges discussed here is not the sole responsibility of RCE programs. The rehabilitation field, in general, is acknowledging its role and accepting the challenges for the overall development of the rehabilitation counseling profession and the preparation of those who seek to enter it.

REFERENCES

Anderson, J. K., & Parente, F. R. (1982). Rehabilitation counselors forecast their future. *Journal of Rehabilitation, 48*(1), 36–42.

Berkowitz, E. D. (1979). The American disability system in historical perspective. In E. D. Berkowitz (Ed.), *Disability policies and government programs* (pp. 78–80). New York: Praeger.

Berven, N. L. (1979). The roles and functions of the rehabilitation counselor revisited. *Rehabilitation Counseling Bulletin, 23,* 84–88.

Bowe, F. (1984). *Employment trends: 1984 and beyond.* Hot Springs: University of Arkansas Rehabilitation Research and Training Center.

Bowe, F. (1985). Future trends and the implications for policy and employment of disabled persons. In R. V. Habeck, D. E. Galvin, W. D. Frey, L. M. Chadderdon, & D. G. Tate (Eds.), *Economics and equity in employment of people with disabilities* (pp. 197–202). East Lansing, MI: University Center for International Rehabilitation.

Brinkman, P., Rabinowitz, V., Karuza, J., Coates, D., Cohen, E., & Kidder, L. (1982). Models of helping and coping. *American Psychologist, 37*(4), 368–384.

Brubaker, D. (1981). Professional status of rehabilitation counseling. In R. M. Parker & C. E. Hansen (Eds.), *Rehabilitation counseling* (pp. 37–58). Boston: Allyn & Bacon.

Burkhead, E. J., & Sampson, J. P. (1985). Computer-assisted assessment in support of the rehabilitation process. *Rehabilitation Counseling Bulletin, 28,* 262–274.

Commission on Rehabilitation Counselor Certification. (1985). *Guide to rehabilitation counselor certification.* Arlington Heights, IL: Author.

Council on Rehabilitation Education, Inc. (1983). *Accreditation manual for rehabilitation counselor education programs.* Chicago: Author.

Danek, M. M., Linkowski, D. C., Power, P., & Mitra, S. (1985). Networking among rehabilitation education programs. *Journal of Rehabilitation, 51*(4), 51–53.

Dickman, F., & Emener, W. G. (1982). Employee assistance programs: An emerging vista for rehabilitation counseling. *Journal of Applied Rehabilitation Counseling, 13*(3), 18–20.

Dietl, D. (1986). Two decades later—C. Esco Obermann: History is on his side. *Journal of Rehabilitation, 52*(1), 10–15.

Emener, W. G. (1985). Rehabilitation counselor education: A state of the art perspective. In E. L. Pan, S. S. Newman, T. E. Backer, & C. L. Vash (Eds.), *Annual review of rehabilitation* (Vol. IV, pp. 55–82). New York: Springer-Verlag.

Emener, W. G., & Rubin, S. E. (1980). Rehabilitation counselor roles and functions and sources of role strain. *Journal of Applied Rehabilitation Counseling, 11*(2), 57–69.

Engram, B. E. (1981). Communication skills training for rehabilitation counselors working with older persons. *Journal of Rehabilitation, 47*(4), 51–56.

Farkas, J., & Anthony, W. A. (1980). Training rehabilitation counselors to work in state agencies, rehabilitation and mental health facilities. *Rehabilitation Counseling Bulletin, 24,* 128–143.

Feinberg, L. B., & McFarlane, F. R. (1979). Setting-based factors in rehabilitation counselor role variability. *Journal of Allied Rehabilitation Counseling, 10*(3), 95–101.

Field, T. F. (1981). The consolidation of the professional rehabilitation associations: Pros and cons. *Journal of Applied Rehabilitation Counseling, 12*(2), 65–68.

Finnerty-Fried, P. (1985). Adapting rehabilitation counseling for older persons. *Rehabilitation Counseling Bulletin, 29,* 135–142.

Fraser, R., & Clowers, M. (1978). Rehabilitation counselor functions: Perceptions of time spent and complexity. *Journal of Applied Rehabilitation Counseling, 9*(2), 31–35.

Geist, G. O., & Emener, W. G. (1981). Rehabilitation counseling and rehabilitation counselor education: Implications for social work and social work education. In J. A. Browne, B. A. Kivlin, & S. Watt (Eds.), *Rehabilitation services and the social work role: Challenge for change* (pp. 125–128). Baltimore: Williams & Wilkins.

Goodwin, L. R., Jr. (1986). Marketing rehabilitation counselor education programs. *Journal of Applied Rehabilitation Counseling, 17*(4), 42–47.

Graves, W. (1979). The impact of federal legislation for handicapped people on the rehabilitation counselor. *Journal of Applied Rehabilitation Counseling, 10*(2), 67–71.

Gutowski, M. (1979). *Rehabilitation in the private sector: Changing the structure of the rehabilitation industry.* Washington, DC: The Urban Institute.

Hahn, H. (1985). Changing perception of disability and the future of rehabilitation. In L. G. Perlman & G. F. Austin (Eds.), *Social influences in rehabilitation planning: Blueprint for the 21st century* (pp. 53–64). Alexandria, VA: National Rehabilitation Association Press.

Hershenson, D. B. (1982). Rehabilitation counseling is a profession. *Rehabilitation Counseling Bulletin, 25,* 251–253.

Kuehn, M. D. (1984). *Manpower studies in rehabilitation.* Unpublished manuscript.

Livingston, R. (1979). The history of rehabilitation counselor certification. *Journal of Applied Rehabilitation Counseling, 10*(3), 111–118.

Luck, R. S., & Rothrock, J. A. (1984). The education and training of rehabilitation counselors. In D. K. Hollingsworth, W. G. Emener, & A. Patrick (Eds.), *Critical issues in rehabilitation counseling* (pp. 85–108). Springfield, IL: Charles C Thomas.

Lynch, R. K. (1984). Certified insurance rehabilitation specialist (CIRS): A certification for just about anyone. *ARCA-NRCA Newsletter, 25,* 4–5.

Lynch, R. K., & Herbert, J. T. (1984). Employment trends for rehabilitation counselors. *Journal of Applied Rehabilitation Counseling, 15*(3), 43–46.

Lynch, R. K., & McSweeney, K. (1981). The professional status of rehabilitation counseling in state/federal vocational rehabilitation agencies. *Journal of Applied Rehabilitation Counseling, 12*(4), 186–190.

Matkin, R. E. (1983). The roles and functions of rehabilitation specialists in the private sector. *Journal of Applied Rehabilitation Counseling, 14*(1), 14–27.

McAlees, D. C., & Schumacher, B. (1975). Toward a new professionalism: Certification and accreditation. *Rehabilitation Counseling Bulletin, 18,* 160–165.

McCollum, P. S., & Chan, F. (1985). Rehabilitation in the information age: Prologue to the future. *Rehabilitation Counseling Bulletin, 28*(4), 211–218.

McMahon, B. T., Matkin, R. E., Growick, B., Mahaffey, D., & Gianforte, G. (1983). Recent trends in private sector rehabilitation. *Rehabilitation Counseling Bulletin, 27,* 32–47.

Muthard, J. E., & Salomone, P. R. (1969). Roles and functions of the rehabilitation counselor. *Rehabilitation Counseling Bulletin, 13,* 81–168.

National Council on the Handicapped. (1986). *Toward independence: An assessment of federal laws and programs affecting persons with disabilities—With legislative recommendations* (GPO Stock No. 052-003-01022-4). Washington, DC: U.S. Government Printing Office.

National Rehabilitation Counseling Association. (1985). *Critical Issues Symposium.* Worcester, MA: Author.

Parker, R. M., & Hansen, C. E. (1981). *Rehabilitation counseling.* Boston: Allyn & Bacon.

Patterson, C. H. (1967). Specialization in rehabilitation counseling. *Rehabilitation Counseling Bulletin, 10,* 147–154.

Rasch, J. D. (1979). The case for an independent association of rehabilitation counselors. *Journal of Applied Rehabilitation Counseling, 10*(4), 171–176.

Rasch, J. D., Hollingsworth, D. K., Saxon, J. P., & Thomas, K. R. (1984). Student recruitment issues in the 1980's. *Rehabilitation Counseling Bulletin, 28,* 46–49.

Rehabilitation Services Administration. (1984). *RSA National Task Force on Training* [Final report, March 21, 1984]. Washington, DC: Author.

Roth, W. (1985). The politics of disability: Future trends as shaped by current realities. In L. G. Perlman & G. F. Austin (Eds.), *Social influences in rehabilitation planning: Blueprint for the 21st century* (pp. 41–48). Alexandria, VA: National Rehabilitation Association Press.

Rubin, S. E., & Emener, W. G. (1979). Recent rehabilitation counselor role changes and role strain—A pilot investigation. *Journal of Applied Rehabilitation Counseling. 10*(3), 142–147.

Rubin, S. E., Matkin, R. E., Ashley, J., Beardsley, M. M., May, V. R., Onstott, K., & Puckett, F. D. (1984). Roles and functions of certified rehabilitation counselors. *Rehabilitation Counseling Bulletin, 27,* 199–224.

Rubin, S. E., & Puckett, F. D. (1984). The changing role and function of the rehabilitation counselor. *Rehabilitation Counseling Bulletin, 27,* 225–231.

Rubin, S. E., & Roessler, R. T. (1983). *Foundations of the vocational rehabilitation process* (2nd. ed.). Baltimore: University Park Press.

Sales, A. (1979). Rehabilitation counseling in the private sector: Implications for graduate education. *Journal of Rehabilitation, 45*(3), 59–61.

Scalia, V. A., & Wolfe, R. R. (1984). Rehabilitation counselor education. *Journal of Applied Rehabilitation Counseling, 15*(3), 34–37.

Smits, S. J., & Ledbetter, J. G. (1979). The practice of rehabilitation counseling within the administrative structure of the state-federal program. *Journal of Applied Rehabilitation Counseling, 10*(2), 78–84.

Szymanski, E. M. (1985). Rehabilitation counseling: A profession with a vision, an identity, and a future. *Rehabilitation Counseling Bulletin, 29,* 2–5.

The Urban Institute. (1980). *Forecasting manpower requirements in the rehabilitation industry.* Washington, DC: Author.

The Urban Institute. (1981). *Changing patterns in manpower.* Washington, DC: Author.

Thomas, K. R. (1982). A critique of trends in rehabilitation counselor education toward specialization. *Journal of Rehabilitation, 48*(1), 49–51.

Thomas, K. R. (1985). Rehabilitation services, training and research: A political analysis. *Journal of Rehabilitation, 51*(4), 17–21.

Ugland, D., Coffey, D., & Menz, F. (1985, May 10). *National Council on Rehabilitation Education (NCRE) graduate follow-up report 1978 through 1984*. Unpublished manuscript.

U.S. Commission on Civil Rights. (1983). *Accommodating the spectrum of individual abilities*. Washington, DC: Author

U.S. Department of Education, Consumer/Parent Committee on Rehabilitation Issues. (1985). *Issues and recommendations for rehabilitation counselor training*. Washington, DC: Author.

Whitehouse, F. A. (1975). The rehabilitation clinician: An emerging role. *Journal of Rehabilitation, 41*(3), 24–26.

Wright, G. N. (1980). *Total rehabilitation*. Boston: Little, Brown.

Wright, G. N. (1982). Contemporary rehabilitation counselor education. *Rehabilitation Counseling Bulletin, 25*, 254–256.

Wright, G. N. (1984). Professional perspectives and planning. *Journal of Applied Rehabilitation Counseling, 15*(3), 5–7.

16

Preparing Rehabilitation Counselors to Deal with Ethical Dilemmas

A Major Challenge for Rehabilitation Education

Stanford E. Rubin, Jorge Garcia, Richard Millard, and Henry Wong

THE FINDINGS OF recent surveys of both rehabilitation counselor educators (Emener & Rasch, 1984) and graduates of rehabilitation education programs (Janes & Emener, 1983) regarding rehabilitation education curricula suggest that both groups would prefer more attention placed in rehabilitation education on ethical issues. The results of two recent studies (Emener & Wright, 1986; Pape & Klein, 1986) suggest that such training is definitely needed for practicing rehabilitation counselors.

While sufficient instructional materials exist for training rehabilitation counselors for the technical aspects of service delivery, there is an absence of rehabilitation education materials available for preparing them to deal with ethical issues. This resource void has probably contributed to the current limited focus on ethical issues in master's-, doctoral-, and continuing rehabilitation education curricula.

Junior authorship of this chapter is shared equally by Jorge Garcia, Richard Millard, and Henry Wong.

This chapter provides a discussion of the conflicts between the recent legislative mandate for full integration of individuals with disabilities, and coexisting policy and attitudinal barriers to its full-fledged implementation in our society (e.g., limited resources, policy containing counterincentives, negative stereotypes, and paternalistic attitudes). These conflicts are seen as sources of ethical dilemma for those rehabilitation professionals who assume responsibility for the full integration of individuals with disabilities into the mainstream of American life. The chapter also discusses the need for ethics education for rehabilitation professionals, and reviews the instructional methods utilized by other helping professions to prepare their members to deal with ethical dilemmas.

THE MANDATE

Over the last 2 decades, a major civil rights movement of consumers with disabilities has emerged. The members of that movement have fought for the right of full integration into the mainstream of American society. Their activity has led to the manifestation of a "full integration" public policy mandate through the passage of three significant pieces of original legislation—the Rehabilitation Act of 1973, the Education for All Handicapped Children Act of 1975, and the Developmental Disabilities Assistance and Bill of Rights Act of 1975—and their subsequent amendments.

The Rehabilitation Act of 1973 (PL 93-112) and its amendments have directed attention toward addressing the rehabilitation needs of individuals with severe disabilities. Attention is placed on expanding the services available to disabled persons whose rehabilitation problems are considered very difficult to overcome (Jenkins, 1981, p. 22). Title V of that act addresses disability rights via nondiscrimination, affirmative action, and environmental accessibility mandates (Rubin & Roessler, 1987). Referred to as the "bill of rights" for disabled persons, its provisions are directed at promoting the full integration of disabled persons into the mainstream of American life. Stimulated by Section 504, which prohibits discrimination on the basis of disability, additional legislation has been subsequently passed that mandates the end of discrimination against disabled persons in education, employment, transportation, and housing by any recipient of federal funds.

When the Education for All Handicapped Children Act (PL 94-142), passed by Congress in 1975, is paired with the Rehabilitation Act of 1973, the federal mandate for the full integration of disabled persons into the mainstream of American society becomes even more evident. Many of the specific mandates concerning the rights of children with disabilities to a free and appropriate elementary and secondary education found in PL 94-142 are closely related to the provisions of Section 504 in regard to right to access and integration.

The Developmental Disabilities Assistance and Bill of Rights Act (PL 94-103) of 1975 and the Developmental Disabilities Act of 1984 (PL 98-527) were directed toward improving the care and increasing the training opportunities for individuals with developmental disabilities. These acts mandate that the states implement plans to assure that individuals with developmental disabilities obtain the necessary services, treatment, and care to allow them to attain their maximum potential. The overall purpose of this legislation is to enable individuals with disabilities to become more independent, productive, and fully integrated into the life of the community.

Support for the "full integration" mandate regarding equal accessibility to transportation can be found in legislation dating back to 1964 (Urban Mass Transportation Act of 1964). A 1970 amendment (Urban Mass Transportation Assistance Act of 1970, Section 16) to the 1964 act mandates equal access for disabled persons to mass transit facilities and services. The latest federal regulations (*Federal Register,* May, 1986, Vol. 51, p. 18994) regarding that mandate allow urban mass transit systems that are recipients of U.S. Department of Transportation financial assistance to meet the accessibility obligations by providing any of the following: a special service (such as dial-a-ride or taxi voucher), a bus system (on-call or regular scheduling), or a combination of an accessible bus system and a special service (Rubin & Roessler, 1987).

The "full integration" mandate has also been reflected in legislation at the state level. For example, state support for the removal of environmental barriers can be found in the Maine Human Rights Act of 1985 and the Illinois Human Rights Act of 1983. Illinois legislation that became law on July 1, 1986 (HB 1953), allows disabled individuals access to gasoline at self-service prices at full-service pumps (Illinois Department of Rehabilitation Services, 1986). This legislation enabling equal access to gasoline at the self-service price may appear insignificant when the savings only amount to 4¢ per gallon. However, access to affordable transportation in a culture dependent on the ability to be mobile is vital to all people.

Litigation outcomes have also provided support for the "full mandate." The case of *Wyatt v. Stickney* in 1972 supported the right of people with disabilities to live in the least restrictive environment. When local communities have opposed the integration of disabled people into community life, the courts have responded in support of the mandate (*City of Cleburne v. Cleburne Living Center,* 1985; *City of White Plains v. Ferraioli,* 1974; *Fitchburg Housing Authority v. Board of Zoning Appeals of Fitchburg,* 1980). In the case of *Halderman v. Pennhurst State School and Hospital* (1977), the court, basing its opinion on Section 504 of the Rehabilitation Act of 1973 and the 14th Amendment's equal protection clause, decreed that the developmentally disabled residents of the institution were to be relocated in small, community-living residential units with supportive community-based services provided (Laski, 1980).

Compatible with the spirit of the mandate is the position recently taken on the provision of health care by the President's Commission for the Study of Ethical Problems and Biomedical and Behavioral Research (1983):

> 1) that society has an ethical obligation to ensure equitable access to health care for all . . . , 2) equitable access. . . requires that all citizens be able to secure an adequate level of care without excessive burdens. . . 3) the ultimate responsibility for ensuring that society's obligation is met. . . rests with the Federal Government. . . 4) the cost of achieving equitable access to health care ought to be shared fairly, and 5) efforts to contain rising health costs are important but should not focus on limiting the attainment of equitable access for the least well served portion of the public. (pp. 3–4)

BARRIERS TO ACHIEVING THE GOALS OF THE MANDATE

Although public policy supports the full participation of disabled persons as active and productive members of society, there are barriers to achieving the goals of that policy. While some of the barriers to full participation are economic, others are attitudinal in nature (Dembo, 1982; Hahn, 1985).

Prejudice and discrimination fostered by negative attitudes toward disabled people in our society, often manifested in paternalistic public policies and models of service delivery, remain a major problem to be confronted and overcome on the road to achieving the goals of the "full integration" mandate. It is slowly being realized that the physical impairment is less handicapping than the barriers of stereotypical attitudes, environmental constraints, and paternalistic public policies (Hahn, 1982; Scotch, 1984).

Attitudinal factors have contributed to the manifestation of contradictions in the public policy that prevent the large scale achievement of the goals of the mandate. For example, there is a large difference between the amount of public funding allocated for paternalistic income support programs (e.g., workers' compensation, SSDI), and those allocated to promote economic self-sufficiency (e.g., those authorized by the Rehabilitation Acts, and The Education for All Handicapped Children Act) (Erlanger & Roth, 1985), with funding tending to favor the former. This imbalance suggests that disabled persons are paternalistically viewed as constituting a population of "deserving poor" with little capacity for self-support and independence (Erlanger & Roth, 1985; Hahn, 1982; Scotch, 1984).

The coexistence of income support/medical benefits and rehabilitation-oriented programs is clearly necessary. Income, medical, and social service programs, like rehabilitation programs, should always be available to severely disabled persons in need. However, when they are based on incompatible philosophies and attitudes (e.g., the existing disability income support system assumes that workers who become disabled cannot or should not work), as well as insufficiently integrated into the disability services system, they play havoc with each other. This is most clearly the case where income support/medical benefits program policies provide disabled persons with a clear disincentive for achieving vocational rehabilitation.

Several solutions to the disincentive problem have been suggested (Berkowitz, 1982; Berkowitz & Berkowitz, 1985). They are based on creating greater internal compatibility within the income support/health benefit/rehabilitation system, in order to provide economic encouragement to persons with disabilities for achieving vocational rehabilitation (Berkowitz, 1982).

An attempt to remove these disincentives can be found in the Employment Opportunities for Disabled Americans Act (PL 99-643) passed in 1986. This act amended Title XVI (Supplemental Security Income for the Aged, Blind and Disabled) of the Social Security Act. Section 1619a of PL 99-643 permits SSI recipients to continue receiving SSI payments when earned income is above the substantial gainful activity (SGA) level (i.e., approximately $300 per month) but below the "spend down" point. The "spend down" point is the point at which earnings reduce an SSI payment to zero dollars (Gorski, 1986). Gorski (1985) provides an example of this process: When a person's income exceeds the SGA of $300 per month, the amount of SSI payments are reduced incrementally as his or her earnings increase. When the person's earnings reach $735 per month, the federal SSI payment of $325 per month is reduced to zero dollars. However, in some states cash benefits may continue even when the person's monthly income exceeds $735, due to allowable deductions (e.g., medically related expenses) and/or state SSI contributions. Although Medicaid eligibility rules vary by state, individuals with disabilities are generally eligible for these benefits as long as they are receiving SSI benefits (Gorski, 1985).

Section 1619b permits continued eligibility for Medicaid when earned income exceeds the "spend down" point, until a person's earnings rise above a certain "threshold" (approximately $12,000 a year). Even when this threshold is passed, the person can continue receiving Medicaid if unable to obtain adequate health coverage from other sources (e.g., denial of medical coverage by private insurance carriers based on a preexisting condition or type of disability) and Medicaid coverage is needed to continue working. While the true effect of this legislation on the counterincentive problem has yet to be determined, it provides a logical attack on the problem (Gorski, 1986).

The attitudes of rehabilitation counselors have been seen as another barrier to achieving the goals of the mandate. Although the professional community expresses the goal of helping disabled persons become active and productive members of society, these professionals have themselves been seen by some disabled consumers as being part of the barrier to their full integration into the mainstream of American society (DeJong, 1979). This consumer perception of the rehabilitation counselor as a "barrier" may stem from observations of conflicting/inconsistent counselor service delivery decisions that could well be the result of attempts to operate within a system governed by an incoherent disability policy. For example, since access to most of the income support, social service, and medical benefits might be lost if the person returns to work (Berkowitz, 1982), rehabilitation counselors are frequently confronted in the case management process by the opposing needs of client economic well-being versus vocational rehabilitation. Inconsistent rehabilitation decisions might also result from a counselor's professional education causing a questioning of the validity of society's expectations for disabled persons, while not sufficiently changing their own attitudes toward disabled persons. This possibility is reflected in claims made by Rubenfeld (Chapter 2, this volume) and Nosek (Chapter 3, this volume). They generally perceive health, social service, and rehabilitation professionals (physicians, nurses, social workers, rehabilitation counselors) as underestimating the ability of disabled individuals to work and live independently.

The economic and attitudinal inconsistencies embodied in a public policy on disability containing both a "full integration" mandate and barriers to its achievement generate conditions for the emergence of many ethical dilemmas faced by the rehabilitation counselors when providing direct services to disabled persons. Rehabilitation counselors must be sensitive to both the presence and source of ethical dilemmas confronted in the service delivery process, and must also become proficient in dealing with these dilemmas. Some examples help illustrate the confusion faced by the rehabilitation practitioner when attempting to provide services according to the mandate:

1. What is meant by "acting in the best interest of the client"?
2. What is meant by "loyalty to all parties involved in the rehabilitation process," and how can the needs of all the parties involved be equitably addressed?
3. How much discretionary behavior does the rehabilitation professional have while still complying with existing disability policies and laws?
4. When is paternalistic behavior appropriate?
5. When should the validity of the estimates of what the person with a disability can do be questioned?

These questions tend to arise when ethical dilemmas are confronted in the service delivery process. While they often lack absolute answers, the rehabilitation counselor's ability to address them is greatly dependent on her or his level of ethical decision-making skills. Rehabilitation counselors who have the ability to apply ethical reasoning to assess the value of incompatible service delivery decision options will be more likely to serve severely disabled persons in a consistently ethical manner.

NEEDED: MORE EMPHASIS ON ETHICS EDUCATION

Rehabilitation education programs currently introduce their students to the content of ethical codes. In this process, students are told to be honest, keep confidences, be faithful to colleagues, do no harm, and respect clients' dignity (Purtilo, 1983, p. 215). While these are proper moral norms, such brief didactic instruction does not prepare the student for the ethical decision making necessary in a challenging situation in the future, when to act according to one moral principle (e.g., beneficence) compromises another (e.g., justice) (Purtilo, 1983, p. 215). Knowing the code of ethics and knowing how to respond to situations containing ethical dilemmas (i.e., situations where a choice must be made between two alternative actions without the ability to discern clearly the superiority of the rationale for the chosen alternative *a priori* [Harding, 1985]) are not necessarily the same (Pape & Klein, 1986). This curriculum deficit has typically been justified on the basis that the extensive need for technique training and general professional information leaves little room in the curriculum for a formal course on ethics (Handelsman, 1986a; Veatch & Sollito, 1976). Handelsman (1986b) has questioned the ethical soundness of this justification by asking, ''Is it ethical to train people to do a variety of skills without training them to perform those skills in an ethical manner?'' (p. 371).

Rest (1982, 1983, 1984) has argued that ethics education should sensitize students to ethical issues by helping them to: 1) become sensitive to needs of others and the consequences of their actions on the lives of other people, 2) develop a sensitivity to ethical principles that stimulate the taking of an appropriate action, and 3) increase their understanding of the consequences of not acting on ethical principles. Five ethical principles are frequently cited as considerations in the reasoning process for resolving ethical dilemmas (Beauchamp & Childress, 1983; Kitchener, 1984). These are: 1) autonomy (the right to make one's decisions and the need to respect others' rights to make free choices); 2) nonmaleficence (not engaging in any intentional harm or in actions that have a high risk of harm); 3) beneficence (engaging in actions that benefit others); 4) justice (treating others impartially and equally); and 5) fidelity (being faithful, keeping promises, being loyal).

Rehabilitation counselors develop relationships with: ''1) the client, 2) the client's family, 3) the client's employer or supervisor, 4) fellow counselors, 5) colleagues in other professions, 6) their own employer or supervisor, 7) the community, [and] 8) other programs, agencies, and institutions''

(Matkin & May, 1981, p. 15). Such a diversity of relationships creates an arena for competing interests among parties that can result in ethical dilemmas.

An example of such an ethical dilemma follows: A 45-year-old woman with a prior back injury has been referred to a rehabilitation counselor by a private insurance carrier. She is motivated to return to work and has chosen to return to a job which is quite different from her prior work and will require placement with a different employer. She does not wish to return to a different job with her former employer. The insurance carrier who referred the case to the rehabilitation counselor and who is covering all rehabilitation costs has recommended several different jobs with the client's former employer. The rehabilitation counselor considers the jobs recommended by the insurance carrier to be inappropriate given the functional limitations of the client. The rehabilitation counselor wants to recommend long-term training for the client, which will cost the insurance carrier more than their proposed plan. The insurance carrier is pressuring the rehabilitation counselor to close the case as early as possible and his supervisor is in agreement with the insurance carrier.

How would the rehabilitation counselor resolve this ethical dilemma where ethical principles such as beneficence, fidelity, and autonomy appear to be involved? Typically, rehabilitation education programs prepare students to address ethical dilemmas by introducing them to the canons, rules, and guidelines found in relevant professional codes of ethics. However, dilemmas such as the one described above would probably require solutions that go beyond the scope of the typical professional code of ethics. The validity of this supposition is somewhat supported by results of recent surveys. In a recent national survey of a random sample of the American Rehabilitation Counseling Association (ARCA) and National Rehabilitation Counseling Association (NRCA) members, Pape and Klein (1986) found that while many respondents had been confronted by ethical dilemmas in their professional practice, over 70% of the respondents indicated never referring to a code of ethics for guidance in resolving such dilemmas. In a subsequent national survey of a random sample of ARCA and NRCA members, Emener and Wright (1986) found similar results. Their findings suggest that when faced with an ethically complex situation, rehabilitation counselors respond at least 75% of the time without consulting a code of ethics.

NEEDED: GUIDANCE ON HOW TO TEACH ETHICS

While sufficient education materials exist for training rehabilitation professionals for the technical aspects of service delivery, there is an absence of rehabilitation education materials available for preparing students to deal with ethical issues. This resource void has probably played a role in restricting both the extent and quality of the current focus on ethical issues in master's-level, doctoral-level, and in-service rehabilitation education curricula. Guidance for filling this void can be obtained from descriptions of ethics education curricula from the literature of other professional disciplines (Purtilo, 1983). A partial review of the contents of that literature follows.

Among ethics education courses designed for professional school curricula, common goals are to help students develop the analytical thinking, problem-solving, and decision-making skills necessary for dealing with ethical dilemmas (Francouer, 1983). These courses typically attempt to increase student: 1) sensitivity to ethical issues, 2) ''ability to reason about ethical issues,'' and 3) tolerance for ambiguity in the ethical decision-making process (Kitchener, 1986, p. 307).

A number of descriptions of ethics education courses in medical and allied health education curriculums have been reported in the literature (Bicknell, 1985; Boyd, Currie, Thompson, & Tierney, 1978; DeWachter, 1978; Fentem, 1985; Law, 1985; Shotter, 1985; Smith, 1985; Welbourn, 1985). Such ethics courses typically utilize a combination of lecture and group discussion formats through which ethical theory and principles are applied to actual dilemmas experienced by physicians in clinical practice.

A relatively typical general structure for an introductory course has been described by Francouer (1983) as containing four levels. At the first level, students are introduced to basic deontological and utilitarian theories of ethics. To help students understand the tenets of these theories, they are presented a case study and asked to identify the predominant ethical issue, propose a solution, and argue in support of that solution from either a deontological or utilitarian position. This approach enables the student to view the ethical issue and related principles from both perspectives. The second level focuses on ethical principles (e.g., autonomy, beneficence, nonmaleficence, fidelity, and justice). These principles are reviewed through an analysis of patient rights and responsibilities. In addition, ethical codes are reviewed regarding their relationship to these ethical principles. The third level addresses ethical rules. At this level, students create a set of ethical guidelines or a code for their profession. Students then move to the fourth level, where they apply problem-solving methods and decision-making techniques to a variety of ethically laden case studies drawn from their profession. The structure of Francouer's course is compatible with recommendations found in the literature by the Hastings Center. The Hastings Center (1980) recommends a balance between case study material and an introduction to ethics theory for ethics instruction in professional schools.

Tymchuk (1982) has also suggested that courses on ethics for human services professionals draw upon vignettes that portray ethical dilemmas. Utilizing those vignettes, students would go through the following seven-step process for making ethical decisions:

Step 1. Describe the parameters of the situation.
Step 2. Describe the potential issues involved.
Step 3. Describe the guidelines already available that might affect each issue (e.g., values, laws, codes, practice, research).
Step 4. Enumerate the alternative decisions for each issue.
Step 5. Enumerate the short term, ongoing, and long term consequences for each alternative.
Step 6. Present evidence (or lack thereof) for those consequences as well as the probability of their occurrence.
Step 7. Rank order and vote on the decision. (Tymchuk, 1982, p. 170)

Tymchuk (1982) has used this simulated model as part of "a formal graduate course for students in psychology, education, and medicine to train them to make ethical decisions" (p. 173). It appears to be highly compatible with the fourth step in the model described by Francouer (1983).

While the best method for teaching ethics to helping professionals has yet to be empirically determined, the references cited have expressed convergent opinions on ethics education. It is generally agreed that while educators may convey and discuss ethical principles and issues in their daily interaction with students in professional training programs, such an "osmosis" approach is insufficient. Students must be systematically taught, through formal training, the use of ethical reasoning to resolve ethical dilemmas (Bicknell, 1985).

The validity of the systematic ethics education position has been supported by several studies demonstrating that ethics training increases students' sensitivity to ethical issues. For example, Baldick (1980) found that clinical and counseling psychology interns who had completed a formal ethics training program are more able to discriminate ethical considerations in an ethical discrimination inventory than those who had not. Morrison and Teta (1979) report that graduate students enrolled in a humanistic psychology course have higher scores on an ethical conflict questionnaire at posttraining and 3-month follow-up than prior to training, indicating that students recognized more of the ethical conflict situations covered by the questionnaire after taking the course.

CONCLUSION

For the past 20 years, individuals with disabilities have fought for inclusion as equal participants in society. One result of the efforts of this emerging disability rights movement is a federal legislative and judicial mandate for the full integration of individuals with disabilities into the mainstream of American life. Coexisting with this mandate are attitudinal barriers, economic constraints, overt paternalism, and a public policy containing counterincentives that impede the full integration of people with disabilities.

Rehabilitation counselors as professionals assume a responsibility to carry out the mandate, assisting individuals with disabilities to achieve full integration. However, conflicts created by the coexistence of the mandate and by numerous barriers result in ethical dilemmas faced by those attempting to meet this responsibility. Ethical codes alone appear to provide insufficient guidance for rehabilitation counselors confronted by ethical dilemmas. It is open to question whether current rehabilitation education programs are emphasizing more than the appropriate code of ethics in their instructional process for preparing rehabilitation counselors to deal with ethically laden situations.

This chapter recommends that rehabilitation education curricula should contain a formal course that includes not only an introduction to ethics theory, ethical principles, and professional codes, but also practice in applied problem-solving and decision-making techniques. The literature suggests that such courses should utilize case studies depicting ethical dilemmas, and ask students to identify the ethical dilemmas and to suggest solutions. With such training, rehabilitation counselors should be at least minimally prepared to deal with ethical dilemmas.

REFERENCES

Baldick, T. (1980). Teaching discrimination ability of intern psychologists: A function of training in ethics. *Professional Psychology, 11,* 276–282.

Beauchamp, T. L., & Childress, J. F. (1983). *Principles of biomedical ethics* (2nd ed.). New York: Oxford University.

Berkowitz, M. (1982). Disincentives and the rehabilitation of disabled persons. In E. L. Pan, T. E. Backer, & C. L. Vash (Eds.), *Annual review of rehabilitation* (pp. 40–57). New York: Springer-Verlag.

Berkowitz, M., & Berkowitz, E. (1985). Widening the field: Economics and history in the study of disability. *American Behavioral Scientist, 28,* 405–417.

Bicknell, D. J. (1985). Current arrangements for teaching medical ethics to undergraduate medical students. *Journal of Medical Ethics, 11,* 25–26.

Boyd, K., Currie, C., Thompson, I., & Tierney, A. (1978). Teaching medical ethics. *Journal of Medical Ethics, 4,* 141–145.

City of Cleburne v. Cleburne Living Center, 105 S.C. 3249, 53, U.S.L.W. 5022 (1985).

City of White Plains v. Ferraioli, 34 N.Y. 2d 71, A.L.R.R. 3d 687 (1974).

DeJong, G. (1979). Independent living: from social movement to analytic paradigm. *Archives of Physical Medicine and Rehabilitation, 60,* 435–446.

Dembo, T. (1982). Some problems in rehabilitation as seen by a Lewinian. *Journal of Social Issues, 38*(1), 131–139.

Developmental Disabilities Act of 1984, PL 98-527, 98 Stat. 2662.

Developmental Disabilities Assistance and Bill of Rights Act of 1975, PL 94-103, 89 Stat. 491.

DeWachter, M. (1978). Teaching medical ethics: University of Nijmegen, The Netherlands. *Journal of Medical Ethics, 4,* 84–88.

Education for All Handicapped Children Act of 1975, PL 94-142, 89 Stat. 773.

Emener, W. B., & Rasch, J. D. (1984). Actual and preferred instructional area in rehabilitation education program. *Rehabilitation Counseling Bulletin, 27,* 269–280.

Emener, W. B. & Wright, T. (1986). *Rules of ethical conduct and rehabilitation counseling: Results of a national survey.* Unpublished manuscript, University of South Florida, Tampa.

Employment Opportunities for Disabled Americans Act, PL 99-643, 100 Stat. 3574.

Erlanger, H., & Roth, W. (1985). Disability policy: The parts and the whole. *American Behavioral Scientist, 28,* 319–345.

Federal Register, May, 1986, Vol. 51, p. 18994.

Fentem, P. H. (1985). Methods of teaching medical ethics at the University of Nottingham. *Journal of Medical Ethics, 11,* 27–28.

Fitchburg Housing Authority v. Board of Zoning Appeals of Fitchburg, 380 Mass. 869, 406 N. E. 2d 1006 (1980).

Francoeur, R. T. (1983). Teaching decision making in biomedical ethics for the allied health student. *Journal of Allied Health, 12*(3), 202–209.

Gorski, R. (1985). 1619: It's a working number! *Disabled USA, No. 1,* 12–15.

Gorski, R. (1986). A capital concern with employment. *Disabled USA, No. 1–2,* 6–7.

Hahn, H. (1982). Disability and rehabilitation policy: Is paternalistic neglect really benign? *Public Administration Review, 42,* 385–390.

Hahn, H. (1985). Introduction: Disability policy and the problem of discrimination. *American Behavioral Scientist, 28,* 293–318.

Halderman v. Pennhurst State School and Hospital, 446 F. Supp. 1295 (E.D. Pa., 1977).

Handelsman, M. M. (1986a). Ethics training at the master's level: A national survey. *Professional Psychology: Research and Training, 17,* 24–26.

Handelsman, M. M. (1986b). Problems with ethics training by "osmosis." *Professional Psychologic Research and Practice, 17,* 371–372.

Harding, C. G. (1985). *Moral dilemmas.* Chicago: Precedent.

Hastings Center. (1980). *The teaching of ethics in higher education.* Hastings-on-Hudson, NY: Author.

Illinois Department of Rehabilitation Services (1986). *From the gallery . . . Legislation of interest.* Springfield: Author.

Illinois Human Rights Act, Illinois Rev. Stats. ch. 68 (1983).

Janes, M. W., & Emener, W. G. (1983). Graduates' views of instructional/competency areas in rehabilitation counselor education programs: A hypothesis generating study. *Journal of Applied Rehabilitation Counseling, 15,* 38–43.

Jenkins, W. M. (1981). History and legislation of the rehabilitation movement. In R. Parker & C. Hansen (Eds.), *Rehabilitation counseling* (pp. 7–37). Boston: Allyn & Bacon.

Kitchener, K. S. (1984). Intuition, critical evaluation, and ethical principles: The foundation for ethical decisions in counseling psychology. *Counseling Psychologist, 12,* 43–55.

Kitchener, K. S. (1986). Teaching applied ethics in counselor education: An integration of psychological processes and philosophical analysis. *Journal of Counseling and Development, 64,* 306–310.

Lasky, F. (1980). Right to services in the community: Implications of the Pennhurst case. In R. J. Flynn & K. E. Nitsch (Eds.), *Normalization, social integration, and community service* (pp. 167–183). Baltimore: University Park Press.

Law, S. A. T. (1985). The teaching of medical ethics from a junior doctor's viewpoint. *Journal of Medical Ethics, 11,* 37–38.

Maine Human Rights Act, ME. Rev Stat. Ann. Tit. 5 Sec 4553 (West Supp. 1985).

Matkin, R. E., & May, R. (1981). Potential conflicts of interest in private rehabilitation: Identification and resolution. *Journal of Applied Rehabilitation Counseling, 12,* 15–18.

Morrison, J. K., & Teta, D. (1979). Impact of a humanistic approach on students' attitudes, attributions, and ethical conflicts. *Psychological Reports, 45,* 863–866.

Pape, E., & Klein, M. (1986). Ethical issues in rehabilitation counseling: A survey of rehabilitation practitioners. *Journal of Applied Rehabilitation Counseling, 17*(4), 8–13.

President's Commission for the Study of Ethical Problems and Biomedical and Behavioral Research. (1983). *Securing access to health care* (Vol. 1). Washington, DC: U.S. Government Printing Office.

Purtilo, R. B. (1983). Ethics in allied health education: State of the art. *Journal of Allied Health, 12,* 210–221.

Rehabilitation Act of 1973, PL 93-112, 87 Stat. 355.

Rest, J. R. (1982). A psychologist looks at the teaching of ethics. *Hastings Center Report, 2,* 29–36.

Rest, J. R. (1983). Morality. In J. Flavell & E. Markman (Eds.), *Cognitive development* (Vol. 4, pp. 556–629). New York: John Wiley & Sons.

Rest, J. R. (1984). Research on moral development: Implications for training counseling psychologists. *Counseling Psychologist, 12,* 19–29.

Rubin, S. E., & Roessler, R. T. (1987). *Foundations of the vocational rehabilitation process* (3rd ed.). Austin, TX: PRO-ED.

Scotch, R. K. (1984). *From good will to civil rights.* Philadelphia: Temple University.

Shotter, E. (1985). Self help in medical ethics. *Journal of Medical Ethics, 11,* 32–34.

Smith, A. (1985). The teaching of medical ethics. *Journal of Medical Ethics, 11,* 35–36.

Tymchuk, A. J. (1982). Strategies for resolving value dilemmas. *American Behavioral Scientist, 26,* 159–175.

Urban Mass Transportation Act of 1964, 49 U.S.C. §1601 et. seq. 1612 (1964).

Urban Mass Transportation Assistance Act of 1970, 16(a), 49 U. S. C. 1612 (1970).

Veatch, R., & Sollito, S. (1976). Medical ethics of teaching: A report of a national medical school survey. *Journal of the American Medical Association, 235,* 1030–1033.

Welbourn, R. B. (1985). A model for teaching medical ethics. *Journal of Medical Ethics, 11,* 29–31.

Wyatt v. Stickney, 344 F. Supp. 387 (M.D. Ala., 1972).

17

The Study of the Future

A Contemporary Challenge for the Rehabilitation Counseling Profession

Charles Victor Arokiasamy, James A. Leja, Gary Austin, and Stanford E. Rubin

WHILE MANKIND HAS always been fascinated with and curious about the future, the 20th century has seen serious scientific study of the future become a popular and accepted facet of contemporary life (Ferkiss, 1977; Fowles, 1978; Hughes, 1985; Jouvenel, 1967; Thompson, 1979). Shocked by the frightening predictions of Orwell's *Nineteen Eighty-four* (1949) and Huxley's *Brave New World* (1932); titillated by more modern, popular, and upbeat scenarios like Toffler's *Future Shock* (1970) and *The Third Wave* (1980), and Naisbitt's *Megatrends* (1982); stretched to the limits of the imagination by science fiction writers such as Arthur C. Clarke, Issac Asimov, and H. G. Wells; and necessitated by the need to forecast for economic planning, the second half of this century has seen an explosion of activity on the study of the future. In the United States alone, there are more than 200 research institutes and numerous other organizations dealing with the future (Dickson, 1977). Entire new magazines like *Futures, The Futurist,* and *Omni* have emerged to meet market demands created by the growing interest in the future.

It is perhaps ironic to have a chapter on the future in a book on contemporary challenges to the rehabilitation counseling profession. Yet, as this

The authors were assisted in writing this chapter by Peggy Sattler.

chapter attempts to establish, taking on the challenge of studying the future is or at least should be a contemporary concern of the rehabilitation counseling profession as well. This discussion of the reasons for studying the future, and the relative absence of futurism studies in the rehabilitation literature, provides a rationale for the involvement of the rehabilitation counseling profession in the study of the future.

WHY STUDY THE FUTURE?

The history of rehabilitation in the United States is replete with examples of reactive program planning and policy making (Berkowitz, 1985; Rubin & Roessler, 1987). Program planning and policy making based solely on past experience and present need result in programs and policy that rapidly become outdated, constantly need adjustment, often carry excess baggage in the form of historical legacies and constraints, and are frequently resistant to change (Berkowitz, 1985; Noble, 1985; Nosek, 1985). Such reactive approaches also "limit creative solutions to massive problems faced by persons with disabilities and perhaps, unconsciously, perpetuate medieval attitudes and methods" (Nosek, 1985, p. 21). If the rehabilitation counseling profession is to avoid such pitfalls, it becomes a crucial and contemporary challenge to shift to proactive planning and explore the future (Lorenz, Larson, & Schumacher, 1981; Spears, 1983).

Futurism literature provides three basic reasons for studying the future: to prepare for inevitable futures, to avoid undesirable futures, and to plan desirable futures. The phenomenon of computer applications in rehabilitation provides an illustration of all three goals. The expanding use of computers as a trend that is here to stay makes it an inevitable future (Crimando & Godley, 1985; Crimando & Sawyer, 1983; Growick, 1983; McCollum & Chan, 1985; Perlman & Austin, 1984; Schmitt & Growick, 1985). The warnings of potentially negative consequences of computer utilization in rehabilitation—the dehumanizing effect on the counseling relationship and ethical concerns regarding confidentiality of computer-stored information (McCollum & Chan, 1985)—represent possible undesirable futures. Finally, the numerous benefits of computer use—efficiency, cost reduction (Chan, McCollum, & Pool, 1985), telecommuting, and home-based employment (Crimando & Godley, 1985)—provide examples of desirable futures.

It is highly likely that if rehabilitation had studied the future in the 1960s, some issues currently being posed as contemporary challenges would have been predicted. Chan, Matkin, Parker, and McCollum's examples of computer applications in rehabilitation (Chapter 14, this volume) provide an example of a current trend that could have been easily predicted. Although less predictable, the issues of consumerism and the independent living movement in Rubenfeld (Chapter 2, this volume) and Nosek (Chapter 3, this volume) could have been seen as inevitable results of the civil rights trends of the 1960s (see DeJong, 1979).

A significant current trend with important implications for rehabilitation is the aging of the baby boom generation, a generation that has had and continues to have a major impact. It can be anticipated that as its members move into old age, they will have an impact on politics (making it more conservative?), recreation (generating demands for more leisurely and less physical recreation?), and medical care and research (increasing the focus on medical and psychological problems of old age?), and that this growing population of older persons will create a serious strain on Social Security. Rehabilitation counselors can expect the range of disabilities to include more age-related disabilities, and they will need to prepare for these developments.

Which of the contemporary challenges presented in this book are likely to be present for another 10–50 years, and which are likely to be passing fads? Which are temporary responses to urgent pressures, and which are genuine innovations that are likely to shape the rehabilitation counseling profession of the future? To the extent that answering such questions is considered important, it becomes important for the rehabilitation counseling profession to study the future.

FUTURE STUDY IN CURRENT REHABILITATION LITERATURE

A number of publications in rehabilitation literature purport to deal with the future, or use futuristic terms like "the information age" (e.g., see Berkowitz, 1985; Bowe, 1985; Hahn, 1985; Levis, Louvet, & Ulstrup, 1985; Lorenz et al., 1981; McCollum & Chan, 1985; Perlman & Austin, 1985; Scadden, 1984; Spears, 1983). However, except for Levis et al. (1985), Lorenz et al. (1981), and Spears (1983), they primarily discuss past and current trends and events (e.g., see McCollum & Chan, 1985; Perlman & Austin, 1985) and therefore differ greatly from the general futurism literature. While not actually forecasting the future, Spears performed the important task of setting an agenda for those who would. He identified three useful areas of future study: the changing natures of disabilities, work, and society. Lorenz et al. (1981) predicted that the concept of disability would change from "an all-or-none phenomenon" to one in which disability will be seen on a continuum (p. 361). They also predicted the demise of private nonprofit agencies, the expansion of private for-profit agencies, growth in professionalism, and the concomitant emergence of rehabilitation technicians. Lorenz et al. saw the need for the development of a cadre of highly competent manager/leaders capable of guiding the profession through these changes. However, they do not provide specific time frames for their projections, though such time frames are strongly recommended by futurists such as Dickson (1977) and Jouvenel (1967).

Levis et al. (1985) make long-range projections about the incidence, prevalence, recovery rates, attrition by death, and distribution of disabled persons in the labor force by age, sex, and year from 1980 to 2020. This study comes closest to those produced by traditional futurists in that it specifies a time frame (2020 A.D.), uses a specific futurism technique (trend extrapolation), states its assumptions, and describes its limitations.

As is evident, the study of the future regarding rehabilitation-related issues has been sparse. There is a need for new research questions and hypotheses about the effect of future changes on the rehabilitation counseling profession, such as the aging of the population; medical and technological advances; and economic, political, cultural and demographic changes. For example, will medical advances eliminate some disabilities? Will technological changes create new disabilities? Will changes in the structure of work affect rehabilitation services? It is certainly to the benefit of the profession to study questions such as these.

TECHNIQUES OF FUTURE STUDY

While future study is still in its infancy, several techniques to study the future have been developed, including: 1) trend extrapolation, 2) the Delphi technique, 3) qualitative historical observations, and 4) scenario writing. Each of these techniques is briefly described below.

Trend Extrapolation

Many activities in daily living are based on anticipated regularities (Hill, 1978). Without realizing it, we count on these "trends" to structure our lives. The technique of trend extrapolation is based on this very premise—that occurrences in the past provide a pattern to future occurrences (Dickson, 1977).

Trend extrapolation is a technique for empirically examining an ongoing event through repeated measurements taken across time (Hill, 1978). The phenomenon of interest is plotted on a graph over time as a solid line and a projection plotted into the future as a dotted line, following the trend of the previously established line (Dickson, 1977). Before trend extrapolation is applied and the data plotted, two conditions should be met: 1) the events must be identified and expressed numerically, and 2) a sufficient time series should be available to reflect significant rather than temporary changes in events (Hill, 1978).

The advantage of trend extrapolation as a forecasting tool is its conceptual simplicity. A major drawback, however, is the assumption that past factors will continue to be important (Dickson, 1977). Unanticipated changes in economics, politics, or technology may invalidate this assumption (Martino, 1978). For further references to trend extrapolation, readers are directed to Hill (1978).

The Delphi Technique

The Delphi technique, aptly named for the site in Greece where Pythia communicated the words of Apollo to priests and supplicants (Linstone, 1978), was developed by the Rand Corporation in the late 1950s on the premise that an organized group of experts could speculate on the future better than an individual or unstructured group of forecasters (Dickson, 1977; Ferkiss, 1977; Linstone, 1978). Though not strictly a forecasting method, it has been used by forecasters as "a method for structuring a group communication process so that the process is effective in allowing a group of individuals as a whole, to deal with complex problems" (Linstone, 1978, p. 274).

In the Delphi technique, invited "experts" who remain anonymous to each other are given general information about the area they are to forecast (Martino, 1978), and then asked to develop and submit a list of possible events that may occur during a specified time frame. These events are then compiled into a questionnaire and resubmitted to the panel, who now attach numerical probabilities for their occurring within a given time frame, and add supporting remarks. In the third step, the panel receives a revised questionnaire based on their responses in the preceding step. They are provided an opportunity to revise their probability estimates and are asked to state the reasons for any changes made. In the final step, this revised list of events, associated probabilities, and remarks are given to the experts for final revision. The end product of this process is a list of possible events, dates by which the events are estimated to occur (median dates given in the last step), information on the relative probability of the forecasted dates, and supportive arguments for accepting, advancing, or delaying the forecasted dates (Martino, 1978). Much of the logic behind the Delphi technique lies in the anonymity of the respondents, which prevents bias due to the influences of any personality; controlled feedback through a questionnaire format; and statistical responses through probability estimates (Hill, 1978; Martino, 1978).

Oddly enough, major criticism of this technique (Sackman, 1975) comes from its developers, the Rand Corporation. Sackman identified 16 negative aspects of methodology and application, including poor questionnaire design and a frequent lack of established measurement reliability and scientific validity. Readers are directed to Sackman for further comments about the Delphi technique.

Qualitative Historical Observations

A more recent approach to forecasting, one that Funkhouser (1984) suggests may improve the ability to make predictions of behavior patterns, societal trends, and hard-to-measure factors within the soft sciences, is qualitative historical observation. Funkhouser notes that if behaviors observed in the past continue to be observed today, it is highly likely that these behaviors will also occur years into the future until influenced by intervening events. The greater the length of time between measurements of past and present events, the greater the certainty when extrapolating.

To describe the logic behind this approach, Funkhouser (1984) uses the analogy of shooting a gun. In order to aim a gun, two sights are used: the rear sight (or past events) and the front sight (or present events). The shorter the distance between the rear and front sights (i.e., the interval of time between past and present events), the less accurate the aim (or the greater the uncertainty in extrapolating events into the future). Conversely, the greater the distance between the two sights, the more accurate the aim. In addition, the bullet in flight is subject to "windage": conditions (societal factors) that alter the flight path of the bullet, such as wind (intervening events or new technologies).

There are three basic steps involved in applying qualitative historical observations. First, the specific behavior to be studied must be defined. Second, careful observations are taken of the present occurrence and nature of this behavior, as well as an analysis of various factors that generate or alter the behavior. Third, sources reputed to be accurate and well respected are used to identify past observations of the behavior. If, as a result of comparing past and present observations, a valid pattern of behavior is identified, further extrapolation of that pattern into the future can be pursued.

This technique requires little sophisticated equipment or training. Many sources of past observations are readily available, such as the Bible, and the writings of philosophers and historians. However, there are also disadvantages. Measurements may be unreliable due to biased or nonfactual sources, generalizations made may not necessarily apply to the behaviors of all individuals exhibiting the forecasted behavior, and the interpretations of trends and the predictions are to some degree a matter of judgment on the part of the researcher (Funkhouser, 1984).

Scenario Writing

Scenario writing, one of the most communicable form of futures conjecture, is described by the Stanford Research Institute (1975) as "an outline of one conceivable state of affairs, given certain assumptions" (p. 193). The scenario has three basic characteristics: 1) it is a hypothetical narrative, 2) it is only a sketch, and 3) it is multifaceted and holistic (Wilson, 1978). Its hypothetical nature is obviously due to the unknowable nature of the future. Since any predicted event, no matter how well based on trends, is nevertheless hypothetical, the best approach may be to examine several detailed alternative futures. The scenario is well suited to generate such alternative futures.

As a brief sketch, the scenario can provide an outline, showing the different directions along which the future may develop, while examining the causes that may divert it in other directions. Scenarios may explore a limited domain like the subsequent computer applications example in this chapter, or broader domains. Broad scenarios may combine variables such as demographic changes, social trends, political events, and economic and technological changes, to reflect the flow of history (and the future) and portray the changeable nature of these variables as they interact.

Zentner (1975) proposed three criteria by which to test the tenability of a scenario: credibility, utility, and intelligibility. The events described in a scenario must appear likely enough or be supported by data or logic to function as a believable picture of the future. If a scenario does not identify possibilities or warnings relevant to the problems of the users, it becomes little more than entertainment. Finally, the scenario must be intelligible, explaining the logic, intuition, data, and so forth behind its conclusions.

Though the scenario has been widely used as a planning tool, it has not escaped criticism. Some believe that the futurist who uses scenarios is attempting to have his or her cake and eat it too, presenting plausible and varied future alternatives that can each also be construed as actual predictions (Ferkiss, 1977, p. 23). Others often see scenarios as merely science fiction, based on no more than a vivid imagination (Wilson, 1978).

APPLICATION OF SCENARIO WRITING TO REHABILITATION TOPICS

As a quick illustration of how future study techniques could be effectively utilized in the rehabilitation field, let us examine two futuristic rehabilitation scenarios. For each scenario, a certain future trend or trends are identified and pertinent questions generated. Scenario I is an example of a limited, middle-range future that deals with the specific question of using computer technology in the intake and evaluation phase of the rehabilitation counseling process in the year 2010. Scenario II is an example of a broader, long-range future that deals with the impact of future developments on the type of disability, service delivery, and life-styles. Futurists commonly use the future or present tense in describing scenarios. Accordingly, Scenario I employs the future tense and Scenario II speaks of the year 2030 as if it were already here. In reading the first scenario, it is helpful to remember that when a futurist says something *will* happen, he or she is really saying that it is likely that X would happen given that A, B, and C develop as expected.

Scenario I

Posited future influence: That the continuing development of computer technology will expand its applications in the rehabilitation service system.
Question: How will computer technology affect the way rehabilitation counselors conduct evaluation and planning with clients?

By the year 2010, the evaluation and planning process in rehabilitation will be greatly shaped by the widespread use of computer technology in the rehabilitation service system. The intake interview will be a very efficient client diagnostic data collection instrument, highly structured, and administered by the rehabilitation counselor in an empathetic, respectful, and sincere way. The interview will be recorded by a computer that has been programmed to process the information (think diagnostically and prognostically) in a manner similar to that used by rehabilitation counselors with the best diagnostic skills. Being portable, the computer will also be taken along for interviews that occur outside the counselor's office, such as those held in the client's home.

The futuristic process will proceed as follows. Upon reaching the decision that the interview has been completed, the rehabilitation counselor will push a button (or perhaps just speak to the computer) and the computer will either concur or provide a list of unanswered questions that should be addressed before the intake interview process ends. When an optimal amount of information has been collected via the intake interview, the computer will: 1) indicate what additional information should be acquired via other evaluation procedures (e.g. medical, psychological, or vocational); 2) provide a list of specific questions to be addressed via those procedures; and 3) provide a list of possible locations and appointment times for those evaluations. The rehabilitation counselor will then explain the purpose of the additional evaluations to the client, and they will jointly select the time for each appointment. Via electronic mail, the computer will set up the necessary appointments and provide each subsequent evaluator with the list of assessment questions that will need to be addressed. Immediately following the completion of the additional evaluations, the evaluation reports will be sent to the rehabilitation counselor, again via electronic mail. The computer will then, like the expert diagnostic rehabilitation counselor, process the following together: 1) all the information on the client; 2) information on available relevant counseling, restoration, and education/vocational training services; and 3) the functional demands of available jobs that would be feasible with or without reasonable accommodation (e.g., affordable job modifications). As a result of this data processing, the computer will provide an integrated summary of the information obtained on the client, as well as a group of potential occupational choices and associated rehabilitation plans, and reasons why each would be supported by the information contained in the data summary. These proposed rehabilitation plans will constitute clinical hypotheses; that is, it would be hypothesized that positive consequences would result for the client from the implementation of such a rehabilitation plan.

To obtain further support for the potential efficacy of each plan, the rehabilitation counselor will ask the local computer to communicate with a larger national computer that houses a data bank of rehabilitation cases. The national computer will report on problems encountered and outcomes achieved by previous clients with similar characteristics and with whom similar rehabilitation plans were carried out. The integration of the first report and the second report by the computer will provide a clinical-actuarial interpretation on the client and his or her rehabilitation feasibility via different alternatives.

When all feasible vocational choices have been identified, the client will use an interactive computer-assisted career guidance system to review comprehensive information on each job, using videotapes acquired from a computerized occupational information library (data base). The system will allow the client to stop the tape and ask for clarification or additional information on any aspect of the job. The computer will respond to such questions by drawing on additional occupational information stored in the data base. All videotapes in the library will show persons with disabilities working at each job. Using a disabled person as the employee model should help clients become more aware of their own potential. That in turn can have a positive effect on the client's vocational self-concept.

Once the diagnostic process is completed and the client has sufficient occupational information from the computer-assisted career guidance system, the counselor and client will discuss the evaluation report containing feasible jobs and components of the rehabilitation plan related to each alternative. During this planning process the counselor will facilitate in-depth client self-exploration of each alternative, with special attention focused on client feelings and concerns. Upon completion of this process, which could require more than one planning interview, a rehabilitation plan will be selected and finely tuned to meet the needs of this specific client. The computer will print a relevant number of copies of an aesthetically designed and illustrative master plan that will specify the goals, objectives, schedules of implementation, deadlines, flow charts, process checks, motivational aids, recordkeeping aids, accountability checks, and contractual components. The counselor, client, and other relevant persons will each receive a copy, and the plan will be implemented. Throughout the rehabilitation process the computer will flag noncompliance with the plan, and necessary changes or revaluation, while simultaneously keeping a record of progress. As a result of computerized aids, the entire process for achieving this goal will be very time efficient, without depriving the client of the experience of a facilitative counseling relationship.

Scenario II

Posited future influences: 1) That technology will continue to develop rapidly and have an impact on every facet of life; 2) that there will initially be a pronounced rise in the percentage of older citizens, followed by a stable leveling off; 3) that public attitudes toward different disabilities will change; and 4) that overall political and economic conditions will continue to be stable and positive.
Questions: Who will the consumers of rehabilitation be in the year 2030? What disabilities will be most common? How will disability be viewed by society at that time? What will rehabilitation services and goals be like in the year 2030?

By 2020, the increase in life expectancy and the aging of the population began leveling off. Currently, in the year 2030, 45% of the population is above 65. They are relatively better educated and healthier than such groups in the past. Members of this group have become accustomed to extra attention given to their needs and interests. Almost 70% of the total health care expenditure is spent on them. As a result of more attention, especially in terms of research and service for the disabilities of aging and elderly persons, many chronic conditions have all but disappeared, and the functional limitations of others have been effectively reduced. Diabetes, hypertension, and heart disease are no longer high prevalence diseases. Orthopaedic problems are also not as functionally debilitating as before, due to developments in prosthetic technology, transplant technology, and barrier-free environments.

Physical disabilities are very common but are normally regarded as nonhandicapping for a number of reasons. First, some physical impairment or other has become an ordinary fact of life for the majority of citizens as they age. Second, technological and medical advances have made functional limitations related to physical disability almost negligible. Medical advances have made limb and tissue regeneration and bionic replacement of body parts possible. Technology has made mobility-enhancing equipment, environmental modification, and hi-tech prosthetics affordable and commonplace. Bionic body parts and hi-tech prosthetics have become commonplace in the same way that contact lenses to correct visual impairment became commonplace during the last century. Some historians have credited the current social acceptance of physical disabilities and efforts at creating an accessible environment to a moral regeneration that began emerging in society during the last quarter of the 1900s. Other historians suggest that such acceptance came about primarily because of political pressure by growing numbers of aged persons and because technology made environmental modification cheaper.

Mental disabilities present the most serious handicaps. Cures have been found for a number of mental disabilities, through drug therapy and nerve and brain segment transplants. Others have become preventable through genetic manipulation. However, this highly ''technologized'' society has sharply enhanced the value of mental ability, just as physical prowess had been highly esteemed in past times. Ordinary life activities, like education, transportation, shipping, banking, and recreation, have become highly computerized. While computerization has simplified these activities for ''normal'' persons, they have made ''computer dropouts'' of those with lesser mental abilities. Functional limitations are also experienced by persons lacking in decision-making ability. Rapid automation and computerization that require conscious decision-making steps for the completion of routine life activities have made them outcasts. For instance, shopping for a dress in the past involved simple visual inspection, selecting one pleasing to the eye, trying it on, and checking to see if it was affordable. Today, a person must answer a long series of computer-generated questions, from the initial ''What can I do for you?'' and ''What would you like to buy?'' to specific questions on dress style, color, size of hem, sleeve, waist, chest, type of fabric, and whether one would like insurance on delivery. Each of these steps require conscious decision making that proves stressful to some.

Emotional disorders are next on the list of disabilities. People with inadequate social skills experience severe functional limitations. They have difficulties with social integration because automation and computers have taken over many of the manually performed jobs and depersonalized many aspects of life, making 21st century society more recreation oriented than any in the past. Those lacking social skills have difficulty participating in socialized recreation and avoid such opportunities. These problems of social integration, coupled with the demand for rapid decision making, have created many stress-related emotional disorders even in the present leisure-oriented society.

Such changes in types of disability and life-style have influenced service delivery. Services are greatly tailored to the individual's goals. The rehabilitation effort consists mainly of the following: 1) training in the acceptance, use, and maintenance of new body parts (some of which surpass the functional abilities and aesthetic qualities of their natural counterparts), which make possible the relearning of old skills and the reengagement in former pursuits; 2) social skills training in the form of group therapy, simulated social situations, and *in vivo* social situation training; and 3) life adjustment and emotional counseling for making choices about the types of prostheses and capacities that the client wants.

Along with the shifts in social life-style and values, rehabilitation goals too have changed. Because of the shift from the work ethic of the 20th century to the social and recreational ethic in the 21st century, leisure goals, social goals, and aesthetic and intellectual enhancement goals have largely replaced the vocational goals of the past.

CONCLUSION

The study of the future, though it has frequently been subjected to a great deal of criticism and skepticism (e.g., see Michael, in preparation), is both necessary and important (Clarke, 1978; 1984; Dickson, 1977; Hightower, 1976; Jouvenel, 1967; Toffler, 1970). Disciplines, organizations, and even individuals who do not prepare for the future run the grave risk of extinction from future shock (Hightower, 1976; Toffler, 1970), or at least of becoming irrelevant. Hence, systematic and disciplined study of the future has become common. Long-range planning committees, 5-year plans, and the like have become common activities. While concern and curiosity about the future have existed since earliest times, methods of divining the future have changed. Instead of the soothsayer, we turn to the futures researcher. Instead of the pools of the Pythia, we use the computer.

The concrete benefits to the rehabilitation counseling profession of availing itself of scientific methods of studying the future go beyond being able to paint a pretty picture. Scholars within the field will be in a better position to defend funding for programs that anticipate future needs. Even obscure influences that bring about sweeping changes may no longer catch the profession by surprise, and academic and public planning can be more sound. Client populations will benefit by program planning that anticipates their long-term needs. The entire rehabilitation counseling profession can enhance its relevance and effectiveness for the 21st century.

This chapter has discussed the necessity for the rehabilitation counseling profession to be concerned with the future, and has outlined various techniques to study the future. It is hoped that there will be greater and more vigorous examination of the future. To help the profession plan and prepare for the future, research is certainly needed in the area of methodology and on the effect of changes in the world of work, economy, technology, leisure patterns, medical practice, public attitudes, life-styles, and politics on disabled persons and the rehabilitation profession.

REFERENCES

Berkowitz, E. D. (1985). Social influences on rehabilitation planning: Introductory remarks. In L. G. Perlman & G. F. Austin (Eds.), *Social influences on rehabilitation planning: Blueprint for the 21st century* [A report of the Ninth Mary E. Switzer Memorial Seminar, November, 1984] (pp. 11–18). Alexandria, VA: National Rehabilitation Association.

Bowe, F. (1985). Employment trends in the information age. *Rehabilitation Counseling Bulletin, 29,* 19–25.

Chan, F., McCollum, P. S., & Pool, D. A. (1985). Computer-assisted rehabilitation services: A preliminary draft of the Texas Casework Model. *Rehabilitation Counseling Bulletin, 28,* 219–232.

Clarke, A. C. (1978). Communications in the future. In J. Fowles (Ed.), *Handbook of futures research* (pp. 637–651). Westport, CT: Greenwood.

Clarke, A. C. (1984). *Profiles of the future*. New York: Holt, Rinehart, and Winston.

Crimando, W., & Godley, S. (1985). The computer's potential in enhancing employment opportunities of persons with disabilities. *Rehabilitation Counseling Bulletin, 28,* 275–282.

Crimando, W., & Sawyer, H. (1983). Microcomputers in private sector rehabilitation. *Rehabilitation Counseling Bulletin, 26,* 26–31.

DeJong, G. (1979). Independent living: From social movement to analytical paradigm. *Archives of Physical Medicine and Rehabilitation, 60,* 435–446.

Dickson, P. (1977). *The future file*. New York: Rawson Associates.

Ferkiss, V. C. (1977). Futurology: Promise, performance, prospects. *The Washington papers, 5*. Beverly Hills: Sage Publications.

Fowles, J. (Ed.). (1978). *Handbook of futures research*. Westport, CT: Greenwood.

Funkhouser, G. (1984). Using qualitative historical observations in predicting the future. *Futures, 16*(2), 173–182.

Growick, B. (1983). Computers in vocational rehabilitation: Current applications and future trends. *Rehabilitation research review*. Washington, DC: Rehabilitation Information Center.

Hahn, H. (1985). Changing perception of disability and the future of rehabilitation. In L. G. Perlman & G. F. Austin (Eds.), *Social influences on rehabilitation planning: Blueprint for the 21st century* [A report of the Ninth Mary E. Switzer Memorial Seminar, November, 1984] (pp. 53–64). Alexandria, VA: National Rehabilitation Association.

Hightower, M. D. (1976). Status quo is certain death. *Journal of Rehabilitation, 42*(2), 32–35, 41–43.

Hill, K. Q. (1978). Trend extrapolation. In J. Fowles (Ed.), *Handbook of futures research* (pp. 249–272). Westport, CT: Greenwood.

Hughes, B. B. (1985). *World futures: A critical analysis of alternatives*. Baltimore: Johns Hopkins University Press.

Huxley, A. (1932). *Brave new world*. New York: Harper & Row.

Jouvenel, B. (1967). *The art of conjecture*. New York: Basic Books.

Levis, A. H., Louvet, A. C., & Ulstrup, L. C. (1985). *A population model of working age disabled individuals* (TMF-P009-13). Topeka, KS: The Menninger Foundation.

Linstone, H. A. (1978). The Delphi technique. In J. Fowles (Ed.), *Handbook of futures research*. Westport, CT: Greenwood.

Lorenz, J. R., Larson, L., & Schumacher, B. (1981). Prologue to the future. In W. G. Emener, R. S. Luck, & S. J. Smith (Eds.), *Rehabilitation administration and supervision* (pp. 355–370). Baltimore: University Park Press.

Martino, J. P. (1978). Technological forecasting. In J. Fowles (Ed.), *Handbook of futures research* (pp. 249–272). Westport, CT: Greenwood.

McCollum, P. S., & Chan, F. (1985). Rehabilitation in the information age: Prologue to the future. *Rehabilitation Counseling Bulletin, 28*(4), 211–218.

Michael, D. N. (in preparation). With both feet planted firmly in mid-air: Reflections on thinking about the future. In M. Marien & L. Jennings (Eds.), *What have I learned?*

Naisbitt, J. (1982). *Megatrends*. New York: Warner Books.

Noble, J. H. (1985). [Excerpts of reviews and comments]. In L. G. Perlman & G. F. Austin (Eds.), *Social influences on rehabilitation planning: Blueprint for the 21st century* [A report of the Ninth Mary E. Switzer Memorial Seminar, November, 1984] (pp. 21–22). Alexandria, VA: National Rehabilitation Association.

Nosek, M. A. (1985). [Excerpts of reviews and comments.]. In L. G. Perlman & G. F. Austin (Eds.), *Social influences on rehabilitation planning: Blueprint for the 21st* [A report of the Ninth Mary E. Switzer Memorial Seminar, November, 1984] (pp/ 21–22). Alexandria, VA: National Rehabilitation Association.

Orwell, G. (1949). *Nineteen eighty-four.* New York: Harcourt, Brace.

Perlman, L. G., & Austin, G. (Eds.). (1984). *Technology and rehabilitation of disabled persons in the information age.* Alexandria, VA: National Rehabilitation Association.

Perlman, L. G., & Austin, G. F. (1985). *Social influences on rehabilitation planning: Blueprint for the 21st century* [A report of the Ninth Mary E. Switzer Memorial Seminar, November, 1984]. Alexandria, VA: National Rehabilitation Association.

Rubin, S. E., & Roessler, R. T. (1987). *Foundations of the vocational rehabilitation process* (3rd ed.). Austin, TX: PRO-ED.

Sackman, H. (1975). *Delphi critique.* Lexington, MA: Lexington.

Scadden, L. (1984). Blinders in the information age: Equality or wrong? *Journal of Visual Impairment and Blindness, 78*(9), 394–400.

Schmitt, P., & Growick, B. (1985). Computer technology in rehabilitation counseling. *Rehabilitation Counseling Bulletin, 28,* 233–241.

Spears, M. (1983). Rehabilitation in the Third Wave. *Journal of Rehabilitation, 49*(3), 4–7.

Stanford Research Institute, Center for the Study of Social Policy. (1975). *Handbook of forecasting techniques.* Fort Belvoir, VA: U.S. Army Corps of Engineers.

Thompson, A. E. (1979). *Understanding futurology: An introduction to future studies.* North Pomfret, VT: David & Charles.

Toffler, A. (1970). *Future shock.* New York: Random House.

Toffler, A. (1980). *The third wave.* New York: William Morrow.

Wilson, I. A. (1978). Scenarios. In J. Fowles (Ed.), *Handbook of futures research.* Westport, CT: Greenwood.

Zenter, R. D. (1975, October 6.). Scenarios in forecasting. *Chemical and Engineers News,* pp. 22–34.

Index

Ability Information System (AIS), 262
ABLEDATA, 262
Accommodation of disabled persons, 15–28
  by ARCA members' employers, 19–22
  by federal contractors, 21–22
  societal, legislation regarding, 15–16
Accreditation, of rehabilitation counselor education programs, 289–290
Acute rehabilitation, for traumatic brain injury patients, 199–200
Adolescents
  learning disabled, vocational outcome, 95–96
  response to family members with cancer, 192
  school-to-work transition, 93–108, 135–149, 158, 159, 160, 161
  sensory impaired, 157–161
Advocacy, role in rehabilitation counseling, 25–27
Affirmative action for disabled persons, legislation concerning, 15–16
Agencies, federal/state
  Centers for Independent Living programs and, 52–53
  and closures in supported employment, 128–129
  cooperation in school-to-work transition, 136–137
  disability accommodation requirements of, 15–16
  policies regarding persons with life-threatening disabilities, 63–64
  and rehabilitation counselor education, 275, 276–277
  and sensory impaired persons, 169–170
  versus private sector employers, 295–296
Aging, and sensory impairments, 171–172, 174
American Rehabilitation Counseling Association (ARCA)
  influence on rehabilitation counselor education, 290–291
  members' employers' attitudes to disabled persons, 19–22
    compared to federal contractors, 21–22
  survey of members, 18–23
    employers' characteristics, 19
    personal characteristics, 18–19
  survey on ethics, 310
  survey on independent living, 57–58
APTICOM, 97
ARCA, see American Rehabilitation Counseling Association

Barden-LaFollette Act (PL 78-113), 274
Behavioral rehabilitation programs, for traumatic brain injury patients, 200, 203–205
Blindness
  computer use for employment, 267
  counseling considerations, 169–170
  definition of, 154–155
  employment considerations, 164–165, 168

Blindness—*continued*
see also Deaf-blindness; Sensory impaired persons; Sensory impairments

CACREP, see Council for the Accreditation of Counseling and Related Educational Programs
Cancer
economic costs, 184
modes of treatment
psychological implications, 185–186
psychobehavioral, 186–188
psychological impact
on the family, 190–192
on the individual, 188–190
and rehabilitation counseling, 193–194
statistics on, 183–184
vocational considerations, 192–193
see also Life-threatening disabilities
Career Maturity Inventory (CMI), 97
Career Planning System (CPS), 99
CARF, *see* Commission on the Accreditation of Rehabilitation Facilities
Case closure
and independent living, 55
in supported employment, 88, 128–129
Case management
computer applications for, 260–263
in rehabilitation of traumatic brain injury patients, 202–203, 222–223
Catastrophic head injury, 221
Centers for Independent Living, legislation regarding, 52–53
see also Independent living
Certification of rehabilitation counselors, influence on education, 288–289
Chemotherapy, 185
Client–rehabilitation counselor relationship, 31–43
Closed head injury, 218
CMI, *see* Career Maturity Inventory
Cognitive retraining, in traumatic head injury patients, 223–225
Coma
Glasgow Coma Scale of, 219
Glasgow Outcome Scale for, 219
rehabilitation objectives for, 199
Co-management approach to rehabilitation counseling, 41
Commission on the Accreditation of Rehabilitation Facilities (CARF)
need for guidelines in sensory impairment rehabilitation, 176
standards specific to traumatic brain injuries, 208
Communication skills
cancer patients and families, 190–191
computer-based assistive devices for, 264
sensory impaired persons and families, 158
Community action role in rehabilitation counseling, 25–27
Comprehensive outpatient rehabilitation facilities, 201
Comprehensive service delivery model, 10
agency cooperation and involvement, 104
employment skills training, 100–102
identification of learning styles in, 98
individualized transition plan, 96–98
job maintenance in, 102–103
parent cooperation and involvement, 103–104
vocational planning in, 98–99
Computer-assisted counseling, 262–263
Computer-based assistive devices, 263–264
Computers, 1, 7
computer-assisted career exploration, 99
in rehabilitation counseling
computer-assisted counseling, 262–263
client employability issues, 267
client-oriented applications, 263–265
counselor-oriented appplications, 260–263
education and training issues, 267–268
ethical considerations, 265–266

research in, 268
in vocational assessment, 97–98
in vocational planning, 99
Conflict management, 100–101
COPA, *see* Council on Post-secondary Accreditation
CORE, *see* Council on Rehabilitation Education
Council for the Accreditation of Counseling and Related Education Programs (CACREP), 289
Council on Post-secondary Accreditation (COPA), 289
Council on Rehabilitation Counselor Certification (CRCC), 278, 290
assessment of counselors, 278
study on adequacy of independent living movement, 57
Council on Rehabilitation Education (CORE)
counselor education requirements
independent living, 57–58
school-to-work transition, 145–146
supported employment, 124–125
influence on professional education, 278–280, 282, 289, 290
Counselor-client relationship, 31–43
CPS, *see* Career Planning System
CRCC, *see* Council on Rehabilitation Counselor Certification

Data management software, use in rehabilitation counseling, 261
DCS, *see* Dilemma Counseling System
Deaf-blindness
counseling considerations, 154, 160–161, 170
definition of, 155–156
employment considerations, 166–167
job placement, 163
see also Sensory impaired persons; Sensory impairments
Deafness, definition of, 154
see also Sensory impaired persons; Sensory impairments
Deep muscle relaxation, in cancer therapy, 186, 187, 188
Delphi technique, in future studies, 321
Developmental deficits, in sensory impaired children, 159–160
Developmental Disabilities Assistance and Bill of Rights Act (PL 94-103), 2, 304, 305
Dilemma Counseling System (DCS), 263
Disability
definition of, 15
changes in, and rehabilitation counselor education, 292–293
life-threatening, 61–73, 183–194
paradigm of disease in, 34–35
sociocultural conceptualization of, 244
Disability models
economic, 3–4
medical, 3–4, 35–36
sociopolitical, 3
Disability rights movement, 2
ethical challenges, 8
newly recognized disability groups, 3–4
Disabled persons
aging of
future studies of, 319
influence on rehabilitation counselor education, 287
attitudes toward disability, 40
attitudes toward rehabilitation counseling, 31–32, 36, 40–41
civil rights for, 304–309
computer-based assistive devices for, 263–265
counselor attitudes toward, 39–40
emphasis on limitations of, 36–37
history of attitudes toward, 33–34
rights of (UN resolutions), 16
transition from school to work, 93–108, 135–149
with life-threatening disabilities, 61–73
see also specific disability
DISCOVER, 99
Discrimination against disabled persons, 16–17
Disease versus disability, 34–35

Early intervention, with sensory impaired persons, 157–158, 159–160
Economic costs of cancer, 184

Education
  postsecondary
    for rehabilitation counselors, 278–280, 281–282, 288–290
    for sensory impaired persons, 162–163
  of rehabilitation counselors, *see* Rehabilitation counselor education
  see also Employment skills training; Job skills training; Vocational planning
Education for All Handicapped Children Act (PL 94-142), 1, 94, 137, 304, 305, 306
Electronic spreadsheet/budgeting software, use in rehabilitation counseling, 261
  see also Computers
ELIZA, 263
Emotional response to life-threatening disability, 68–69, 189–192
Employment
  of ARCA members, 19
  computer applications in, 265, 267
  considerations for cancer patients, 192–193
  outcomes in supported, 122–123
  potential for
    in persons with life-threatening disabilities, 65–66
    in traumatic brain injury patients, 210–212
  of sensory impaired persons, issues in, 164–166
  skills training for, 100–103
  supported, 79, 111–112
  transitional, 78–79
  trends, for rehabilitation counselors, 294–296
Employment Opportunities for Disabled Americans Act (PL 99-643), 307
Employment services
  job development, 89, 121
  job maintenance, 90, 122, 238
  training and assistance, 89–90, 121–122
  transitional, 127
Employment skills training, 100–102
  computerized, 265
  job-seeking skills, 102–103
  for sensory impaired persons, 162–164
Employment training specialists, 83, 85–86, 115, 128
Enclave, in supported employment, 115
Environmental/interactional approach to rehabilitation, 4–5
Ethics
  in computer applications to rehabilitation counseling, 265–266
  in rehabilitation counseling education, 309–312
  see also Professional values
Extended care programs, for traumatic brain injury patients, 199–200, 222–223

Family response to disability
  cancer, 190–192
  current theories on, 245–247
  rehabilitation counselor's role in, 247–248, 255–256
    assessing family functioning, 248–252
    developing support systems, 253–254
    facilitating transition, 254–255
  providing information, 253
  traumatic brain injury, 205–207
Federal contractors, accommodation of disabled persons by, 21–22
Federal legislation
  effect on rehabilitation counselor education, 274–277
  and "full integration" mandate, 304–309
Federal/state agencies, *see* Agencies, federal/state
"Full integration" mandate, and public policy, 304–306
  barriers to achievement, 306–309
Functional limitations approach to rehabilitation, 4
Funding, academic, effect on rehabilitation counselor education, 293–294
Future studies
  application of scenario writing to rehabilitation, 323–327
  in current literature, 319–320
  techniques, 320–323
  use in rehabilitation counseling, 318–319

Glasgow Coma Scale, 219
Glasgow Outcome Scale, 219
Group therapy, and traumatic brain injury patients, 235
Guided imagery, in cancer therapy, 186, 187

Handicap, definition of, 15
Hard-of-hearing, definition of, 154
Head injury, *see* Traumatic brain injury
Hearing impairment
  definition of, 154
  see also Sensory impaired persons; Sensory impairments
Heart disease, 64, 67
Helen Keller National Center
  definition of deaf-blindness, 157, 161
  definition of visual impairment, 156
  national registry of deaf-blind children, 160–161
History taking, for traumatic brain injury rehabilitation, 227–228
HOMEBOUND program, 267
Hypnosis, in cancer therapy, 187

Income support programs, as barrier to "full integration" mandate, 306–307
Independent living, 45–47
  congressional support for, 49
  history of, 47–50
  legislation regarding, 50–53
  professional service providers for, 53–54
  program types, 48–49
  and rehabilitation counseling, 54–57
  rehabilitation counselor education in, 57–58, 287
  for sensory impaired persons, 166–168
  support services for, 46–47
  see also Centers for Independent Living
Individual supported competitive employment, 115
Individualized education programs (IEPs), rehabilitation counselor's role in, 142
Individualized transition plan, for persons with learning disabilities, 96–98
Individualized written rehabilitation programs (IWRPs)
  agency cooperation to develop, 176
  assignment of responsibility for, 84
  educating counselors about, 145
  rehabilitation counselor's role in, 142
  supported employment as goal, 128
In-service training
  in services for sensory impaired clients, 175
  for supported employment counseling, 126–127
Intensive retraining programs, for traumatic brain injury patients, 200

Job Accommodation Network, 262
Job coach, *see* Employment training specialists
Job-seeking skills
  for sensory impaired persons, 163–164
  training in, 102–103

Learning disabilities
  adolescent problems with, 95–96
  comprehensive service delivery model for, 96–104
  employment skills training for, 100–102
  legislation pertaining to, 94–95
Least restrictive environment, relation to school-to-work transition, 144–145
Life-threatening disabilities
  barriers to rehabilitation in
    agency policy, 63–64, 71, 72
    client's physical condition, 62–63
    client's psychosocial adjustment, 67–79
    employer attitude, 64–67
    the rehabilitation counselor, 70–71
  incidence and prevalence of, 61–62
  psychological impact of
    in family, 190–192
    in individual, 188–190
  public education regarding, 72–73
  see also Cancer

Medical benefits programs, as barriers to "full integration" mandate, 306–307

Mild head injury, 220
Millon Clinical Multiaxial Inventory, 231
Minnesota Multiphasic Personality Inventory, 231
Mobile crew, in supported employment, 115
Moderate head injury, 220
Models of disability
  economic, 304
  medical, 3–4, 35–36
  sociopolitical, 3
MORTON, 263
Multiple disabilities, and sensory impairments, 173–174
Myocardial infarction, role of emotions in recovery, 69

National Council on the Handicapped
  policy on independent living, 50
  statements on accommodation, 16
National data bases, computer access to, 262
National Head Injury Foundation, 197, 201, 229
  estimates of injured who have not been rehabilitated, 201
  goals, 197–198
  guidelines for rehabilitation programs, 209–210
  source of information on specialists, 229
National Institute for Handicapped Research, 77
  funding study of counselor certification, 289
National Institute on Neurological Diseases and Blindness, statistics on blindness, 156
National Rehabilitation Counseling Association (NRCA), 276, 290
National Society for the Prevention of Blindness, definition of blindness, 155
Neoplastic disease, *see* Cancer
Neuropsychological testing, of traumatic brain injury patients, 229–231

Occupational Outlook Handbook, 297
Office of Special Education and Rehabilitation Services (OSERS), 136–137
  initiative on behalf of hearing impaired persons, 158
  promotion of multidisciplinary skills training, 141–142
  school-to-work transition initiatives, 136

Parents
  involvement in school-to-work transition, 103–104
  as participants in supported employment programs, 81, 87
  see also Family response to disability
Partial sensory impairment, problems in, 172–173, 174
Participating Life-long Plan for Affecting Needs (P.L.A.N.), 170
Penetrating head injury, 218
Professional identity, in rehabilitation counseling, 277–278
  and counselor education, 278–288
Professional values, 17, 22–23, 24–25
  see also Ethics
Project PERT, 142, 144
Psychobehavioral treatment modalities, in cancer therapy, 186–188
Psychological assessment, of traumatic brain injured patient, 231
Psychosocial adjustment to disability
  cancer patients, 185–186
  family, 245–247, 248–255
  in life-threatening conditions, 67–70
  after traumatic brain injury, 204–205

Qualitative historical observation, as future studies technique, 321–322

Radiation therapy, for cancer, 185
Regional centers for deaf-blind children, definition of deaf-blindness, 155
Regional rehabilitation continuing education programs (RRCEP), 58

Rehabilitation
approaches to, 4–5, 8
values in, 15–17
Rehabilitation Act of 1973 (PL 93-112), 2, 31, 49, 304
affirmative action/nondiscrimination sections, 15
definition of learning disabilities in, 94–95
effect on rehabilitation counselor education, 275
1978 amendments, 2, 166, 304
see also Title VII—Comprehensive Services for Independent Living
Rehabilitation Act of 1973—1978 amendments, *see* Title VII—Comprehensive Services for Independent Living
Rehabilitation counseling
barriers to, in persons with life-threatening disabilities, 62–71
co-management approach to, 41
definition of, 6
employment trends in, 294–296
future of the profession, 317–320, 323–328
and independent living, 54–57
models of disability for, 3–4, 8
professional challenges in, 5–7, 24–28
professional organizations, 290–291
professional values in, 24–25
range of theory and practice in, 28
role of advocacy/community action in, 25–27
specialization within, 280–283
traditional service delivery versus supported employment, 112–114
trends in, 1–5
utilitarianism theory in, 27–28
Rehabilitation counselor education
accreditation of, 289–290
certification standards, 288–289
in computer technology, 267–268
definition of disability, 292–293
effect of employment trends on, 294–296
effect of perceptions of the profession, 291–292
in ethics, 309–312
funding concerns, 293–294
in independent living, 57–58
influence of federal legislation, 274–275
change in service population, 275–276
political/bureaucratic priorities, 276–277
in life-threatening disabilities, 70–71, 72
and professional identity, 277–278
emerging concerns, 286–288
professional education, 278–280
roles and functions, 283–286
specialization, 280–283
professional organizations and, 290–291
in school-to-work transition, 145–146
in sensory impairment, 175
specialization in, 280–283
student recruitment into, 294
in supported employment, 123–127
Rehabilitation counselors
attitudes of, 22–23
as barrier to "full integration" mandate, 307–308
disability limitations emphasis, 36–37
expectations of disabled persons, 37–38
negative stereotyping in, 39–40
toward disabled persons, 35, 41–43
toward independent living, 56
certification of, 288–289
changing roles and functions, and education of, 382–286
and client with life-threatening disabilities, 70–71
ethics education of, 309–312
expectations of clients, 37–38
opportunities in traumatic brain injury rehabilitation, 212–213
professional challenges to, 24–28
relationship with client, 31–43
role in school-to-work transition, 140–145
role in supported employment, 86, 118–122

Rehabilitation counselors—*continued*
roles and functions in working with families, 247–256
use of computers by, 260–263
see also Rehabilitation counselor education
REHABIT system, 224
Rehabilitation Services Administration (RSA)
funding of rehabilitation employment projects, 90–91
reduction in financial program support, 293
report on federal funding, 274
report on lack of family support, 243
role in expansion of supported employment, 85
standards for counselor education, 279
steps to enhance qualification of counselors, 297
Residential community reentry programs, for traumatic brain injury patients, 200–201
issues in, 207–208
RRCEP, *see* Regional Rehabilitation Continuing Education Programs
RSA, *see* Rehabilitation Services Administration

Scenario writing, as future studies technique, 322–323
applications to rehabilitation, 323–327
Sensory impaired persons
education/job skills training for, 162–163
elderly, 171–172, 174
employment issues for, 164–166
and independent living, 166–168
job placement for, 163–164
and multiple disability, 173–174
prevocational and transitional issues for, 157–161
problems in partial impairment, 172–173
in rural populations, 172, 174
service delivery to, 168–170, 174
vocational evaluation of, 161
Sensory impairments
definitions of, 154–156
epidemiology of, 156–157
rehabilitation counselor education in, 175
research needs in, 175–177
Service delivery
comprehensive model, 10, 96–194
for sensory impaired persons, 168–170, 174
Severe functional vision, definition of, 155
Severe head injury, 221
Sickle cell anemia, 64, 67
Social service programs, as barrier to "full integration" mandate, 306–307
Societal accommodation of disabled persons
legislation regarding, 15–16
prejudice and discrimination as barriers to, 16, 306
Software for rehabilitation counseling, 260–263
see also Computers
Special educators, role in school-to-work transitions, 82, 139–140, 141–142, 146–148, 160
Specialization, in rehabilitation counseling field, 280–283
State legislation, and "full integration" mandate, 305–306
Stress management, in cancer therapy, 186, 187, 188
Supervised living programs, for traumatic brain injury patients, 200
Supported employment
case management in, 87–88
definition and criteria, 79, 127–128
models of, 79–80,114–122
outcomes in, 122–123
participants in
consumer, 81–82
relations among, 83–86
service provider, 82–83
program components in, 80
rehabilitation counselor education in, 123–127
role of rehabilitation counselor in, 86, 118–122

service delivery
model for, 10
phases in, 116–118
services for, 88–90
for traumatic brain injury patients, 237–238
versus traditional rehabilitation services, 112–114
Surgery, for cancer, 185

Team approach to rehabilitation for traumatic brain injury patients, 202–203
Title VII—Comprehensive Services for Independent Living, 26, 49
Centers for Independent Living authorization, 52–53
comprehensive services authorization, 51–52
independent living services for older blind persons authorization, 53
Transition
employment, 78–79
services for, 127
from school to work, 93–94, 135–137
comprehensive services delivery model for, 96–104
factors negatively affecting, 139
issues in, 146–148
for sensory impaired persons, 158, 159, 160, 161
vocational, 127
Transition employment services, 127
Transition services, current issues, 146–148
Transitional living programs, for traumatic brain injury patients, 200–201
Transportation, equal access legislation, 305
Traumatic brain injury
biomechanics of, 218
case finding considerations, 201–202
cognitive retraining after, 223–225
early assessment, 219
employment potential after, 210–212
problem checklists for, 221–222
rehabilitation counseling opportunities in, 212–213
rehabilitation programs for, 198–199
acute, 199–200
behavioral problems and intervention, 203–205
community reentry issues, 207–208
comprehensive outpatient rehabilitation facilities, 201
family education/therapy, 205–207
residential or transitional, 200–201
staffing patterns, 222–223
standards for evaluation of, 208–210
team approach/case management concepts in, 202–203
resultant disability, 219–221
vocational rehabilitation process in, 225–227
client history, 227–228
employment services, 237–238
neuropsychological assessment, 229–231
planning and counseling, 233–236
psychological assessment, 231
specification of deficits, 228–229
support system analysis, 229
vocational evaluation, 231–233
Trend extrapolation, 320–321

United Nations
Declaration on the Rights of Disabled Persons, 16
resolutions regarding disabled persons, 15–16
Utilitarianism, 27–28

Visual impairment, definition of, 155
see also Blindness; sensory impaired persons; Sensory impairment
Vocational educators, role in school-to-work transitions, 86, 139–140
Vocational evaluation
for sensory impaired persons, 161–162
for traumatic brain injury patients, 231–233
use of computers in, 97–98, 262–263

Vocational planning
for persons with learning disabilities, 98–99
in school-to-work transition, 143–144
for traumatic brain injury patients, 234
Vocational rehabilitation
in school-to-work transition, 139–140, 141–142, 146–148
for traumatic brain injury patients, 200–201, 225–238
Vocational transition, 127
VOCOMP, 262

Work Readiness Inventory, 98
World Health Organization
definition of blindness, 155
resolutions concerning disabled persons, 15